YIN YANG
BALANCE

FOR

MENOPAUSE

"*Yin Yang Balance for Menopause* provides a fascinating way to customize your journey through this transition. By making fine distinctions among different body types, Gary Wagman helps to establish treatment protocols for common complaints that will really work for each individual. No more, 'but I'm doing everything right, so why do I still feel so bad?' Once you have established your yin yang body type, you can learn your physical and emotional strengths and weaknesses and how to balance them. This book is a unique addition to the body of menopausal management strategies."

WENDY WARNER, M.D., ABIHM, INTERNATIONAL LECTURER
AND EDUCATOR, FACULTY AT THE INSTITUTE FOR FUNCTIONAL
MEDICINE, PRIOR PRESIDENT OF THE AMERICAN BOARD OF
INTEGRATIVE HOLISTIC MEDICINE, AND AUTHOR OF
BOOSTING YOUR IMMUNITY FOR DUMMIES

"*Yin Yang Balance for Menopause* is a great gift for all those experiencing menopause. It is a fresh, new, and innovative look at the normal conditions women experience during this time in their life. Based on Sasang medicine, a traditional Korean constitutional medicine, Wagman delivers a practical solution, including diet, herbs, and exercises, to remedy the effects of menopause—from hot flashes and depression to insomnia and decreased libido. All healing is self-healing and begins with self-understanding. *Yin Yang Balance for Menopause* will take you on a step-by-step journey to health, well-being, and a greater understanding of yourself. I am certain that readers will thoroughly enjoy reading this book, as Gary Wagman writes in a clear, easy-to-follow, and witty manner."

JOSEPH K. KIM, O.M.D., PH.D., THIRD-GENERATION PRACTITIONER, FORMER CHAIR OF THE DEPARTMENT OF ORIENTAL MEDICINE AT EMPEROR'S COLLEGE, AUTHOR OF *COMPASS OF HEALTH,* AND COAUTHOR OF *YIN AND YANG OF LIFE*

"A uniquely sensitive and compassionate book that speaks to the natural healing power within our own bodies. Written from the perspective of Eastern and Western therapies, with a mind and body integrative approach, *Yin Yang Balance for Menopause* shows that our emotional balance is the essence of menopausal well-being. This profound and highly informative book is suitable for all women—even long before menopause—as it encourages us to develop a positive perception of the changes occurring naturally within our bodies."

DIANA RICHARDSON, AUTHOR OF *TANTRIC SEX AND MENOPAUSE, SLOW SEX, TANTRIC ORGASM FOR WOMEN,* AND *TANTRIC SEX FOR MEN*

YIN YANG BALANCE FOR MENOPAUSE

The Korean Tradition
of Sasang Medicine

GARY WAGMAN, Ph.D., L.Ac.

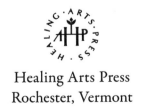

Healing Arts Press
Rochester, Vermont

Healing Arts Press
One Park Street
Rochester, Vermont 05767
www.HealingArtsPress.com

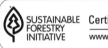

SUSTAINABLE FORESTRY INITIATIVE · Certified Sourcing · www.sfiprogram.org · SFI-00854

Text stock is SFI certified

Healing Arts Press is a division of Inner Traditions International

Note to the reader: *This book is intended as an informational guide. The
remedies, approaches, and techniques described herein are meant to supplement,
and not to be a substitute for, professional medical care or treatment. They should
not be used to treat a serious ailment without prior consultation with a qualified
health care professional.*

Cataloging-in-Publication Data for this title is available from the Library of Congress

ISBN 978-1-62055-848-5 (print)
ISBN 978-1-62055-849-2 (ebook)

Printed and bound in the United States by Lake Book Manufacturing, Inc.
The text stock is SFI certified. The Sustainable Forestry Initiative® program
promotes sustainable forest management.

10 9 8 7 6 5 4 3 2 1

Text design and layout by Virginia Scott Bowman
This book was typeset in Garamond Premier Pro with Online and Myriad Pro
used as display typefaces

To send correspondence to the author of this book, mail a first-class letter to the
author c/o Inner Traditions • Bear & Company, One Park Street, Rochester, VT
05767, and we will forward the communication, or contact the author directly at
http://sasangmedicine.com.

Contents

Foreword by Ann Louise Gittleman, Ph.D, CNS   vii

Acknowledgments   ix

INTRODUCTION   1
Myths and Misconceptions about Menopause
and How Sasang Medicine Can Help

PART ONE
Beginning the Sasang Journey

1 Setting Sail   12
The Basics of Menopause and Sasang Medicine

2 Discovering Your Yin Yang Body Type   36
Physical and Personality Tests to Uncover Your Type

3 Weathering the Storms   74
Emotions and Menopause

PART TWO
Addressing Nine Common
Menopause-Related Challenges

4 Fire Aboard   115
Hot Flashes

5 Sealing the Portholes   143
   Osteoporosis

6 Woman Overboard   167
   The Depths of Depression

7 No Wake Zone   189
   Improving Your Sleep

8 Minding the Waterline   221
   Urinary Health

9 Untangling the Fishing Net   255
   Uterine Fibroids

10 Shouldering the Ropes   274
    Frozen Shoulder

11 Rocking the Boat   293
    Libido

12 Sailing through the Mist   314
    Brain Fog

Continuing the Voyage   335
Useful Resources for Your Menopausal Journey

APPENDIX   338
Five Nutritional Guidelines for Optimum
Menopausal Health

Notes   352

Bibliography   356

Index   365

Foreword

By Ann Louise Gittleman, Ph.D., CNS

The truth is, no one-size-fits-all menopause plan works for everyone. But there is a custom-tailored program that meets your body's special needs, and it is masterfully laid out in Dr. Gary Wagman's *Yin Yang Balance for Menopause: The Korean Tradition of Sasang Medicine*.

Having written several menopause books and gone through "The Change" myself, I only wish I had had Dr. Wagman's priceless resource at my fingertips. He tackles menopausal myths, the most common menopausal symptoms, and current health challenges with the most balanced and individualized solutions for each one based upon four distinct body types. The beauty of his work lies in the realization that every one of us comes into this world with unique physical and emotional strengths and weaknesses. Figuring out your personal body type allows you to make more appropriate diet, supplement, herb, and exercise choices not just during menopause but also for the rest of your life. Based on the Korean Sasang medical system, identifying personal body type is a powerful tool in helping to treat hot flashes, loss of libido, and weight gain as well as dealing with more serious challenges like osteoporosis, heart disease, diabetes, and cancer.

I am particularly struck by Dr. Wagman's insightful knowledge of the underappreciated impact of emotions on physical well-being and structural issues. His description of a client with frozen shoulder syndrome—which he connects with the emotion of grief (connected to the lung meridian)—spoke to me personally, having experienced great sorrow after my father's death and an immobile shoulder since then. Gems like that make this book one you will want to read over and over again.

Not only are the menopausal years a time when we endure power surges—otherwise known as hot flashes—and other changes in our bodies, they are also a time when many of us truly come into our own. I encourage everyone to use this book as a body, mind, and spirit guide to all with menopausal and aging concerns. Dr. Wagman's understanding of herbal medicine and its application is particularly extraordinary.

It is my hope that this book will empower women from adolescence to the menopausal transition to continue the self-health and self-improvement movement that has changed the way we view and now treat menopause. Attention to proper diet, exercise, lifestyle changes, and what the body is actually telling us will make the journey into midlife a time of great freedom and renewed energy. The postmenopausal years should be the time of a woman's life free of child rearing and responsibilities that is rewarded with nothing but good health. As Margaret Meade put it, "The most creative force in the world is a menopausal woman with zest!" Certainly keeping our bodies in biochemical balance is a lifetime adventure that will ensure our passage through each stage of life is filled with zest. The time to repair is now, and with Dr. Wagman's expert advice by our side we can't help but sail through menopause and into a second spring.

Ann Louise Gittleman, Ph.D., CNS, is a New York Times bestselling author of more than thirty books on diet, detox, the environment, and women's health. Beloved by many, she is regarded as a nutritional visionary and health pioneer who has fearlessly stood on the front lines of holistic and integrative medicine. A Columbia University graduate, Gittleman has been recognized as one of the top ten nutritionists in the country by *Self* magazine and has received the American Medical Writers Association award for excellence and the Humanitarian Award from the Cancer Control Society.

Acknowledgments

Yin Yang Balance for Menopause is dedicated to my grandmother, whose heart was filled with enough love to fill the universe. To my mother, who inherited her inner strength and raised my sister and me with profound forbearance and maternal love. To my wife, who is the sail on my ship, and my eleven-year-old daughter, illustrator of all of the meridian drawings herein, who brings joy and meaning to the journey. Without these incredible women in my life, *Yin Yang Balance for Menopause* would never have manifested.

My deep gratitude also extends to Karen Christensen, my editor, friend, and in many ways teacher. Her ongoing encouragement, willingness to contribute, and special way with words brought with them a spark that ignited life into *Yin Yang Balance for Menopause* and my previous book, *Your Yin Yang Body Type*. It is this spark that makes my books playful yet informative introductions to Sasang medicine.

A sincere appreciation also goes to my patients, whom I treasure as one would a family. With Sasang medicine as our navigation system, we've sailed through countless storms, only to grow stronger and healthier along the way. Not a day goes by in the clinic without a reminder of how deep our mutually enhancing relationship runs.

I would never have traveled my path in life if it weren't for Lee Je-ma and his profound understanding of Eastern philosophy and medicine. As the originator of Sasang medicine, he contributed greatly to the start of a new era of self-empowering medicine. I extend this gratitude to my mentor, No Kyung Mun, for his unconditional guidance, and to my colleagues of the Yeon Kyoung Won (Society for the Study of the Classics) for capturing the essence of Lee Je-ma's teaching and devoting their lives to preserving ancient wisdom.

Lastly, I would like to thank life itself for giving me the opportunity to follow my dreams.

INTRODUCTION

Myths and Misconceptions about Menopause and How Sasang Medicine Can Help

With Sasang medicine as your guide and the knowledge of your yin yang body type, navigating the way through the rugged waves of hot flashes, insomnia, depression, pain, and so on is about to become an easier, self-enhancing process. Instead of relying on what the latest remedy is for this or that symptom, you'll soon be able to determine what is appropriate for *you* and *your* body. Sasang medicine introduces four yin yang body types that are based on which of your organs are more or less developed from birth. Our developed organs are the source of the fuel that sends blood and energy to the less developed ones. Most of us have plenty of fuel, readily available within our stronger, more developed organs, but without an effective navigation system, we burn it up without getting far. Sasang medicine enhances your fuel efficiency by introducing body-type-specific foods, herbs, exercises, and emotional balancing techniques to encourage energy flow and enhance well-being.

more than 80 percent of my patients were women of menopausal age. After inquiring about pain, I'd routinely ask my patients if there was anything else they would like to address. It was like I had opened up a Pandora's box! I was asked, "What can you do for hot flashes . . . insomnia . . . depression . . . libido . . . a lazy husband." Despite feeling a bit overwhelmed at first, and admitting that I didn't have a cure for lazy husbands (since I myself have been accused of being one), I felt deep inside that the body-type-specific approach of Sasang medicine could offer tremendous relief during menopause, and I was right! Now, fifteen years later, I have a thriving practice and have successfully addressed the menopausal concerns of thousands of patients.

Before I studied Sasang medicine, my background in traditional Chinese medicine left me trapped in a symptomatically focused perspective, emphasizing the use of herbs and acupuncture for symptoms like hot flashes, depression, insomnia, and so forth. "What about herbs and acupuncture to utilize the strengths and support the weaknesses of the *individual* behind the symptoms?" I'd ask myself. "My patients aren't giant hot flash ovens or blobs of depression; they are people!" As an intern, I remember being surprised when a formula had no effect or made a patient feel worse, even though it was chock-full of ingredients that addressed the patient's symptoms. Sasang medicine explains how each of the yin yang body types has its own emotional and physiological strengths and weaknesses—the strengths giving them a natural advantage, the weaknesses leaving them prone to this or that symptom. This information, hidden beneath layer upon layer of coping skills, is often obscured. The discovery of your yin yang body type empowers you to make accurate health choices, avoid incompatible/unnecessary remedies, and focus on *you*.

Before discussing the yin yang body types further, let's take a moment to discuss five of the most common misconceptions that add to menopausal confusion regardless of your body type. No matter how much you try to avoid it, it's easy to get trapped in one or more of these misconceptions, especially when you are suffering from pain or other discomfort. A smooth menopause transition depends on the ability to release fear and accept that you are entering a new phase of life, steering clear of dread, hopelessness, and despair.

FIVE COMMON MISCONCEPTIONS OF MENOPAUSE

1. My body is making me feel this way. This is perhaps the most obvious misconception about menopause because Western philosophy and medicine have historically perpetuated a mechanical way of thinking about our body. Hormone levels may indeed be out of whack, but this is not what is causing you to feel uncomfortable. Don't blame your body for how you feel; it is not your enemy. Many women pass through menopause relatively symptom-free despite the fact that their estrogen levels have spiked and plummeted throughout the process. Sasang medicine emphasizes the significance of a mind and body integrative approach to addressing menopausal discomfort. Your menopause comfort level depends entirely on your *perception* of the changes occurring within your body. Each of the yin yang body types has its own perception trap. For instance, the Yin Type A has a tendency to disconnect or turn away from pain and discomfort, while the Yin Type B may crouch in fear. The discovery of your yin yang body type makes it easier to recognize these tendencies and redirect them.

2. There must be an easy way out. There may certainly be an easier way, but not an easy way out. The temptation to take a prescription drug or other quick fix remedy may be overwhelming when one is feeling miserable. As we'll see later, there is a place for both Western and Eastern therapies in addressing the symptoms of menopause. Yet along with the assistance of herbs and/or prescriptions comes the responsibility of balancing emotions—a key component of Sasang medicine.

3. There's something wrong with me that I just can't figure out. By eliminating the notion of "wrong," there's a much better chance that you'll figure it out. Keep in mind that menopause is not an illness or disease but a new phase of life. It is less important to "figure it out" than it is to take your time and learn from the new experience, letting go of the "fix it" approach. There isn't necessarily an answer to menopause; rather, it is a process of self-discovery that unfolds differently for each individual.

4. This does not have to do with me; it's something/someone else that's making me feel this way. Menopause has everything to do with you; after all, it's your journey! Granted, the menopausal phase often brings heightened sensitivity to stress, noise, emotion, and touch, but others are not to blame for these changes. Actually, sensitivity can be used to your advantage, inspiring the decision to set up a different sleeping arrangement or take an alternative route to work, encouraging more balance in life. Don't wait for life itself to accommodate you!

5. My emotions have nothing to do with menopausal symptoms. Sasang medicine holds that there's an emotional component to everything we experience in life, including pain. It doesn't claim that discomfort is simply "in your head," but that the mind is capable of reducing and even eliminating pain and discomfort. True, this takes a tremendous amount of work, but it's the ultimate path to optimizing health and well-being. Sasang medicine describes how each of the yin yang body types has its own emotional tendencies that either contribute to misery or enhance our overall health. It emphasizes the ability of our emotional center, the heart, to change misery into joy, and pain into comfort.

THE FIVE PREMISES OF SASANG MEDICINE

If any of the above misconceptions apply to your menopausal experience, then welcome to the club! About half of all women participating in a study at the University of Manitoba believed that menopause is a medical condition requiring medical intervention.[3] It's easy to fall into despair if you face menopause with the belief that you are ill and in need of medication. Simply willing yourself free of the above misconceptions doesn't make things easier. Keep in mind that falling into one or more of them will exacerbate menopausal symptoms. As you become familiar with the teachings of Sasang medicine, the ability to steer clear of these misconceptions will come naturally—as a process that unfolds slowly and consistently. So take ample time to get familiar with your yin yang body type and enhance your menopausal health, day after day.

Sasang medicine proposes a fundamental shift in thinking that emphasizes the power to change how we feel through self-understanding and self-cultivation. The following five premises of Sasang medicine can be applied not only to menopause but to any health situation.

1. The way you respond to menopause depends on the inborn inclinations of your mind and body. Each of us has different physical and emotional tendencies depending on which of our organs are hyper- and hypodeveloped at birth. Our hyperdeveloped organs correlate with stronger emotional tendencies, and the hypodeveloped ones with sensitized, less developed emotions. The Yin Type A, for example, radiates toward joy or cheerfulness, which is associated with her stronger liver, but if she cannot achieve or control this emotion, sadness, which correlates with her weaker lungs, will suffocate it.

2. Emotions move energy. Each of the yin yang body types has its own emotional inclination that determines how energy flows within the body. Balancing these emotions actually enhances the body's ability to transition through menopause, encouraging hormone balance. Anger, for example, sends warm energy upward, while calmness guides cool energy downward. Since the yang types are prone to anger, flow to the upper body is stronger than flow to the lower body. If the yang types have difficulty controlling anger, weakness of the lower body ensues, while upper body pressure increases. This situation is referred to as *hwa seung su gang*, which means "heat ascending and cold descending"—the reversal of healthy energy flow. Lee Je-ma, the founder of Sasang medicine, emphasized the importance of *su seung hwa gang*, "coolness ascending and warmth descending"—where energy flows smoothly throughout the body. Menopause is particularly challenging for the angry yang type, whose excessive upper body energies instigate hot flashes, anxiety, headaches, and high blood pressure. The calmer yang type is able to send ample cool energy down to her weaker lower body, cooling hot flashes and decreasing other menopause symptoms.

3. Each menopausal symptom has its own body-type-specific emotional and physiological source. According to Sasang medicine, every nook and cranny of the body has its own unique emotional affiliation. The lungs, for example, correlate with sorrow, the spleen with anger, the liver with joy, and the kidneys with calm. Emotions associated with our stronger organs are easier to control, while those correlating with our weaker organs easily lose their footing. Lurking underneath symptoms like hot flashes, insomnia, headaches, and so on are emotions such as anxiety, anger, and/or sadness. Ignoring underlying emotions may be the reason why a particular symptom doesn't improve despite our earnest effort. The first step in dealing with any chronic condition is to balance our emotions and expectations surrounding it. Fear feeds pain, and expectation almost always leads to disappointment. Our symptoms aren't the enemy. Don't panic! Step back for a moment and reflect on your yin yang body type's strengths and weaknesses, discovering how they influence your reaction to each menopausal symptom. Knowing why you feel a certain way makes it easier to take the appropriate action.

4. By getting to know your body-type-specific tendencies and making an effort to balance your innate energies, you are capable of alleviating menopausal symptoms. In the midst of despair, it is easier to believe in a doctor, pill, or tonic before trusting in our own natural ability to heal. There are numerous situations where medications and tonics come in handy, but even these cannot help without the support of the natural healing power within our bodies. The first step to self-healing is self-knowledge, or the discovery of what our natural strengths and weaknesses are. Sometimes my patients resort to tonics like ashwagandha or ginseng for the sake of combating fatigue. These herbs stimulate the Yin Type B's hypodeveloped spleen system but could harm the other types. After taking them, my Yin Type B patients not only feel energized but overall healthier too! But those who aren't Yin Type Bs, even if they experience more short-term energy, eventually start to show signs of high blood pressure, palpitations, and/or anxiety. With the knowledge of your yin yang body type, these common missteps can be avoided.

5. Balance, and nothing else, is the essence of well-being. No matter how intense your hot flashes are, they will eventually go away once estrogen and progesterone reach an agreement within your body. During menopause, many women experience a dive in estrogen, and the other hormones are left to figure things out on their own. As the disparities between hormones increase, so does the frequency and intensity of menopausal symptoms. Eventually estrogen and progesterone both decline significantly, closing the gap. Even at a bare minimum, estrogen, progesterone, and testosterone are fully capable of getting along despite the spats along the way. Hot-flash relief comes sooner for some and later for others, depending not on body type or genetics, but on the ability to balance one's body-type-specific emotional and physiological tendencies. True, estrogen and progesterone have an effect on your emotions, but how you feel emotionally also directly affects your hormone levels. The choice of whether to be controlled by or in control of your hormones is yours!

Familiarizing yourself with the misconceptions about menopause is like studying road signs in a driver education class. Even after years of driving, we may lose track of, take for granted, or simply ignore road signs or proper driving etiquette. While reading through the following chapters, it wouldn't hurt to occasionally return to the misconceptions and premises, just to make sure that you're on the right track.

JOURNEYING ONWARD

Now that we've discussed the basics, it's time to discover how to apply Sasang medicine to your own menopausal journey. Chapter 1 introduces yin and yang theory and how it applies to each of the yin yang body types. Here we'll look at the connection between Eastern and Western approaches to menopause and explain how yin and yang correlate with different hormones. We'll then explore how yin and yang relate to the physiological and psychological tendencies of each yin yang body type.

The discovery of your own yin yang body type awaits you in the second chapter, which includes a detailed questionnaire about your emotional and physical tendencies. Since emotional balance is the center of all Sasang medicine healing processes, the journey continues with the third chapter, in which you will find out how to balance your emotions during menopause. Navigating these waters can be a bit tricky because our true nature often lurks under layer upon layer of coping strategy.

Chapters 4 through 12 discuss nine of the most common symptoms of menopause. Many of you will be tempted to read only the sections that apply to your situation. I recommend, however, that you take ample time to jump in and explore them all. The deeper you dive, the more you'll understand.

Yin Yang Balance for Menopause concludes with several appendices, introducing body-type-specific exercise and food guidelines to help you on your journey.

Bon voyage!

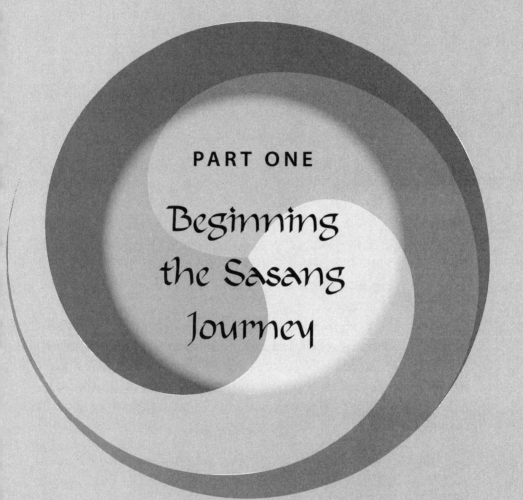

PART ONE

Beginning the Sasang Journey

1

Setting Sail

The Basics of Menopause and Sasang Medicine

Why do some women serenely sail through menopause while others seem to suffer through every symptom? Why does Brook, who is in great physical shape, suffer from hot flashes and insomnia, while Cindy, who does not exercise and eats everything in sight, makes menopause look easy? Shouldn't optimum physical and emotional health guarantee a smooth transition? For many women, menopausal symptoms are unpredictable, often catching them off guard. While the female body has been transitioning through menopause since the beginning of humankind, the menopausal experience varies according to the individual.

MENOPAUSE AND YOUR BODY TYPE

Because innate emotional and physical strengths and weaknesses influence how a woman reacts to menopause, every woman responds to the menopause transition in her own unique way. Discovering your body type can help you identify your strengths and weaknesses, and making modifications according to your type can help you adapt to hormonal changes within your body and within your environment.

Even though some women are born healthier or take better care of themselves than others, health alone does not account for the differences described above. I've seen numerous patients who are otherwise in great physical and emotional shape experience intense hot flashes, fatigue, insomnia, and/or depression. These individuals often explain how, out of the blue, emotions start to spiral out of control, or sweat pours from their skin for no apparent reason. Trying our best to stay healthy can make any change in life relatively easier, but sometimes this just isn't enough to ensure a smooth transition.

There is no "secret" to optimizing your menopausal health and ensuring that you'll be symptom-free, but there are effective ways to help you navigate your way through the choppy waters. You are about to embark on a journey of self-discovery in which a deeper understanding of your emotional and physical strengths and weaknesses unfolds. Through this discovery comes the ability to control how your mind and body feel at any given moment.

Yin Yang Balance for Menopause emphasizes the ability to address menopausal issues naturally, by balancing your mind and body. It does not offer ways to increase your estrogen or progesterone or ensure a symptom-free menopause; rather, it guides you through the process of balancing the hormones already within you and provides the tools necessary to recognize and address changes along the way. This book isn't designed as an alternative to hormone treatment or as a companion to it. Instead, it focuses on optimizing emotional and physical health, whether you are receiving hormone treatment or not.

With the introduction of a four-body-type system, the Sasang medical approach offers insight into why and how your menopausal journey is the way it is. It explains why hot flashes occur when they do, why insomnia is suddenly an issue, or why depression has taken over. As the upcoming pages unfold, you'll discover the different psychological and physiological aspects of each body type and how they affect the menopausal transition and learn about body-type-specific foods, herbs, and exercises.

WHAT EXACTLY IS MENOPAUSE?

The quick answer to the above question is in the name: *meno* is Latin for "menses" and *pause* refers to a cessation. Yet there is nothing "quick" about menopause, since it is a process that takes up to seven years as the body's yin energy, in the form of estrogen, starts to decline, potentially causing physiological and psychological changes along the way. Officially, however, it occurs after a woman's monthly cycle has been absent for twelve months, and it cannot be explained by other health issues.

In Sasang medicine, health is dependent on the ability to adapt to our surroundings by harmonizing our inner environment, which is influenced by the relative strength of our organ energies. During the menopausal transition, our stronger and weaker organs have to reassess their relationship, just as marriage asks us to do every now and then to keep love alive. This relationship is tested every seven years for women and every eight years for men during a time when the body's circadian clock resets its rhythm. Menopause is considered the seventh of seven (7 x 7) phases, and at age forty-nine, a female undergoes the most significant change in her lifetime—the closing of one door and opening of another.

In the East, this is viewed as a "year of renewal," which is in stark contrast to the predominant Western idea that menopause is simply another step closer to death as the body loses its precious hormones and their ability to support our biological functions. In the East, life is not interpreted as a linear process from birth to death but rather as a continuous cycle in which the death of one phase brings life to a new one. The Sasang approach is not based on artificially reversing the aging process but on balancing and adapting harmoniously to each of life's phases.

Accordingly, menopause is an opportunity to reignite one's passion for life, as the time and energy devoted to producing and then raising a newborn is transferred into energy to *be* reborn and discover oneself anew. As with most cultures, seven signifies rest and rejuvenation. In Chinese culture, it signifies the end of one cycle and the beginning of another. The seventh day of the week, for example, is an opportunity to recharge and gear oneself up for the following week. Hence seven multiplied by seven is a significant time in a woman's life when she can take a step back and reevaluate, rediscover what is precious, and shed unnecessary fears and unhealthy thoughts. It is an opportunity to reflect on and distinguish between what is precious and what is expendable.

Menopause is often blamed for the anguish women may feel during an intense time in life when their nest is emptied, their parents are getting older or have passed away, they no longer have a day job, and/or they are left to grope their way through all of this without anyone to guide them. But keep in mind that, as I just mentioned, it is all about adjusting, and the guide you need in such times is nowhere else but within you. Yet simply telling yourself that everything is going to be all right usually doesn't cut it when you are in the midst of a hot flash or experiencing emotional ups and downs. Adjustment requires deep insight into your situation and the ability to detect why you react the way you do. The Sasang approach goes beyond the image of menopause as a roller coaster of fluctuating hormones and delineates how women react and adjust in different ways depending on their innate strengths and weaknesses.

WHAT IS SASANG MEDICINE?

The Korean word *sasang* means "four types" in English and signifies the classification of all people into four major body types. This medical system was first established by a Korean doctor named Lee Je-ma (1837–1900), who was well versed in the Eastern medical tradition, which is a system that focuses on the balance of yin and yang energy to treat emotional and/or physical illness. He was distraught from seeing that certain patients suffering from the same symptoms improved quickly, while others suffered longer despite adequate treatment. Sasang medicine was born from his ability to cater to these differences while emphasizing the unique constitutional requirements of each patient.

As previously mentioned, the Sasang medical system is based on the idea that each individual is born with varying emotional and physical strengths and weaknesses depending on his/her body type. These tendencies have a direct influence on how we react to the external world and our body's internal environment. It holds that the hormonal changes and fluctuating energies that a woman experiences during menopause aren't what make her feel this way or that; rather, it is a woman's *response* to these changes that dictates how she feels. For instance, it is easy to claim that depression is caused by a drop in estrogen and relative excess of progesterone. Actually, depression is an inability to adapt to these changes. How do we know this? Because, to put it simply, not everyone who experiences these changes in hormone levels is depressed!

According to Sasang medicine, our response to life's changes highly depends on how we relate to our own innate emotional and physical strengths and weaknesses. A child with anger issues may eventually learn how to curb that anger. An individual with an introverted nature may choose to interact with others more often rather than feel alone. We do not have to be experts in Sasang medicine to recognize, strengthen, and modify these traits. Yet these innate strengths and weaknesses are often difficult to detect, and even if we do detect them, it may be difficult to know how to proceed in handling them. We all have unique but untapped strengths that are hidden within, awaiting an opportunity to come out. Yet other traits, which often manifest too easily, require modification, restructuring, or disregarding, especially when we are experiencing difficulties or going through a vulnerable time in life. Menopause may be the perfect excuse for emotions like anger and sadness to appear. It may also unlock the door for excessive heat or stored emotions to find their way to the surface. When accumulated energy within works its way outward, you need to be prepared or else be in for a rude awakening!

Yin Yang Balance for Menopause is a key that unlocks your greatest potential by facilitating deeper insight and giving you the tools to modify your unique body-type-specific strengths and weaknesses.

After getting to know the Sasang approach, you'll be able to do the following:

- Avoid the emotional ups and downs of menopause and strengthen your inner self.
- Recognize your innate strengths and weaknesses and make the most of "now."
- Make wiser choices about which foods to eat for an easier transition through menopause.
- Avoid guessing whether or not this or that supplement works for your type.
- Choose the right herbs and forms of exercise.

YIN AND YANG THEORY

Before we jump into the discovery of your body type, let's take a deeper look at a few basic Sasang concepts. First of all, with 7.3 billion people on the Earth, you may be wondering why they fall into only four body types. To answer this, we first have to return to the basics of Asian philosophy, which holds that all things emerge from a central source, referred to as the Taiji, which then branches into yin and yang or two opposing energies, and then again into the so-called Four Manifestations, also known as the Four Symbols, which we will discuss shortly.

Even though yin and yang are often referred to as opposites, it is only when they are used in a specific context that we grasp their meaning. If we say the moon is yin, then we are only comparing it to things that are more yang, like the sun. If we say the sun is yang, we mean that it is relatively more yang than the moon. Actually, our sun may be more yin compared to the sun of a different galaxy! Dark describes a degree of darkness rather than the complete absence of light. When we say that something is moving slowly, we are comparing it to something in faster motion. Yet there are surely things that move more slowly! Hence yin and yang serve as symbolic images that help express the different degrees of relativity and how all things are intricately related rather than existing in isolation. Table 1.1 provides several natural phenomena that are represented by either yin or yang.

TABLE 1.1. YIN AND YANG NATURAL PHENOMENA

Yin	Yang
Moon	Sun
Dark	Light
Night	Day
Cold	Hot
Down	Up
Moist	Dry
Back	Front
Slow	Fast
Feminine	Masculine

YIN YANG BODY TYPES

Yin and yang do not have any meaning in themselves, since there is no such thing as pure this or pure that. Only when they merge and dance together do they have meaning. This dance begins when yin mingles with yang and yang with yin, giving rise to four possibilities—referred to as the Four Symbols, or Sasang (four types): yin within yang, yang within yang, yin within yin, and yang within yin. These represent the most fundamental division of all things that exist in time and space, such as the four seasons, four cardinal directions, four basic DNA proteins that produce every gene in the body, and so on. In Sasang medicine there are four body types: two yin types and two yang types. Each of these body types represents one of the above yin and yang combinations. Table 1.2 lists each of the types in English and Korean.

TABLE 1.2. YIN YANG BODY TYPES

Body Type (in English)	Korean Name	Translation
Yang Type A (yin within yang)	So Yang	Lesser Yang
Yang Type B (yang within yang)	Tae Yang	Greater Yang
Yin Type A (yin within yin)	Tae Eum	Greater Eum
Yin Type B (yang within yin)	So Eum	Lesser Eum

Pronunciation Key
So is pronounced like the English word *so.*
Ya in *yang* is pronounced as it is in *yacht.*
Tae rhymes with *day. Eum* rhymes with *loom.*

Because of the intermingling of yin and yang, figuring out your body type is not as simple as black and white. The yin and yang body types all have different degrees of yin and yang. Although, as would be expected, the two yang types share more yang traits, and the two yin types share more yin traits, the yang types always have yin traits, and the yin types naturally have certain yang traits. By now you may be asking yourself, what exactly are yin and yang traits? Table 1.3 provides some answers.

TABLE 1.3. YIN AND YANG TRAITS

Yin	Yang
Complacent	Active
Gets cold more easily	Gets hot more easily
Stronger lower body	Stronger upper body
Relaxed	Tense
Night owl	Morning person
Slow metabolism	Fast metabolism
Slow motion	Quick motion
Follower	Leader
Higher estrogen, lower progesterone levels	Lower estrogen, higher progesterone levels

YIN YANG AND THE THREE HORMONES

Menopause-related books often discuss the decline of estrogen and progesterone levels within the body. Yet the pitfalls of hormone therapy show us that simply toggling these hormones does not always provide an untethered solution. According to Sasang medicine, menopausal health is primarily dependent upon the balance of yin and yang energy rather than hormone quantity. Modern research has led many of us to think that fluctuations in hormone levels automatically cause our mind and body to react this way or that. Yet less-mentioned studies demonstrate how the opposite is also true and that happiness, meditation, joy, anger, and so forth cause the secretion and suppression of various hormones in the body. Estrogen levels are also affected by exercise and emotional state.

Sasang medicine explains how our emotions and hormones affect one another but emphasizes that our innate emotional inclinations have a greater effect on how we feel than our hormone levels. Hormones may be considered environmental—as opposed to constitutional—factors that influence us but don't control how we feel. Among the various hormones within the body, estrogen and progesterone are arguably the most influential of menopause's environmental factors.

Each has specific yin and yang qualities that vary according to each body type and individual.

Estrogen, or the "female" hormone, correlates with yin and is associated with cold, moisture, nourishment, and softness. Its main function is to develop female sexual characteristics, such as the breasts and the inner lining of the uterus—a yin (feminine) quality. Progesterone exhibits both yin and yang traits and is primarily responsible for preparing the uterus for pregnancy by thickening and vascularizing the wall of the uterus—a yin (nourishing) quality—and for increasing the body temperature to enhance fertility—a yang (warming) quality. Testosterone, or the "male" hormone, is the least discussed hormone of the female body because of its role in developing male sexual characteristics. Yet keep in mind that every woman has a significant amount of this hormone, and it is associated with increasing her libido—a yang characteristic—at the beginning of the monthly cycle.

From the standpoint of Eastern medicine, estrogen is considered to be more yin compared to progesterone, and progesterone to be more yin than testosterone, which is almost purely yang. As estrogen decreases after menopause, testosterone is reduced at a slower pace and thus is given a chance to flex its muscles. A pronounced decrease in estrogen often results in testosterone-dominant, heat-related symptoms such as hot flashes, dry skin and hair, osteoporosis, muscle and tendon tightness, and even acne—considered in Eastern medicine to be a result of excess heat within the body rebelling upward. Rising heat may also cause red blotches on the skin that occasionally burst, like a bubble rising to the surface of boiling water. Anger is also an example of excessive heat within the body that rises from the spleen, its source.

Excessive moisture and stagnation of fluid are the result of yin dominance—a common occurrence when estrogen levels increase in one's teens and right before they start to plunge during perimenopause. This condition is often balanced by increasing yang through the release of progesterone and/or testosterone, yet during the menopausal transition, these hormones may also be on the decline.

In Eastern medicine, hormonal imbalance is seen as an internal battle between yin and yang. Yet all hope is not lost! Asian philosophy interprets this battle as a phase that inevitably precedes balance and harmony. And before you throw in the towel, know that there are other ways to increase and balance yin and yang during and after the menopausal transition, such as balancing your emotions and consuming yin/yang energy foods and herbs. These methods will be discussed in detail in the following chapters.

Table 1.4 provides a number of other examples of symptoms that can occur when one hormone is dominant (present in higher amounts than the other hormones).

TABLE 1.4. SYMPTOMS THAT MAY OCCUR WHEN ONE HORMONE IS DOMINANT

Estrogen-Dominant Symptoms (Yin Dominant)	Progesterone-Dominant Symptoms (More Yang, Less Yin)	Testosterone-Dominant Symptoms (Yang Dominant)
Cold (especially hands and feet), weight gain, fibroid/cyst growth, sadness/depression, muscle weakness, delayed menopause, longer menstrual cycles	Heat (hot flashes), excessive weight loss, muscle tightness, depression/anxiety, mild acne, mood swings, breast tenderness, loss of libido	Absence of menstrual cycle/shorter cycles, infertility, moderate/severe acne, excessive hair growth, anger/rage, early menopause, headaches

YIN YANG AND THE HORMONE PHASES

Estrogen and progesterone levels fluctuate extensively throughout the monthly cycle and as we age. The first half of a cycle, starting from the first day of menses, is said to be estrogen dominant, and the latter half is progesterone dominant. In between these hormonal fluctuations is ovulation, a phase in which yin transforms into yang, marked by a sudden decrease of estrogen and increase of progesterone, causing the release of an egg (ovum) from the ovary. The fluctuation of hormone levels during the cycle (see fig. 1.1, page 22)—estrogen yielding to progesterone and progesterone handing its authority back to estrogen—closely resembles the ebb and flow of yin and yang, where yin gives rise to yang and yang gives rise to yin. When yin and yang are balanced, this process goes smoothly, but when one abuses its power or the other stages a coup d'état, uncomfortable symptoms arise. For instance, higher levels of progesterone (yang) may cause sudden flashes of heat after ovulation or during perimenopause, a time when estrogen (yin) drops rapidly. Excessive levels of estrogen may instigate sudden bouts of depression during the first fourteen days of the cycle or during early to mid-stage perimenopause, when progesterone is comparably lower.

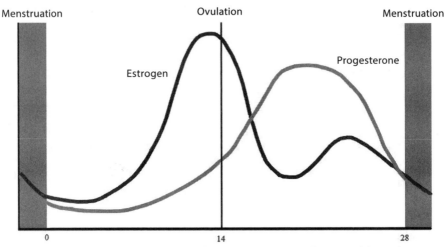

Fig. 1.1. The ebb and flow of hormones during the monthly cycle

Both estrogen and progesterone levels increase rapidly in a female's teenage years, with estrogen levels relatively higher. They peak in adulthood, with progesterone occasionally higher than estrogen, and in later years they steadily decrease, with progesterone decreasing faster. This pattern is also seen with yin and yang, which increase significantly during menarche (one's first menstrual period and the second of the seven-year cycles), reach their prime in one's twenties (the third of the seven-year cycles), and decline during and after perimenopause (the sixth and seventh of the seven-year cycles). Estrogen and progesterone levels tend to fluctuate rapidly during puberty and perimenopause, often contributing to both yin- and yang-related symptoms such as depression, breast tenderness, cramps, and weight gain, which are associated with yin, and hot flashes, flushing, and irritability, which are associated with yang. The continuous fluctuation of hormone levels within the body may give you the feeling that you are at the mercy of their ups and downs. Thankfully, however, you are more than just a collection of chemical reactions. Your mind (or heart, as we say in Sasang medicine) inevitably calls the shots, and if you learn to control your mind, then you can learn to balance the flow of hormones, blood, energy—you name it!

HORMONES AND
THE YIN YANG BODY TYPES

Since the body types have varying levels of yin and yang, they also have differing levels of estrogen, progesterone, and testosterone. Generally speaking, the yin types have greater relative levels of estrogen, while the yang types have more testosterone and progesterone. Hence the yin types tend toward estrogen-dominant symptoms such as sensitivity to cold, gaining weight, and so on, while the yang types have more progesterone/testosterone-dominant symptoms such as sensitivity to heat, anger, and acne. With more estrogen, the yin types often experience later menopausal onset than the yang types. There are more cases of estrogen-fed fibroids among the yin types, and progesterone-related issues such as amenorrhea or lack of ovulation among the yang types. Yet as we mentioned above, yin and yang are not absolute, and hence the yin types may occasionally experience testosterone-dominant symptoms, and the yang types estrogen-dominant symptoms. The trick is to discover the underlying cause of dominance by familiarizing yourself with the ebb and flow of yin and yang within your body, which you'll do as the following chapters unfold.

OUR ORGAN SYSTEMS DETERMINE
OUR BODY TYPE

As shown above, each body type is born with different degrees of yin and yang: the yang types with more yang, the yin types with more yin. Also mentioned was the concept of yang correlating with the upper body and yin with the lower body. Sasang medicine identifies four major organ systems within the body: lungs, spleen, liver, and kidneys. The lungs and the spleen are considered yang organ systems because they govern the function of the upper body, while the liver and kidneys are considered yin organ systems because they control the lower body functions.

The lungs, as the uppermost of the four major organs, have the most yang and are the strongest organ of the Yang Type B. This organ controls the flow of energy and blood to the chest, neck, and brain. The spleen, situated directly below the lungs, is the strongest organ of the Yang Type A and governs the flow of energy and blood through the upper digestive tract, such as the pancreas, stomach, and spleen area. The liver, situated below and to the right of the spleen, is the strongest organ of the Yin Type A and controls the gallbladder and small intestine functions. Finally, the kidneys, residing below the liver, are the Yin Type B's strongest organs and govern the function of the bladder, kidney, and large intestines. Table 1.5 shows a breakdown of the organ systems, their functions in Sasang medicine, and their corresponding body types.

TABLE 1.5. ORGAN SYSTEMS' FUNCTIONS AND BODY TYPES

Organ System	Function	Body Type for Which It Is the Strongest Organ	Body Type for Which It Is the Weakest Organ
Spleen	Supports the digestive function of the stomach and controls the flow of energy to the epigastric area	Yang Type A	Yin Type B
Lungs	Fortify and nourish the heart and control the flow of energy to the head and chest	Yang Type B	Yin Type A
Liver	Controls the function of the gallbladder and small intestine and regulates the flow of energy to the abdomen	Yin Type A	Yang Type B
Kidneys	Govern the function of the bladder and large intestines and control the flow of energy to the lower body	Yin Type B	Yang Type A

Since yin and yang oppose one another, the stronger a yang organ system is, the weaker its correlating yin organ system becomes, and the stronger a yin organ system is, the weaker its correlating yang organ system becomes. Hence the Yang Type A, born with a stronger spleen system, has weaker kidneys, and the Yin Type B, born with stronger kidneys, has a weaker spleen system. The Yang Type B, born with stronger lungs, has a weaker liver, but the Yin Type A, born with a stronger liver, has weaker lungs. The relative strengths and weaknesses of the lungs, spleen, liver, and kidneys determine our body type and play a major role in menopause. The different levels of organ strength are what contribute to energy flow within the body. Health depends on the smooth flow of energy from our stronger to our weaker organs. Life's challenges may cause our stronger organs to greedily hoard their energies, leaving the weaker organs to fend for themselves.

Do our organ energies equalize when we are healthy? Actually, energy couldn't flow from one place to another within the body if all of our organs were created equal. Just as particles in areas of high pressure flow to areas of low pressure, energy naturally flows from the stronger organs to the weaker ones. It's only when the higher pressure of our stronger organ groups accumulates and explodes or when the lower pressure of our weaker organs collapses that our health is impeded. Let's take a deeper look at how each of these organs influences our everyday life and menopause.

According to Sasang medicine, our emotional inclinations—namely, anger, sorrow, joy, and calmness, referred to herein as "predominant emotions"—are what determine which organ systems are stronger and weaker. Sorrow, for instance, sends energy to the lungs, and a propensity toward sorrow produces a stronger lung. Too much sorrow, however, can injure the lungs. Anger feeds the spleen, and an inclination toward anger gives rise to a stronger spleen. Yet if anger gets out of hand, it destroys the health of the spleen. Joy nourishes the liver but can also injure it, and calmness pumps up the kidneys but can congest them too. In our culture, joy and calmness are usually interpreted as positive emotions. Yet, as illustrated in our discussion of yin and yang, our emotions also need to be balanced in order for energy to flow smoothly. Anxiety, for instance, is only a small step away from joy, since they both may cause our heart to race and palms to sweat. Calmness can easily morph into complacency if the family room couch is too enticing!

The four predominant emotions determine how we feel from moment to moment. Stress, trauma, and—you guessed it—menopause influence our predominant emotions in different ways depending on our type. Table 1.6 shows the temperament of each body type.

TABLE 1.6. YIN YANG BODY TYPES AND THEIR PREDOMINANT EMOTION

Body Type	Predominant Emotion
Yang Type A	Anger
Yang Type B	Sorrow
Yin Type A	Joy
Yin Type B	Calmness

Can My Body Type Change?

For better or for worse, your body type is here to stay. Think of it as a diamond in the rough that shines abundantly after being polished. Sure, it may be a bit dirty at first, but that doesn't mean you have to throw it out and exchange it for a new one. Our body type is a precious gift that never gets overused or outdated; it is the source of renewed energy and health. Listen to it and it will teach you; ignore it and it will still teach you—the hard way. The menopausal years are a time when, once again, you must take a deeper look at yourself, your body type, and your inner world. The more you discover about yourself, the more you can improve and modify your response to the menopausal transition. This happens naturally when we discover aspects of ourselves that don't serve us well. Sometimes we may feel too "yingy" or "yangy" and decide to become a yin-like yang type or a yang-like yin type. Nothing is wrong with challenging yourself in this way as long as you don't lose track of who you are. Cultivating your strengths instead of getting caught up with your weaknesses brings about profound change.

Let's review a few key Sasang principles:

- While fluctuating hormone levels contribute to menopausal discomfort, they do not cause it.
- How our mind and body *react* to hormonal fluctuation is what determines the intensity and frequency of our discomfort.
- No matter how uncomfortable your menopausal symptoms are, you can improve your condition significantly by balancing how you react to your environment.
- How we react to hormone changes is influenced by our inherent organ energies and their correlating emotions.
- The recognition of our innate strengths and weaknesses is the first step toward a smooth transition.
- The next step is the modification of our lifestyle through body-type-specific foods and herbs and balancing our predominant emotions.

MENOPAUSE AND
THE FOUR ORGAN SYSTEMS

Each of the four organ systems plays a major role throughout every moment of our entire lives, influencing how we feel emotionally and physically. Menopause is a time when these systems undergo significant changes and it becomes crucial for women to keep their stronger and weaker organs in balance. The stronger lungs of the Yang Type B, for example, have a tendency to steal energy from the rest of the body during menopause, making shortness of breath and chest fullness a common issue as excessive pressure accumulates there. The Yin Type B's stronger kidneys tend to rob energy from the other organs, often leading to urinary discomfort during the menopausal transition.

Menopause-related symptoms are not always body-type specific. The Yin Type As and Yang Type As, for instance, can both experience hot flashes. Yet each body type has its own underlying cause and method of treatment. The Yin Type A's hot flashes are a result of a hyper-developed liver, whereas the Yang Type A's hot flashes are from a hyper-developed spleen. When addressing hot flashes, the Yin

Type As are routinely prescribed herbs that address liver heat and the Yang Type As herbs that cool spleen heat. If herbs that clear spleen heat were given to the Yin Type A or herbs that clear liver heat to the Yang Type A, they may experience temporary relief, but hot flash symptoms would eventually worsen.

As discussed earlier, perimenopause marks the time in a woman's life when yin and yang energy rapidly fluctuate back and forth. While some may experience this process as an unpleasant shock, others may view it as an awakening, as if their life were shifted into high gear. Each of the body types responds differently when yin estrogen or yang progesterone/testosterone energy dominates. When yang energy dominates, it may feel like a double whammy of heat and anger for the yang types, while the yin types suddenly feel bouts of energy they haven't felt before, occasionally propelling them into drastic action. When yin energy dominates, the yin types may feel groggy, bloated, and depressed, while for the yang types, it may help them slow down a bit. When all is said and done, if you can't beat it, well . . . I guess you have to join it.

An ancient Chinese story tells of Yu the Great, a sage who was the only one in more than one hundred years who could tame the raging Yellow River and stop it from flooding. His simple but effective solution was to respect the river and dig it a path around a large mountain standing in its way, instead of building trenches as his forefathers had done. Menopause does not require trenches; it needs to be honored and respected and allowed to flow smoothly. Knowing about the four organ systems is like observing the Yellow River and seeking guidance from it.

Let's take a look at each organ system to see how it may affect the menopausal experience.

The Lung System

Table 1.7 provides a snapshot of the lung system's functions along with its balanced and imbalanced effects during menopause.

TABLE 1.7. FUNCTIONS OF THE LUNG SYSTEM

Function	Balanced Effects	Imbalanced Effects
Controls the opening and closing of skin pores	Sufficient sweating with exercise	Uncontrollable sweating or not enough sweating
Controls the immune system	Prevention of common colds and influenza	Frequent chills and fever, common colds, viral influence
Controls the flow of energy to the brain	Ability to focus and remember things easily	Lack of mental clarity, forgetfulness
Controls sorrow	Ability to feel sad and sympathize with others but not be overwhelmed by it	Depression, utter wretchedness

Born with weaker lungs, Yin Type As often have difficulty sweating. Yet the tides change during perimenopause, when excessive heat accumulation in the body escapes from their hyperactive liver, pushing through the skin's pores. During this phase, the Yin Type A may go from being a nonsweater to a sweat factory. Trauma to the lungs from smoking or other irritants can also be a culprit behind excessive or deficient sweating, no matter what the body type. Weakened lungs may encourage the onset of immune-related disorders during perimenopause or after menopause, such as common colds, rashes, joint inflammation, or allergies. "Foggy brain," or a lack of mental clarity and loss of memory, is another common symptom of lung deficiency during menopause. Whereas Western medicine equates this with menopause-related hormone loss, Sasang medicine relates it to a deficiency of the lungs and their ability to pump energy upward to the brain. See chapter 12, "Sailing through the Mist," for more details on foggy brain.

Each emotion, according to Eastern medicine, has its important role to play in encouraging energy to flow within the body. Excessive emotions, however, cause energy to either flow too quickly or stagnate and accumulate. As we've seen, sorrow is the basis of the Yang Type B's actions. When balanced, sorrow helps the lungs push energy upward to fill the upper body and brain. Yet unbalanced sorrow can send shockwaves of energy upward, interfering with brain function and leading to depression and lack of clarity. If Yang Type Bs learn to control their sorrow, then optimum health awaits them.

The Spleen System

Table 1.8 provides a snapshot of the spleen system's functions along with its balanced and imbalanced effects during menopause.

TABLE 1.8. FUNCTIONS OF THE SPLEEN SYSTEM

Function	Balanced Effects	Imbalanced Effects
Controls metabolic function	Sufficient digestion and transformation of food into energy	Fatigue after meals, diarrhea and/or constipation
Regulates body temperature—heats the body up	Just enough warmth in the body	Hot flashes (excessive heat), facial redness, acne
Controls the flow of energy to the shoulders, upper back, and chest	Sufficient shoulder mobility and sturdy upper back posture	Tightness and lack of mobility of the shoulder joint, postural issues (slouching)
Controls anger	Ability to express anger and stand up for oneself/ others	Rage, animosity, or the inability to express anger

Weight gain is another common occurrence during the menopausal years. Hormone loss, by itself, cannot be blamed since other factors such as emotion, diet, and exercise play a significant role. In Sasang medicine, the spleen is in charge of metabolism and hence its weakness may result in weight gain or other digestive issues such as stomachaches, a sensation of fullness after meals, and/or diarrhea. Both yin types have a tendency to gain weight and suffer from digestive issues as a result of a weaker spleen system, especially around menopausal age, when metabolism switches into low gear. The spleen is also responsible for keeping our body warm, causing the Yang Type A to overheat easily and the Yin Type B, born with a weaker spleen, to freeze. The other body types tend to flip-flop between feeling hot and cold, pushing off the covers after a hot flash only to shiver with cold shortly afterward.

Anger originates from the spleen, assisting in the circulation of energy throughout the chest. Yet unbalanced anger in the form of rage can cause energy to stagnate in the chest, interfering with heart and stomach function. If Yang Type As learn to control their predominant emotion of anger, then optimum health will be theirs.

The Liver System

Table 1.9 provides a snapshot of the liver system's functions along with its balanced and imbalanced effects during menopause.

TABLE 1.9. FUNCTIONS OF THE LIVER SYSTEM

Function	Balanced Effects	Imbalanced Effects
Controls the detoxification of blood	Adequate blood flow, prevention of inflammation and buildup of oxidants	Toxic accumulation and thickening of blood, causing circulatory issues
Regulates the digestion of fatty foods and protein	Sufficient breakdown of fatty foods and utilization of protein	Accumulation of fat tissue in the abdomen
Controls the flow of energy to the abdomen	Smooth bowel flow through the intestines	Constipation and/or diarrhea
Controls joy	Ability to feel joyful and share one's joy with others	Twisted joy, finding joy in taking advantage of others

For the most part, the Yin Type A's stronger liver does an efficient job of filtering toxins from the blood. Yet excessive strength often throws things off, since enhanced liver absorption soaks up everything in sight. During perimenopause, our stronger organ may go berserk, frantically attempting to balance rapidly shifting hormones and bodily energies. The stronger liver will eventually respond by becoming engorged with the very toxins it is supposed to let go of, resulting in fat accumulation in the lower abdomen—its home. Excessive absorption may also cause the bowels to stagnate or harden. Weight gain and constipation are often the culprits behind an uncomfortable menopause transition for the Yin Type A.

Joy is associated with the liver and helps it to fill the upper abdomen with fresh blood and energy. Yet unbalanced joy can lead to congestion and abdominal issues. Excessive joy, or the extreme desire for joy, can also cause liver toxicity. If Yin Type As learn to balance their predominant emotion of joy, then they can experience optimum health. Born with a weaker liver system, Yang Type Bs have difficulty seeing the light at the end of the tunnel; hence sorrow rather than joy is their predominant emotion. For Yang Type Bs, menopause is often a time when they come face-to-face with sadness as it works its way to the surface. While Yin

Type As may also have to clean a few sorrowful skeletons out of their menopausal closet, unexpected moments of profound joy also manifest. The key is to strike a balance between joy and sorrow and not let either emotion steer you astray.

The Kidney System

Table 1.10 provides a snapshot of the kidney system's functions along with its balanced and imbalanced effects during menopause.

TABLE 1.10. FUNCTIONS OF THE KIDNEY SYSTEM

Function	Balanced Effects	Imbalanced Effects
Controls urinary output and water metabolism	Sufficient urine output without urgency	Frequent and/or incomplete urinary output
Regulates body temperature—cools the body down	Cooling of the body just enough to prevent overheating	Constant feeling of cold
Controls the flow of energy to the hips, lumbar spine, and lower body	Rapid healing of lower body injuries, sufficient strength of lower body	Weakness and lack of mobility of the lower back, hips, or legs, balance issues
Controls calmness	Ability to feel calm in most, if not all, situations	Anxiety, isolation, desperate desire to feel calm

The kidneys are the Yin Type B's strongest organ, providing strong legs and a healthy urinary system and lumbar spine area. They come in handy during menopause by cooling the body to resolve hot flashes. Yet if the other organs have trouble getting along with one another, the kidneys may struggle to mediate the situation, resulting in kidney-related symptoms. During the change of life, even Yin Type Bs may notice a reduction of energy in their lower body or have urinary difficulties, but the kidneys are usually the last organ to give them trouble. The Yang Type A's weaker kidneys, on the other hand, are prone to chronic urinary issues such as difficult or frequent urination or recurring urinary tract infections (UTIs) that may worsen during the menopausal transition. Thus, Yin Type Bs have to be significantly ill before they experience kidney-weakness-related symptoms, while for Yang Type As they may be commonplace.

Calmness, associated with the kidneys, helps fill the lower body with fresh blood and energy. Yet unbalanced calmness, or the extreme desire for it, can sink the energy downward, causing diarrhea and extreme fatigue. If Yin Type Bs learn to control their predominant emotion of calmness, then optimum health awaits, but if they try too hard to achieve it, then even their stronger kidneys cannot escape illness. Born with a weaker kidney system, Yang Type As have difficulty calming down; hence anger rather than calmness is their predominant emotion. For the Yang Type A, menopause is a time when anger often rages out of control. While the Yin Type B may also experience bouts of anger during menopause, an overall sense of calmness always seems to cool things down. The key is to strike a balance between calmness and anger and not let either emotion get the best of you.

THE FOUR SENSES AND MENOPAUSE

Did you know that many women experience a heightened sense of smell during perimenopause? This phenomenon, which is seldom discussed in the literature, also tends to occur during the early stages of pregnancy and may have to do with your body type! In Sasang medicine, the sense of smell correlates with the liver. Since Yin Type As are born with a stronger liver, they have a stronger sense of smell. Actually, the sense of smell is how they relate to the world around them. The Yin Type A can "smell a rat" when others are not truthful, or be attracted to someone because of how they smell. Whenever the mind and body go through a major transition (such as pregnancy or menopause), our strongest organ has to work harder to keep us on our toes, so its correlating emotion and sense are enhanced. The Yin Type A's predominant emotion of joy, which is associated with the liver, is also enhanced during the change of life and offers bouts of utter delight and rejuvenation. Despite these benefits, unfortunate circumstances and rancid odors are unavoidable, and unsustainable joy or stinky perfume may drive the Yin Type A crazy. The nose is also a great conduit for healing, as it is a portal through which the introduction of pleasant scents can enter weaker lungs and make them stronger.

The Yin Type B's stronger kidneys provide them with an enhanced sense of taste, which increases during perimenopause. This can do funny things to a Yin Type B's taste buds. In some cases it may give them a renewed interest in food, but in others it can induce food sensitivities and an aversion to certain flavors. The Yin Type B's sense of taste extends beyond food, providing them with a sensitive "taste" in music, theater, photography, and so forth. For this type, menopause may be a chance to enhance an interest in the arts and further natural abilities.

A stronger spleen gives the Yang Type A keen eyesight that heightens during menopause. We're not talking about the ability to see with the eyes per se, but rather to see with the mind, or with insight. Even if their eyesight fails them, Yang Type As are still capable of "seeing through" people or "reading between the lines," an ability that comes from the eyes, according to Sasang medicine, which are associated with the spleen.

Thanks to a pair of stronger lungs, the Yang Type B can hear the sound of the Earth rotating on its axis . . . well, metaphorically at least. The lungs, associated with the ears, connect us with the universe and heavens above. Menopause for Yang Type Bs is a time of enhanced intuition and psychic capability as their stronger lung energy gets a boost. Yet it's also a time when they have difficulty keeping their feet on the ground and relating to others. They may "hear" voices in their head or be extremely sensitive to certain sounds.

Table 1.11 provides each body type's strongest sense and correlating organ.

TABLE 1.11. STRONGEST SENSES AND CORRELATING ORGANS OF EACH BODY TYPE

Body Type	Strongest Organ System	Correlating Sense Organ	Strongest Sense
Yang Type A	Spleen	Eyes	Sight
Yang Type B	Lungs	Ears	Hearing
Yin Type A	Liver	Nose	Smell
Yin Type B	Kidneys	Mouth	Taste

We are more than just a vessel of hormones lost at sea, fighting the rough waves of menopause. Instead, we carry a unique combination of yin and yang, emotional and physical strengths, and heightened sensitivities. By providing us with a map and compass and the coordinates to determine where we are, the Sasang approach offers abundant opportunities for self-discovery and well-being along the way.

Now that we've dipped our feet into the basics of Sasang medicine, it's time to figure out your body type and apply these concepts to your own menopausal journey.

2

Discovering Your Yin Yang Body Type

Physical and Personality Tests to Uncover Your Type

Our body type is reflected in everything we do and determines how we react to pain, illness, joy, love, stress, and the like. Getting to know your body type requires a significant amount of self-reflection. In Korea, Sasang medicine continues to evolve as researchers identify new and innovative ways to distinguish each body type from the others. Anything from skin and voice tone to facial features can give you hints about your body type. None of these methods by themselves, however, are 100 percent accurate. Body type discovery is often a challenging process that can take a considerable amount of time because what is expressed outwardly may actually be only a fraction of what is felt deep inside. We also develop traits that are not necessarily associated with our body type. These traits become ingrained over time as we observe how others approach life. Acquiring traits from other body types is necessary for our survival and to balance our own weaknesses. Menopause may catch us by surprise, bringing out aspects of mind and body that do not fit the paradigm of life we are accustomed to. The body type is the core matrix of our mind and body; it lurks beneath layer upon layer of who we are on the outside. Each phase in life brings an opportunity to discover untapped physiological and psychological traits that come to the surface, demanding our attention.

Yin Yang Balance for Menopause utilizes three of the most efficient, time-tested ways to determine your body type. The combination of these different techniques ensures the accuracy of your body type reading. The first technique helps you determine whether you tend more to yin or to yang. The second technique has two parts: method A focuses on the relative size and shape of your bodily features, since each body type has its own hyper- and hypodeveloped areas of the body, and method B is trait-specific, focusing on your daily physical and emotional tendencies. The third technique is unique to the premise of this book and aims to clarify your type further by including menopause-specific questions.

UNDERSTANDING THE THREE PARTS OF THE BODY TYPE TEST

It is generally pretty easy to respond to the body shape statements, as they solely involve examination of external features. The other techniques, however, are less tangible and often require considerable self-reflection. Let's examine each in detail.

Part 1: Am I a Yin or a Yang Type?

First we begin with a test to determine if you have more yin or yang traits, as the knowledge of whether you are a yin or yang type is half the battle. The test consists of a number of statements that you will rate according to how much or how little they reflect your true nature. Although these statements are relatively easy to respond to compared to the rest of the test, be extremely careful when considering them. Your stronger nature—yin or yang—as determined by this test will guide which subsequent portions of the test you will take to determine whether you are an A or B body type within that nature. If these statements aren't rated accurately, then your body type results won't be accurate.

No matter how much research goes into making this kind of survey, any test that requires us to reflect on traits that we ourselves may not be aware of can often prove difficult to take. If you are having trouble completing the yin yang body type test, try one or more of the following tips:

> **Tip #1:** Take each test over again to make sure you did not overlook anything.
>
> **Tip #2:** Ask someone close to you to go over the results and reflect on them a second time to confirm that your answers are accurate.
>
> **Tip #3:** Keep in mind that a tendency is not something acquired but a natural inclination. When taking the test, ask yourself if this or that trait or reaction comes naturally for you or not. A trait that takes significant effort to acquire is not associated with your body type. Sure, we may still have to work hard to develop a specific trait that correlates with our type, but this is different than trying to build one that was never there to begin with.

Part 2: Which Yin or Yang Type Am I?

Part 2 of the yin yang body type test consists of two sections. The first section, "Outward Appearance," involves a careful examination of your outward body features, while the second section looks at your emotional and physiological traits.

Method A: Outward Appearance

The shape and ratio of the different parts of the body hint at our body type. Researchers are beginning to take notice of how these features influence how we interact socially. Take, for instance, a recent study that discovered how specific facial features, such as the distance between the cheekbones, has a direct effect on how our personality is interpreted.[1] A wider distance implies a greater degree of dominance, and a narrower distance implies a submissive, gentle quality of character. Interestingly, wider distances have been recorded to coincide with a higher rate of penalties among ice hockey players.[2] These findings also coincide with how the Yin Type B, considered to have a narrower facial width compared to the other types, is more submissive and gentle than the others.

In another study done in 1966, participants were asked to judge the

character of others based solely on a facial photo. Amusingly, their immediate judgment was spot-on when it came to three traits—extroversion,
conscientiousness, and openness—as determined by personality test
results.[3] As we discovered earlier, yang types have a tendency to be more
open and extroverted than the yin types. Studies such as these suggest
that we may actually have the built-in capability of detecting certain
body-type characteristics and their corresponding traits immediately
after meeting others for the first time. They also show just how inter-
connected appearance and character may actually be.

In Eastern medicine, not just the face but the entire surface of our
body is a direct reflection of what occurs inside. Each organ in our body
communicates with the surface in its own way. The lungs, for example,
control the opening and closing of the skin pores, the spleen main-
tains muscle tone, the liver keeps our tendons elastic, and the kidneys
uphold the integrity of our hair and skin. If any of these organs begin
to fail, their corresponding body parts will also be affected. As we saw
earlier, not only does trauma or illness affect our organs, but our emotions do, too. Anger, which is associated with the spleen, can also have
an effect on the contraction of our muscles. Excessive anger, associated
with excessive spleen energy, can therefore easily lead to muscle spasms.
Weakness of the spleen and the inability to express anger, on the other
hand, can result in a weakened or hunched-over appearance.

The development of different parts of our body is also affected by
our stronger (hyperdeveloped) and weaker (hypodeveloped) organs.
Yang types are born with stronger yang organs. Since yang corresponds
to the upper body, these organs cause the muscles, tendons, and bones
of the upper body to be better developed than those in the lower body.
Yin types, on the other hand, have stronger yin organs and hence are
relatively better developed in their lower body.

In addition to these general differences, there are also body-type-
specific differences in appearance. Yang Type As often have protruding
cheekbones and broad shoulders, characteristics that correspond to a
stronger spleen. Yet not all Yang Type As have protruding cheekbones.
This is where things get a bit tricky. If you're heavyset, your face may look
rounded no matter what body type you are. In such cases, you might need
to look at a childhood picture to see if your face changed as you got older.

If so, there may be a Yang Type A lurking within you! Taking a good look in the mirror or asking a friend may also help if you are simply not sure. Generally speaking, our body-type-specific features tend to appear more clearly as we reach middle age. Yet in our youth and later years our body type is often obscured due to age-related physiological changes.

Weight often causes confusion when determining your body type. It is common for budding Sasang experts to believe that Yin Type As are the "heavyset" body type, since their features are often rounded. While most obese people have this body type, there are many exceptions to this rule. Some of the skinniest people I have met are Yin Type As. Don't fret! There are plenty of other clues at your disposal. The lower two or three ribs of skinny Yin Type As, for example, often flare outward on both sides of the rib cage as if to prepare them to develop a large abdomen, even if there is absolutely no other sign of impending weight gain. This is also because the lowermost ribs cover the liver, which, in the Yin Type A's case, is the largest, strongest, most developed organ in the body.

Keep in mind the following tips to help ensure the accuracy of your outward appearance results:

Tip #1: Observe your body closely and take the time to assess every detail. Keep in mind that certain body-type features are less obvious than others.

Tip #2: It is often helpful to use a mirror when examining your body-type features.

Tip #3: Some features may not be apparent when you are clothed, so you may need to disrobe.

Tip #4: If you are not sure whether a certain body-type feature applies to you, ask a close friend, spouse, or family member.

Tip #5: We do not always manifest all the features of our body type. Even though most Yin Type Bs have a short stature, for example, there may be tall people with this body type, too. Even if you don't look like a particular body type, it doesn't necessarily mean that it's not yours. The remaining sections of the yin yang body type test, involving emotional and physiological traits, are even more significant than outward appearance.

Method B: Emotional and Physiological Traits

Our external appearance can be altered cosmetically or by experience, food intake, trauma, and so on, sometimes obscuring our body-type-related appearance. The emotional and physiological traits section of the test digs deeper into the characteristics of each type that are less easily affected by the above factors. While this section is more accurate in determining your body type, it is also more challenging since our emotions are not always easy to interpret. Emotions are often layered, and getting down to how we feel at the core can be a bit tricky. Sadness, for example, may be hiding under layer upon layer of anger, while anxiety may be nothing but joy getting out of hand. This section requires a lot of self-reflection and deep thought, and by completing it, you will have gained deeper insight into the inner workings of your mind and body.

Try your best to rate as many statements as possible, either by yourself or with the help of a close friend or family member to get another perspective. While completing this section, keep the following tips in mind:

Tip #1: If you are not sure of an answer, it may be helpful to consult someone who is close to you, such as your spouse, a parent, a sibling, or a best friend.

Tip #2: Focus on overall tendencies; certain tendencies may change from day to day or throughout the years, making a statement difficult to rate. For the sake of the yin yang body type test it is sometimes helpful to reflect on how things used to be when you were growing up, since our body type never changes.

Tip #3: Some statements may require close self-examination. For instance, you may have to take a good look in the mirror or examine how you walk.

Tip #4: Do not rate the statement if, no matter how much you try, you cannot decide on how relevant it is to you. It is better to leave it blank than to muddle the test results.

Tip #5: If you are not sure how to rate a particular statement, refer to the clarification keys at the end of each section. They offer explanations of the statements, making them easier to assess.

Tip #6: Did you score a tie between two body types? Is your score for one body type only slightly higher than your score for another? If either of these occurs, go over the test again to make sure of your answers. You may also ask for assistance from others who know you well. If, after taking the test again, the difference between two body types remains slight, go with the higher score.

Tip #7: The discovery of your body type often takes a considerable amount of time and self-reflection. A single statement included in the yin yang body type test may take hours, days, or even weeks of careful observation to evaluate correctly. One of the greatest challenges of discovering your body type is the ability to determine whether a particular trait is a reflection of your body type (a core part of who you are) or simply a fleeting characteristic. It is easy to feel angered, for example, if someone cuts in front of you in line, no matter what body type you are. If you rarely get angry, then this feeling may come as a surprise as you may think, "Wow! I must be an angry-natured Yang Type A." Even though anger is a predominant emotion of the Yang Type A, it does not mean that anger makes you a member of this body type. There are often other emotions that lurk beneath our feeling of anger. For Yin Type As, it may be a feeling of "Why can't he be friendly?" since friendship and care are so important to them. For Yang Type As, anger in this situation is a result of feeling disrespected and looked down upon as they think, "How can he treat *me* like this?" Take ample time getting to the root of your emotional and physical characteristics.

Tip #8: If you are still finding the yin yang body type quest to be a challenge, contact our team of Sasang specialists at sasangmedicine.com for additional assistance.

Part 3: Menopause-Specific Indicators

Your body type will most likely have revealed itself by the time you reach this section of the test. The menopause symptoms survey aims to add clarity to the process of body-type discovery. This section is separated into the menopause-related symptoms you may be experiencing. If you don't experience any of the symptoms mentioned in this section, simply leave the statements blank. While completing this section, keep the following tips in mind:

Tip #1: Leave sections blank if they do not apply to your menopausal situation.

Tip #2: Even if you are not currently experiencing a particular menopause-related symptom, try to answer the section if you remember how it felt in the past.

Tip #3: Don't forget to add the points gained in this section to the table at the end of the chapter.

Tip #4: If the test scores between body types are similar by the time you reach this section, then this may be the only way to determine which type you are. If the scores are still similar after you complete this section, I recommend redoing the test from the beginning and following the tips in part 2, methods A and B.

Discovering your body type opens up a whole new spectrum of relationship and health opportunities. Even with the discovery of your body type, however, harmony and balance may feel elusive. There may be aspects of your body type that you wish to change and others that you desire to cling to. Getting to know your body type is a firm step toward navigating through life's challenges and reaching your true potential. Yet it is also accompanied with the responsibility to modify and/or accept who you are physically and emotionally in order to become a healthier and more balanced person. Identifying your body type is the first step toward revealing the infinite potential that lies deep within you.

Take ample time to carefully read through the sections below and answer each question as accurately as possible.

PART I: AM I A YIN OR A YANG TYPE?

This section consists of eight statements that will help you determine whether you are more yin or yang. For each statement in table 2.1 on page 44, choose the response that most accurately reflects who you are. Tally up your score at the end of this section to find out which test to take next. If you have a higher yang score, then only complete the Yang Type A and Yang Type B tests. If you have a higher yin score, then only complete the Yin Type A and Yin Type B tests. If the total scores for each body type, yin and yang, are equal or insignificantly different (by two or less points), then assess both yin and yang body type statements (Yang Type A, Yang Type B, Yin Type A, Yin Type B) in the next part. Following this test section is a clarification key that elaborates on the statements to better help you find your own true response to those you are struggling with.

TABLE 2.1. YIN OR YANG TEST

	All of the Time	Most of the Time	Rarely	Never
1. I naturally enjoy getting up early.	Yang: +2	Yang: +1	Yin: 0	Yin: 0
2. I am exhausted in the evening.	Yang: +2	Yang: +1	Yin: 0	Yin: 0
3. I am easily agitated.	Yang: +2	Yang: +1	Yin: 0	Yin: 0
4. I have more strength in my upper body than my lower body.	Yang: +2	Yang: +1	Yin: 0	Yin: 0
5. I am calm-natured.	Yin: +2	Yin: +1	Yang: 0	Yang: 0
6. I have a slow metabolism.	Yin: +2	Yin: +1	Yang: 0	Yang: 0
7. I am introverted.	Yin: +2	Yin: +1	Yang: 0	Yang: 0
8. I prefer being warm to being cold.	Yin: +2	Yin: +1	Yang: 0	Yang: 0

Yin or Yang Test Clarification Key

Statement 1: The morning correlates with yang, and the yang types often find it easier to function during this part of the day. The yin types have more energy in the evening, during the yin phase of the day. The yin types may also become morning people through motivation and persistence, so be careful and think intensely when assessing this statement, referring to your natural, untouched tendencies.

Statement 2: Evening is the territory of the yin types. The otherwise upbeat and active yang types often become dysfunctional as the evening progresses.

Statement 3: Anger and sorrow are yang emotions, while joy and comfort/calmness are yin emotions, according to Sasang medicine.

Note: Abundant anger is the source of sorrow for the yang types, just as abundant sorrow morphs into anger.

Statement 4: The upper body organ systems of the lungs and spleen are more developed and stronger among the yang types. Hence, the muscles, tendons, ligaments, and bone structure of the upper body are hyperdeveloped, while their lower body is hypodeveloped. The opposite is true for the yin types, whose lower-body liver and kidney systems are stronger. The upper body of the yang types tends to heal from injury more quickly than their lower body, whereas the lower body of the yin types recovers faster than the upper.

Statement 5: Calmness correlates with the kidneys, the strongest organ of the Yin Type B and second-strongest of the Yin Type A. Because the yin types are comfort-prone, they prioritize calmness more than the yang types. The yin types are almost always aware of feeling anxious or stressed, whereas the yang types rarely have a clue even though they may be experiencing it.

Statement 6: Blood and energy flow more easily for the yang types thanks to abundant yang energy, whereas the yin types often have to work harder to lose weight, improve cardiovascular health, and/or boost their metabolism due to excessive yin energy. Even the thin yin type may be plagued with a sluggish metabolism and feel bloated and heavy after eating. Yang correlates with quick movement and yin with stagnation, slow movement, and even motionlessness.

Statement 7: The yang types tend to be more outgoing and less shy than the yin types because yang is associated with outward-flowing energy and yin corresponds to inward-flowing energy. The Yang Type A tends to be the most outgoing of the bunch, while the Yin Type B is introverted, shy, and timid. Caution! Yang Type As may also feel anxious around others, but they still feel it is their duty, or responsibility, to engage with them and rarely think twice about it. Yin Type Bs' social anxiety often keeps them from engaging, giving them a preference for being alone.

Statement 8: Although for some this sounds like an easy statement to evaluate, others who find both hot and cold comfortable and/or unbearable might find it challenging. So think carefully when responding to this statement! It is easier for Yin Type Bs to figure out, because they clearly detest being cold, and for Yang Type As, who particularly dislike overheating. The Yin Type A and Yang Type B, however, may have a tougher time with this statement. Yet even though Yin Type As may also dislike being hot, unlike the yang types, they still enjoy the warmth of a hot shower or bath or hot tea in warmer weather or after exercise. And even though Yang Type Bs may dislike being cold, unlike the yin types, they still enjoy drinking colder fluids, even in bitter cold weather.

Use table 2.2 to tally up your total yin and yang scores.

TABLE 2.2. TOTAL SCORES FOR PART 1

Total Yin Score	Total Yang Score

PART 2: METHOD A—OUTWARD APPEARANCE

If you received a higher yin score in part 1, then respond *only* to the Yin Types A and B statements in the following section. If you received a higher yang score in part 1, then respond *only* to the Yang Types A and B statements in the following section. If your score was tied between the two types or there was a negligible difference (two points or less) between them, feel free to take both the yin and yang tests to continue to get a sense of which traits are stronger.

Add one point for each body feature that applies to you in tables 2.3 through 2.6 on pages 47–52, and add your total score to table 2.16 on page 73 at the end of the chapter.

TABLE 2.3. YANG TYPE A BODY FEATURE SCORE CHART

Body Feature	Points
Broad forehead	
Sunrise-shaped eyelids	
Prominent cheekbones	
Narrow chin	
Broad shoulders	
Developed chest and upper body	
Tapered waist	
Small buttocks	
Total points	

TABLE 2.4. YANG TYPE B BODY FEATURE SCORE CHART

Body Feature	Points
Pointy head vertex	
Pointy/large ears	
Bulging chin	
Thick neck	
Developed upper body	
Narrow waist	
Narrow thighs	
Overall intense/powerful appearance	
Total points	

YANG TYPE A FEMALE

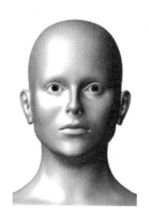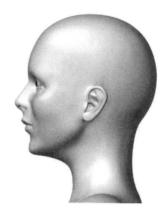

Broad forehead, prominent cheekbones, narrow chin, sunrise-shaped
eyes that arch upward like the sun rising above a mountain

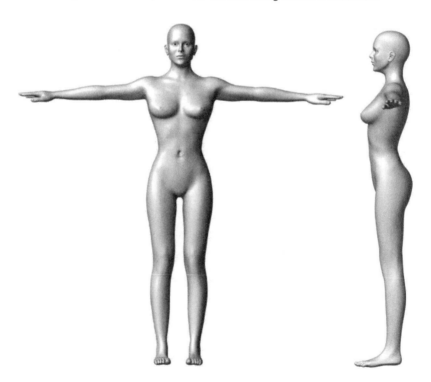

Broad shoulders, developed chest and breast area, tapered waist, smaller buttocks

YANG TYPE B FEMALE

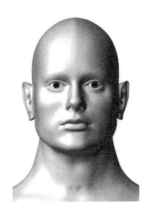
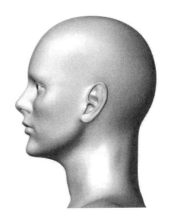

Head has pointy vertex, pointy large ears, bulging chin, thicker neck

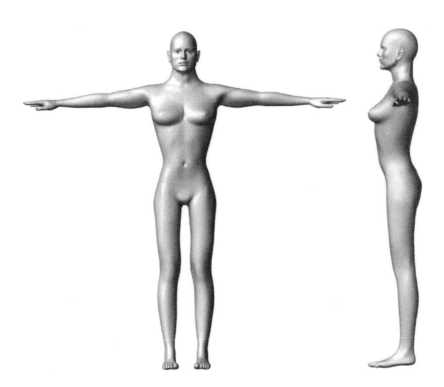

Narrow waist, developed upper body, narrow thighs,
overall intense/powerful appearance

TABLE 2.5. YIN TYPE A BODY FEATURE SCORE CHART

Body Feature	Points
Roundish head	
Roundish eyes	
Large facial features	
Overall calm appearance	
Lower few ribs flare outward	
Protruding abdomen	
Large feet (in proportion to rest of body)	
Developed buttocks	
Total points	

TABLE 2.6. YIN TYPE B BODY FEATURE SCORE CHART

Body Feature	Points
Small head	
Small facial features	
Narrow head shape	
Narrow neck	
Shorter height	
Narrow chest	
Developed buttocks	
Frail appearance	
Total points	

YIN TYPE A FEMALE

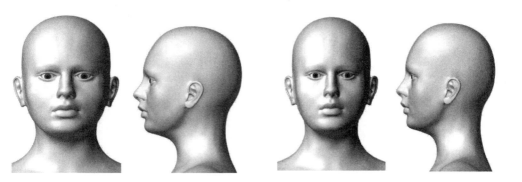

Roundish eyes and head, larger facial features,
overall calm/relaxed appearance

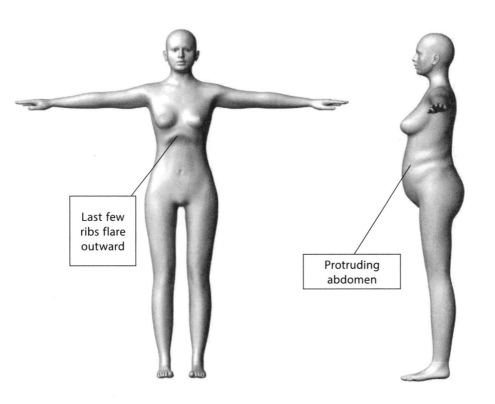

Last few
ribs flare
outward

Protruding
abdomen

Thick and/or rough skin, large foot size

YIN TYPE B FEMALE

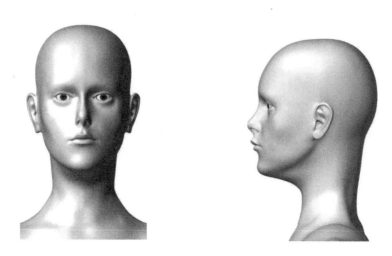

Smaller and narrow-shaped head, narrow neck, smaller facial features

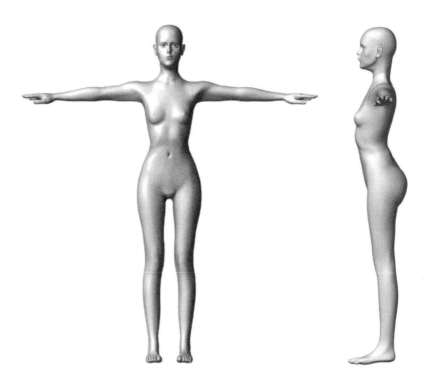

Shorter height, narrow chest, developed buttocks, overall frail appearance

PART 2: METHOD B—EMOTIONAL AND PHYSIOLOGICAL TRAITS

If you received a higher yang score in part 1, then respond *only* to the Yang Types A and B statements (see tables 2.7 and 2.8 on pages 54 and 57, respectively) in the following section. If you received a higher yin score in part 1, then respond *only* to the Yin Types A and B statements (see tables 2.9 and 2.10 on pages 60 and 63, respectively) in the following section. If your score was tied between two types or there was a negligible difference (two points or less) between them, feel free to take both the yin and yang tests to continue to get a sense of which traits are stronger.

Again, following each test section are elaborations on each statement to better help you respond to the ones you are struggling with and provide an explanation about why you have this or that tendency. Most of us don't bother to question why our body and mind react a particular way to a given situation. If you are not certain of how to respond to a statement, be sure to read the clarification key for that statement for further explanation before skipping it. Add your total scores to the table at the end of the chapter.

TABLE 2.7. YANG TYPE A STATEMENTS

	Never (Not True)	Sometimes True (Maybe)	Often True (Likely)	Always True (Definitely)
1. Skipping a bowel movement for several days causes other issues for me (headache, stomachache, bloating, etc.).	0	2	4	6
2. My feet feel hot at night.	0	2	4	6
3. I am very direct with others, often offending them as a result.	0	2	4	6
4. I get easily agitated when I'm hungry.	0	2	4	6
5. I tend to be very judgmental of others.	0	2	4	6
6a. I am good at multitasking . . . (If you circled 2 or higher, then respond to part b of this statement.)	0	1	2	3
6b. . . . but I'm not accurate/thorough.	0	1	2	3
7a. My anger has a tendency to explode . . . (If you circled 2 or higher, respond to part b of this statement.)	0	1	2	3
7b. . . . but my energy feels drained once the anger is released.	0	1	2	3
8. I gain *and* lose weight quickly. (Answer "not true" if only half of this statement is true.)	0	1	2	3
9. I dislike conforming to others but enjoy when others follow me.	0	1	2	3
10. One or more of the following symptoms occur after eating a portion (4 grams) or more of chicken: stomachache, bowel issues (diarrhea/constipation), body aches, vomiting.	0	1	2	3
Total score (per column)				
Grand total score (all columns combined)				

Yang Type A Clarification Key

Statement 1: According to Sasang medicine, yin represents the downward movement of energy within the body, while yang represents the upward movement. Yang types often have trouble taming their yang energy, as it desires to go up, up, and away. Bowel movements help release excess yang from the body. If Yang Type As skip bowel movements for a few days, pressure starts to accumulate due to blocked yang energy, eventually leading to a situation referred to as "yang rebellion" in which it bursts upward, quickly causing headaches, chest pain, or other acute discomfort.

Statement 2: Because yang corresponds to heat, yang types tend to feel hotter than yin types. Sleep is a way to release excess tension and heat from the body. With so much heat already brewing within, yang types often sweat or otherwise feel hot at night, as they release even more heat. Yang Type As, therefore, usually sleep without the covers over their feet in order to stay cooler. Be aware! We're not talking hot flashes here. If feeling hot at night is only a recent phenomenon and you're going through the change, then the answer is "Never/Not True."

Statement 3: Yang Type As are very direct with others as a result of their tendency to be quick-witted and straight to the point without thinking of the consequences. At times, this trait may give them the appearance of being tough, as they go straight for the gut, or otherwise rash and impolite.

Statement 4: Born with a stronger stomach, Yang Type As need to eat often or consume hearty foods to keep their overactive digestive system busy. Hunger causes a rapid accumulation of stomach acid or, in Eastern medicine terms, "stomach fire," which rebels upward and bombards the heart, leading to agitation and anger. Most of the Yang Type A's digestive and emotional issues can be addressed by avoiding long stretches without food and eating body-type-compatible foods.

Statement 5: Yang Type As are quick to judge others without truly giving them a chance. However, quick judgment also has its advantages. Quick-witted and wise Yang Type As are superior at "figuring out" other people and are often sought after for relationship advice. Yang Type As appear intuitive to some and harsh to others.

Statement 6: Yang correlates with action, while yin correlates with inaction. Therefore, yang body types tend to become hyperactive and have a tendency to take on several tasks at once. While yang types are good at multitasking, they tend not to focus on detail. Thus, Yang Type As have a reputation of being too hasty, which often leads to inaccuracy and inconsistency.

Statement 7: According to Sasang medicine, Yang Type As may easily grow impatient when things do not go their way. As a result, Yang Type As often appear angry. This explosive anger may be expressed toward one person or society at large. Yang Type As must work to control their anger because, unchecked, it eventually morphs into acute sadness, which could eventually destroy their health.

Statement 8: The Yang Type As' metabolism is fast and efficient—a yang quality—making it difficult to gain and easy to lose fatty tissue. Yet their weaker kidneys may cause water retention and water-related weight gain from stress and/or fatigue. Water comes and goes much faster than fatty tissue.

Statement 9: Yang Type As are usually the ones to start a trend rather than follow it. They make friends by attracting others to their innovative and trendy ways.

Statement 10: Chicken is considered a hot-natured food, and despite being an excellent source of warmth for the cold Yin Type B stomach, it can lead to stomachaches, bowel issues, body aches, and/or vomiting by scorching Yang Type A's hot stomach. Shellfish, which is a cold-natured food, helps quench the stomach heat of Yang Type As, making it particularly appetizing for them.

TABLE 2.8. YANG TYPE B STATEMENTS

	Never (Not True)	Sometimes True (Maybe)	Often True (Likely)	Always True (Definitely)
1. My neck is larger in proportion to the rest of my body.	0	2	4	6
2. I cannot stand it when others aren't being straightforward/direct.	0	2	4	6
3. I tend to lose my balance and have since childhood.	0	2	4	6
4. I feel the need to be in charge and tell others what to do.	0	2	4	6
5. I push myself to the point of collapsing from exhaustion.	0	2	4	6
6. I have or used to have a tendency to vomit after eating meat.	0	2	4	6
7. I make friends easily but am difficult to get close to.	0	1	2	3
8a. I experience episodes of sadness . . . (If you circled 3, then respond to part b of this statement.)	0	1	2	3
8b. . . . but my sadness turns into explosive anger.	0	1	2	3
9. I make it my business to be social and to make as many friends as possible.	0	1	2	3
10. I have to keep moving.	0	1	2	3
Total score (per column)				
Grand total score (all columns combined)				

Yang Type B Clarification Key

Statement 1: Since yang represents the upper body, yang types have a better-developed upper body than lower body, and Yang Type Bs have more upper-body strength and development than any of the other three types. Most Yang Type Bs have a thicker neck and a larger head, which are out of proportion with the rest of their body.

Statement 2: Yang Type Bs are easily angered when others keep secrets or do not express themselves openly. This is because of a strong concern with public affairs, associated with Yang Type Bs' hyperdeveloped lungs, and weaker interest in intimate group affiliation, correlated with their hypodeveloped liver. With group affiliation, it's okay to hold back one's emotions and/or true intent to avoid offending others or maintaining peace, but not in public affairs, where holding on to one's original objective takes priority.

Statement 3: The weaker lower body of Yang Type Bs, especially the hip area, causes a loss of balance and clumsiness. Yang Type Bs often trip over their own feet!

Statement 4: The more yang you have, the less you are able to take orders from others. This is because yang is active and ambitious while yin is inactive and apathetic. Yang Type Bs have to be in charge and make the rules rather than abiding by them. If they do not assume a leadership position, sickness and/or depression often ensue.

Statement 5: With so much yang energy, Yang Type Bs have trouble slowing down. They easily ignore basic necessities like daily hygiene, sleep, and relaxation. Instead they push themselves to the point of exhaustion.

Statement 6: Yang Type Bs are born with a weaker liver and gallbladder. The liver and gallbladder are in charge of breaking down fat from meat and other high-protein foods. Yang Type Bs often vomit after eating meat because of their weak liver, which can easily get overwhelmed. As strange as it may seem, Yang Type Bs rarely complain of indigestion, stomach pain, or other symptoms, despite the inability to keep meat down. Their body simply rejects and repels what it cannot handle.

Statement 7: As natural-born leaders, Yang Type Bs often come across as powerful and charismatic. Yet they are at a loss when it comes to intimacy. Yang Type Bs have trouble being courteous to their close friends or family members, and they are often clueless when it comes to sustaining a close relationship, even though they make friends easily. Close friends and/or family members often complain about their domineering behavior.

Statement 8: Sadness is the predominant emotion of Yang Type Bs because it is related to their strongest organ—the lungs. Yang Type Bs often look and feel sad about everything. If the Yang Type B's profound sadness gets out of hand, then it will morph into explosive anger, which causes direct injury to the lungs.

Statement 9: Yang Type Bs find more comfort being in larger groups than being one-on-one with another person. The larger the group, the better they feel. Unlike Yin Type As, however, Yang Type Bs prefer being in charge rather than part of a group.

Statement 10: Yang Type Bs are constantly in motion and rarely have enough time to sleep, which interestingly doesn't seem to have an effect on their energy level, except when there's absolutely nothing left to spare.

TABLE 2.9. YIN TYPE A STATEMENTS

	Never (Not True)	Sometimes True (Maybe)	Often True (Likely)	Always True (Definitely)
1. I have difficulty sweating (I sweat less than others around me).	0	2	4	6
2. My abdomen tends to protrude outward and/or fat accumulates or begins in my abdomen.	0	2	4	6
3. I tend to walk with one foot or both feet pointed outward forty-five degrees or more.	0	2	4	6
4. Relaxation is more appealing to me than physical activity.	0	2	4	6
5. I do not feel well after drinking milk and/or eating wheat products.	0	2	4	6
6. I am sensitive to smell (when my nose is not congested).	0	2	4	6
7. If I do not take action, common colds tend to last a long time for me.	0	2	4	6
8. As a child, I suffered from one or more of the following illnesses: tonsillitis, asthma, ear infections.	0	2	4	6
9. My body features are roundish rather than narrow.	0	1	2	3
10. I get a second wind of energy from (approx.) 11:00 p.m. onward.	0	1	2	3
Total score (per column)				
Grand total score (all columns combined)				

Yin Type A Clarification Key

Statement 1: Yin Type As are born with thicker and/or harder skin, which can be a blessing and a curse. Thicker skin protects their weaker lungs, which are responsible for controlling and supporting immune activity. This trait helps guard against otherwise easily contracted colds and flu. Thicker skin, however, also makes it difficult for sweat to push its way through the pores. Sweating is a way to expel unwanted bacteria and toxins from the body. The inability to sweat often results in prolonged colds and other illnesses. Keep in mind that not all Yin Type As have thick skin or trouble sweating.

Statement 2: The liver controls the flow of blood and energy through the abdominal area. As the Yin Type A's strongest organ, the liver can easily become congested and stagnant from excessive activity. When this happens, fat has a tendency to accumulate in the abdominal area. Skinnier Yin Type As will notice that their abdomen is where the skin feels more abundant and full, even if fat has not accumulated there. Heavier Yin Type As may notice that their abdomen tends to protrude outward. It may be difficult to detect whether or not fat has a tendency to initially accumulate in your abdomen if it has done so already in other areas as well.

Statement 3: Every body type has its own way of walking. Let's take a look at some of the other body types. Yin Type Bs tend to look bashful when they walk. Yang Type As look confident when they walk as they swing their shoulders from side to side. Yang Type Bs have a clumsy walk and often lose their balance. Yin Type As walk with their feet pointed outward, making them appear relaxed and bottom-heavy.

Statement 4: Yin Type As often have a lazy nature because laziness corresponds to the liver, their strongest organ. Laziness and inactivity are also yin attributes, while yang is active and ambitious. Yang types may actually become too active and have trouble slowing down. Yin types tend to be less active and face health issues due to an underactive circulatory system. Not all yin types are lazy, though! Many yin types choose to challenge themselves and keep themselves busy. If you ask diligent yin types what they truly desire to do with their time, however, they will most likely say something like take it easy, relax, or do nothing.

Statement 5: Yin Type As are generally sensitive to wheat and dairy products because these foods overstimulate their strong liver. Each body type benefits from eating foods that stimulate their weaker, rather than stronger, organ systems. According to yin and yang theory, if yang gets stronger, then yin will naturally get weaker. Since the strongest and weakest organs form a yin/yang relationship, stimulation of the stronger organ will further weaken the weaker organ. In the Yin Type A's case, stimulation of the liver will lead to weakness of the lungs. Thus, ingesting dairy and wheat products often leads to the accumulation of phlegm, sinus congestion, fatigue, allergy symptoms, and/or frequent colds.

Statement 6: Yin Type As have an acute sense of smell, thanks to their stronger liver.

Statement 7: The lungs of Yin Type As are the weakest organ in their body. Since the lungs regulate and support the immune system, weaker lungs often lead to frequent and/or long-term colds, which seem to last forever. Cardiovascular exercises, which are extremely beneficial for the health of the lungs, help prevent Yin Type A colds.

Statement 8: The weaker and hypodeveloped lungs of Yin Type As make them vulnerable to childhood infections.

Statement 9: Approximately 80 percent of all Yin Type As have roundish body features. This is because Yin Type As have an abundant amount of yin. According to Asian philosophy, yin is round while yang is narrow. Approximately 70 to 80 percent of all Yin Type As suffer from obesity as a result of having abundant yin. Even if they are not overweight, Yin Type As often have rounder features compared to the other body types. Some yang type individuals, however, may also have roundish features, and some yin types narrower features. The Yin Type B, for example, has a narrow neck and chest because these areas are least developed. The Yang Type A's more developed chest and neck may be rounder than that of the Yin Type B.

Statement 10: Yin is associated with nighttime, while yang is associated with daytime. Yang types tend to have more energy during the day, while yin types have more energy at night. Yin Type As often say that they have difficulty getting to sleep because they feel like reading a book, writing, or using the computer late into the night.

TABLE 2.10. YIN TYPE B STATEMENTS

	Never (Not True)	Sometimes True (Maybe)	Often True (Likely)	Always True (Definitely)
1. I have a tendency to develop digestion-related issues.	0	2	4	6
2. One or more of the following help my digestion: ginger (raw, as tea, or as a condiment), warm fluid, heat on my abdomen.	0	2	4	6
3. I am a picky/finicky eater.	0	2	4	6
4. I prefer to have only one or two (close) friends.	0	2	4	6
5. I am delicate/fragile.	0	2	4	6
6. Fat accumulation usually begins in my buttocks and/or hips.	0	2	4	6
7. Chilled foods often give me indigestion.	0	2	4	6
8. I like to take long, warm baths or showers even on hot summer days.	0	2	4	6
9. I am happiest when I'm alone.	0	1	2	3
10. One or more of the following symptoms occur after eating a portion (4 grams) or more of shellfish (e.g., oysters, clams, crab): stomachache, diarrhea, body aches, vomiting.	0	1	2	3
Total score (per column)				
Grand total score (all columns combined)				

Yin Type B Clarification Key

Statement 1: Yin Type Bs are born with a weaker spleen—the source of body heat. In Sasang medicine, the spleen's heat helps the stomach metabolize food. Because they have a weaker spleen, it is challenging for Yin Type Bs' stomach to break down and digest food, making them very cautious about eating. Issues such as indigestion, stomach flu, or food poisoning could easily and quickly become serious for Yin Type Bs, who often compensate for this weakness by becoming picky eaters. Yin Type Bs can enhance their ability to digest foods with ginger, warm water, and/or heat placed on the abdomen.

Statement 2: Yin represents cold, while yang represents heat. Therefore, excessive coldness tends to affect the digestive system of Yin Type Bs. Ginger is very spicy, and its warm energy counters the cold-infested digestive system of Yin Type Bs. Actually, ginger is one of the most beneficial foods for Yin Type Bs.

Statement 3: The Yin Type B's diet is often limited to safe, nonthreatening foods that support rather than interfere with digestion. Unlike Yin Type As, Yin Type Bs aren't necessarily allergic to this or that food but instead are prone to acute illness such as sudden loss of energy, severe diarrhea, acute abdominal discomfort/pain, and even loss of consciousness from eating incompatible foods. Hence they are naturally and rightfully picky eaters.

Statement 4: The shy nature of Yin Type Bs makes it challenging for them to open up to strangers. They can often be seen with their head down, as if to avoid talking to others. With close friends, however, they may jabber away, as if to make up for lost time.

Statement 5: Yin Type Bs have a timid nature and are hypersensitive to what others think and say about them. They are the first to walk away from a fight and make safety a first priority.

Statement 6: Yin represents the lower body, which in yin types is more developed than the upper body. The abdomen of the Yin Type A and the buttocks of the Yin Type B are the best-developed parts of the body. Fat and muscle tend to accumulate in these areas.

Statement 7: Yin body types benefit from and digest yang (warmer-natured) foods much more easily than yang types, who benefit from and digest yin (cooler-natured) foods much more easily than their yin counterparts. Chicken is one of the most yang of the yang foods and is therefore easier to digest for Yin Type Bs. Chicken has so much yang energy that it may cause indigestion or excess heat in Yang Type As.

Statement 8: With so little yang, Yin Type Bs easily get cold and therefore enjoy warming themselves up from the core outward by taking long, warm baths or showers, which often become a daily ritual needed to kick-start their day. It is very challenging for Yin Type Bs to retain heat, so they often desire to sunbathe or find alternative methods of warming themselves up daily. While other body types may complain of having cold hands and feet, Yin Type Bs often feel cold at the core. Cold is what initiates or exacerbates practically every health issue of the Yin Type B.

Statement 9: Yin Type Bs feel most comfortable when they're alone. They tend to think more clearly and dream away while hiking alone or simply shutting themselves into a locked room. Yin Type Bs are the most self-sufficient of all four body types. While the other body types may be independent or need time alone, they will eventually get lonely and need others to comfort them. Yin Type Bs may also get lonely at times, but that does not mean being in the presence of others will offer them comfort.

Statement 10: Yin represents cold, and with so much yin already lurking in their strong kidneys, Yin Type Bs are quickly affected by cold foods. Yin also represents the deeper parts of the ocean, and according to Eastern medicine, shellfish is said to have a very cold nature, since it is often found lurking on the ocean floor, munching on yin foods. Despite shellfish being a refreshing food for the Yang Type A's stomach heat, if Yin Type Bs eat a substantial amount of shellfish, they will experience symptoms such as stomach pain, lethargy, muscle aches, and/or dark-colored diarrhea. If you like and digest shellfish well, then chances are that you are (a) a very healthy Yin Type B or (b) not a Yin Type B at all.

PART 3: MENOPAUSE-SPECIFIC INDICATORS

If you are still in doubt or interested in further clarifying your body type, then read through the following bonus section and respond only to the statements that pertain to your menopausal experience—hot flashes, libido issues, depression, and/or insomnia (see tables 2.12 through 2.15 on pages 67–71). For example, if you experience hot flashes, complete the hot flash statements, but if you don't, skip over that section and move on to one that applies to you. For each section that you complete, add the total scores for each body type to the scoring table (see table 2.16 on page 73) at the end of the chapter. Then add these to the total score for each body type from the previous part. The final score will indicate your body type. (See the example in table 2.11 below.)

Note: You do not have to continue with this bonus section if part 2 already clearly revealed your body type.

TABLE 2.11. EXAMPLE STATEMENT

	Most of the Time	Sometimes	Rarely	Never
My sexual stamina is not as strong as my desire.	Yin Type A: +2	Yin Type B: +1	Yang Type B: 0	Yang Type A: 0

If you chose "most of the time," then add two points to the Yin Type A test; if you choose "sometimes," then add one point to the Yin Type B test, and for "rarely" or "never," do not add any points. *Caution! The body type order may be different according to the statement, so make sure to apply points to the correct type.*

TABLE 2.12. HOT FLASHES

	Most of the Time	Sometimes	Rarely	Never
1. The warmth of a hot flash makes me feel comfortable.	Yin Type A: +1	Yin Type B: +2	Yang Type A: 0	Yang Type B: 0
2. I feel relief while sweating from a hot flash.	Yin Type A: +2	Yin Type B: +1	Yang Type A: 0	Yang Type B: 0
3. Anger can trigger a hot flash.	Yang Type A: +2	Yang Type B: +1	Yin Type A: 0	Yin Type B: 0
4. One or more of the following occur when I get hot flashes: vomiting, acid regurgitation, dry heaves, excessive salivation.	Yang Type B: +2	Yang Type A: +1	Yin Type A: 0	Yin Type B: 0

Hot Flashes Clarification Key

Statement 1: Yin Type Bs are born with excessive yin cold energy and the least yang heat energy of the four types, so hot flashes may actually give them comfort. Yin Type As are often warmer than Yin Type Bs but may occasionally enjoy the heat of a hot flash because they also have more yin than the yang types, who have plenty of heat lurking within them already. Hot flashes can easily exhaust and overheat the yang types.

Statement 2: Yin Type A is the only body type that benefits from abundant sweating because it flushes the body of toxins entrapped by a hyperdeveloped liver. Occasional sweating, as long as it doesn't leave them drenched, may also benefit Yin Type Bs. Since sweat itself is yin, the yin-deficient yang types cannot afford to lose it. Sweating can easily exhaust the yang types.

Statement 3: Anger, the predominant emotion of the Yang Type A, can easily trigger hot flashes. Although not as strong or as frequently expressed by Yang Type Bs, it is still capable of producing hot flashes in them, albeit with less intensity. The yin types may feel angry at times, but rarely enough to produce a hot flash. The anger of the yin types isn't pure anger, which slices like a sharp knife with the yang types. Instead it is usually rooted in other emotions like stress, anxiety, a lack of joy, or feeling uncared for or unprotected.

Statement 4: Born with excessive yang energy, the yang types tend to overheat easily. The Yang Type B's hot flashes indicate extreme accumulation of heat rising up to the head from the upper stomach (fundus) and esophagus. Stomach fluid is often pushed upward when this happens, resulting in vomit, acid regurgitation, dry heaves, and/or excessive saliva.

TABLE 2.13. LIBIDO

	Most of the Time	Sometimes	Rarely	Never
1. No matter how tired I am, there is always enough energy for sex.	Yin Type B: +2	Yin Type A: +1	Yang Type B: 0	Yang Type A: 0
2. I have a high sex drive but have trouble getting physically aroused.	Yin Type A: +2 (high sex drive/ difficult arousal)	Yin Type B: +1 (sex drive/ arousal not an issue)	Yang Type A: 0 (low/ absent sex drive)	Yang Type B: 0 (low/ absent sex drive)
3. I'd feel fine without engaging in sexual intercourse or masturbating.	Yang Type A: +2	Yang Type B: +1	Yin Type A: 0	Yin Type B: 0
4. My mind is in other places during sex.	Yang Type B: +2	Yang Type A: +1	Yin Type A: 0	Yin Type B: 0

Libido Clarification Key

Statement 1: Born with ample kidney energy, which sends energy to the genitals, Yin Type Bs rarely feel too tired to engage in sexual activity. This means not that they are always easily sexually aroused, but that it doesn't take much to get them going once the signal is turned on. The Yin Type B's shy and timid nature, however, may get in the way of expressing and engaging in sexual activity even if the desire is there and the situation is ripe. Since the kidneys are the second strongest system of Yin Type As, sexual energy comes more easily to them than to the yang types, and they can occasionally get aroused even when tired. With little interest in sex to begin with, getting a yang type aroused isn't easy.

Statement 2: Although a stronger liver system contributes to the Yin Type A's sexual desire and arousal, liver stagnation from stress and tension easily interfere. Some Yin Type As have a strong desire that is not matched by their ability to engage in sex without (1) quickly losing interest, (2) getting distracted, and/or (3) having difficulty getting physically aroused. Yin Type As have a natural appetite for sex, but it is easily affected by the stress of daily life. The stressed Yin Type B may also have this issue before engaging in sexual activity, but all it takes is a little stimulation to get things rolling again. Sexual desire *and* arousal usually run low for the yang types since most of their energy is hanging out in the upper body.

Statement 3: Born with a weaker liver and kidneys, the yang types rarely have enough energy flowing to the genitals, placing the desire to engage in sex on the back burner. Even if the desire is somewhat present, it is rarely strong enough to cause them to take action, and if they do, it's usually gone in a flash. To make matters worse, Yang Type B men are often impotent and the women sterile (accounting for about 2 percent of the general population). According to a recent study, 12 percent of all menopausal women (ages forty-five to sixty-four) report a reduction in sexual desire.[4] Moreover, between 17 and 45 percent of all postmenopausal women find sexual intercourse painful, which may also contribute to a lack of sexual desire.[5] Therefore, when responding to this statement, try referring to how things were before age forty-five or before intercourse became painful.

Statement 4: Yang Type Bs constantly focus on the future and don't have time to dwell in the present.

TABLE 2.14. DEPRESSION

	Most of the Time	Sometimes	Rarely	Never
1. I wish I could live on my own, away from others.	Yin Type A: +1	Yin Type B: +2	Yang Type A: 0	Yang Type B: 0
2. It is difficult for me to get going.	Yin Type A: +2	Yin Type B: +1	Yang Type A: 0	Yang Type B: 0
3. My anger easily morphs into depression.	Yang Type A: +2	Yang Type B: +1	Yin Type A: 0	Yin Type B: 0
4. Sadness motivates me.	Yang Type B: +2	Yang Type A: +1	Yin Type B: 0	Yin Type A: 0

Depression Clarification Key

Statement 1: While the other body types may enjoy being alone from time to time, Yin Type Bs crave it and cannot function without substantial time in solitude. Yin Type As may also feel the need to be alone but draw energy from those who are close to them or who share the same values. The yang types need to engage themselves with others on a daily basis to feel balanced and whole. When alone, the yang types feel incomplete, potentially driving themselves crazy.

Statement 2: The stronger liver of the Yin Type A often bites off more than it can chew, bringing about stagnation and congestion of the abdomen. The accumulation of excess energy there is like a weight that makes it challenging for Yin Type Bs to stay active and in motion. Their constant desire for comfort also may get in the way of movement, as a comfortable couch may be more appealing than the outdoors. The yang types don't think twice before making a move and are naturally inclined to stay in motion.

Statement 3: Anger is the predominant emotion of Yang Type As, while sorrow is the outward expression of their anger. Uncontrolled anger can easily morph into depression for the Yang Type A. The Yang Type A's and Yang Type B's depression is a yang type of depression, which is different from the yin type of depression. The former involves a desire to keep going but feeling stuck, while the latter has little or no desire to keep going. Depression for the yin types is due to an imbalance of their own predominant emotions: the Yin Type A's depression is the result of her unaccomplished joy, and the Yin Type B's, a lack of calmness.

Statement 4: For most of us, sadness is rarely a source of motivation, but for Yang Type Bs, it constantly ruffles their feathers, giving them a reason to take action. They are easily saddened by societal affairs, especially when others are not honest with one another. Their sadness can induce outbursts of anger when it is imbalanced, or a desire to support and assist others when it is cultivated. Sadness frequently robs the yin types of motivation, making it difficult for them to participate in public affairs.

TABLE 2.15. INSOMNIA

	Most of the Time	Sometimes	Rarely	Never
1. I feel groggy in the morning.	Yin Type B: +2	Yin Type A: +1	Yang Type A: 0	Yang Type B: 0
2. I wake up between 1:30 and 3:30 a.m.	Yin Type A: +2	Yin Type B: +1	Yang Type A: 0	Yang Type B: 0
3. My energy crashes soon after it gets dark.	Yang Type A: +2	Yang Type B: +1	Yin Type A: 0	Yin Type B: 0
4. I still have ample energy even without sleep.	Yang Type B: +2	Yang Type A: +1	Yin Type A: 0	Yin Type B: 0

Insomnia Clarification Key

Statement 1: Yin Type Bs have the least yang energy of the four body types, and so it takes them more time to get warmed up and ready to go in the morning. In Eastern philosophy, morning is equated with yang, and since the yin types are lacking in this category, they need more stimulation to set the day in motion. The yang types, on the other hand, jump out of bed and are ready to start the day in a flash, yet they often crash in the early evening, when yin time kicks in.

Statement 2: The lungs, being the first organ in the body's circadian energy cycle, receive energy from the liver, the last organ in the cycle, between the hours of 1:30 and 3:30 a.m. Born with weaker lungs, Yin Type As may wake during this hour as the lungs struggle to absorb energy from their liver, which hoards it away. The stronger lungs of the yang types, and their ability to absorb plenty of energy, make it easier for them to stay asleep at this hour.

Statement 3: Yang Type As often feel a sudden loss of energy during kidney time, between 5:30 and 7:30 p.m., and Yang Type Bs lose energy during liver time, starting at 11:30 p.m.

Statement 4: Yang Type Bs just keep going and going until they use up every ounce of energy, in which case they may be bedridden for days. Yang Type As also push themselves beyond their limits but often crash in the evenings, recovering the following day. The yin types require more sleep than the yang types, making seven to nine hours a night a requirement in order for them to function adequately the next day. Peculiarly, they are also more energetic in the evenings and are tempted to sacrifice sleep for other nighttime stimuli.

CONCLUDING YOUR BODY TYPE

We're now ready to tally up the scores from parts 2 and 3 and explore the essential role that emotional balance plays along the menopausal journey. The column with the highest total score indicates your yin yang body type. If after you total your scores one type still doesn't stand out, then try reviewing and fine-tuning your answers to parts 1 and 2 after taking a break. Still not sure after retaking the test? Check out the "Continuing the Voyage" resources section for further assistance.

TABLE 2.16. FINAL BODY TYPE SCORES

	Yang Type A	Yang Type B	Yin Type A	Yin Type B
Part 2: Method A—Outward Appearance				
Part 2: Method B—Emotional and Physiological Traits				
Part 3: Menopause-Specific Indicators				
Grand total score				

3

Weathering
the Storms

Emotions and Menopause

Lee Je-ma, the founder of Sasang medicine, provided detailed treatments for numerous disorders, some of which were life-threatening and others that were more of the day-to-day variety, such as common colds, stress, and insomnia. He offered over a hundred herbal formulas for each body type, covering issues as diverse as malaria and dysentery, with miraculous results. Yet he repeatedly emphasized how it was his patients' focus on healing and cultivating themselves that inevitably determined whether or not they fully recovered. Herbal treatment, according to Lee Je-ma, may get us out of the red, but a "healing attitude" is what inevitably nurtures us back to health. Emotional balance is our best weapon against illness; it's even more powerful than the strongest medicine. Yet as humans, avoiding the use of medicine is not always possible because as soon as we lay down our shield, illness can quickly make its way in. Each of us has emotional and physical Achilles' heels that make us vulnerable to opportunistic infections and toxic emotions. We all have inherently stronger physiological and emotional aspects, too, which prevent us from getting sick. This chapter introduces the emotional strengths and weaknesses of each yin yang body type.

BALANCING EMOTIONS TO AVOID ILLNESS

This book would be only a few pages long if avoiding illness were as simple a matter as saying, "Just balance your emotions and all will turn out fine!" But we all have different emotional tendencies and different ideas about what it means to balance them. We each have excessive emotional tendencies that emerge from our stronger organs and more emotions that lie dormant within our weaker organs. Balancing these emotional tendencies is what promotes the smooth and harmonious flow of energy from our stronger to our weaker organs.

To put it simply, emotions move energy. Hence each emotion has its own role to play in encouraging energy to flow from one part of the body to another. Anger and sorrow promote upward flow; joy and calmness promote downward flow. Excessive anger and/or sorrow causes energy to burst upward, leading to headaches, hot flashes, high blood pressure, and so on. Excessive energy in the upper body leads to weakness of the lower body and the obstruction of flow to the liver, kidneys, bladder, lower back, and legs. Too much joy and complacency sink energy, bringing about diarrhea, organ prolapse, lower body water retention, and a sensation of heaviness, obstructing flow to the upper body (lungs, heart, upper back, and brain). Excessive upward flow results in weakness of the lower back and extremities, and dominant downward flow causes weakness of the upper body and extremities. Lee Je-ma equated health with the ability to balance our emotions, preventing them from bombarding and/or vacating the upper, middle, or lower body.

The flow of energy within the body is controlled not only by our emotions but by each food and herb we consume as well. Foods and herbs in Sasang medicine are classified according to which organ they affect after being digested. Just like the emotion of sorrow, foods and herbs that travel to the lungs promote the upward movement of energy from the chest. While supporting the physiological function of the lungs, these foods also help us cope with and process sadness. Foods and herbs therefore have an effect on our emotions too. Have you ever felt unusually sad or angry after a meal? Foods that promote excessive upward movement of energy may promote such emotions. Food and herbs can also promote emotions like joy and calmness, like the feeling some people get after eating foods that stimulate digestion or bring back fond memories. Along the Sasang journey and within the following chapters you will discover various herbs that benefit the stronger and weaker organs of each body type, supporting the flow of harmonious energy throughout the body.

THE FOUR PREDOMINANT EMOTIONS

As discussed in chapter 1, our emotional inclinations, or predominant emotions, are what determine which organ systems are stronger and weaker, which in turn determines our body type. There are four predominant emotions, one for each of the four body types: anger (Yang Type A), sorrow (Yang Type B), joy (Yin Type A), and calmness (Yin Type B). Obviously, we humans are capable of having more than just four emotions, and each of these four actually encompasses several other emotions (see figs. 3.1 through 3.4).

Fun Fact

After carefully analyzing a total of forty-two facial expressions among 720 participants, researchers recently concluded the existence of only four basic human emotions: happiness, sadness, fear, and anger. This study also discusses how each facial expression has its own physiological advantage, where widening the eyes during fear and surprise increase the visual field, making escape easier. Anger and disgust cause the skin of the nose to wrinkle, narrowing the airways and "inhibiting inspiration of potentially harmful particles."* From the perspective of Sasang medicine, happiness is viewed as the predominant emotion of Yin Type A; sadness, Yang Type B; and anger, Yang Type A. Fear can be interpreted as lack of comfort, the predominant emotion of Yin Type B.

*Jack et al., "Dynamic Facial Expressions."

Yang emotions are generally more active, intense, and sharp, while yin emotions are more subtle, less intense, and softer. Anger is more easily imagined as a yang emotion, being more intense and active than

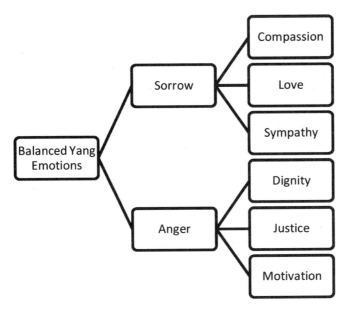

Fig. 3.1. Balanced yang emotions and their correlates

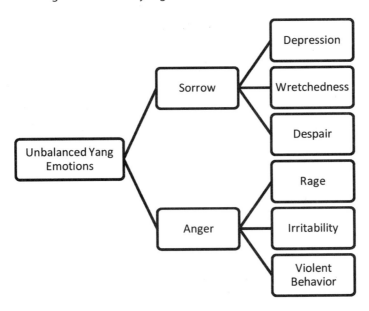

Fig. 3.2. Unbalanced yang emotions and their correlates

calmness, but how about if we compare sorrow and joy? At first glance, joy may seem more active than sorrow, but joy is actually an emotion felt when life slows down or when we are living in the moment—both yin

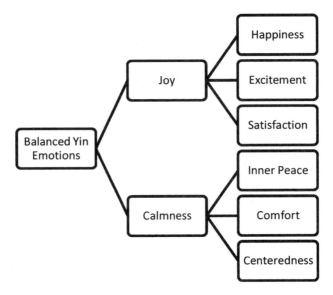

Fig. 3.3. Balanced yin emotions and their correlates

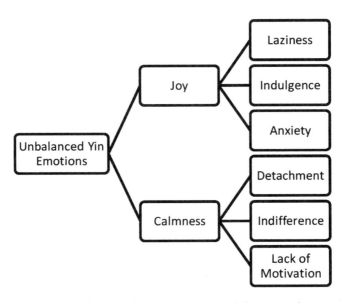

Fig. 3.4. Unbalanced yin emotions and their correlates

traits. Sorrow, on the other hand, is felt when life is active and flowing one minute and then *bang!*, before we know it an obstacle gets in our way. The yang types have difficulty slowing down and react abruptly when someone or something interferes with their progress.

Menopause and the Four Predominant Emotions

Each woman responds to menopause differently, depending on her temperament and body type. For example, the Yin Type A could experience bouts of anger, anxiety, sadness, frustration, and so on as she goes through menopause, but what it all boils down to is whether or not she balances her joy, the emotion associated with her stronger liver. Without joy, she loses her sense of direction, causing the other emotions to get out of hand. When the Yin Type A's temperament of joy is not balanced, the other predominant emotions of sorrow, anger, and calmness are also expressed inappropriately. Imbalanced sorrow morphs into depression, anger into rage, joy into anxiety, and calmness into laziness (see fig. 3.5 on page 80). When the Yin Type A's temperament of joy is balanced, then the other predominant emotions of sorrow, anger, and calmness are also expressed appropriately (see fig. 3.6 on page 80). The challenge is always to make room for joy even in the most challenging of circumstances that can occur on your menopause journey.

The same principle applies to the other types. The Yin Type B is after calmness and a sense of relaxation. An angry or sad Yin Type B is someone who has lost her footing and is unable to find her sense of profound calmness and quietness within—a feeling that she deeply treasures.

Imbalance of the Yang Type A's angry nature impedes her ability to balance sorrow, joy, and calmness. It is particularly challenging for the Yang Type A to control her anger, which makes it difficult for her to experience the same level of joy or calmness as the yin types. By avoiding the pull of her anger, the Yang Type A is capable of enjoyment and calmness, but if her anger goes overboard, she'll fall into an abyss of sadness. This type of sadness rarely leads to depression, which is more prevalent among the yin types (as discussed in chapter 6, "Woman Overboard"). Sorrow for the Yang Type A is often described as a feeling of suppressed anger, waiting to explode.

The Yang Type B also battles with anger, but unlike the Yang Type A, her anger comes from deeply embedded sorrow. The balanced Yang Type B convinces herself that life on earth isn't the pits and that, by accepting and embracing others, she can find joy and calmness while avoiding explosive episodes of anger. This accomplishment is easier said

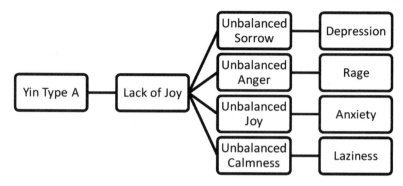

Fig 3.5. Imbalanced joy of the Yin Type A

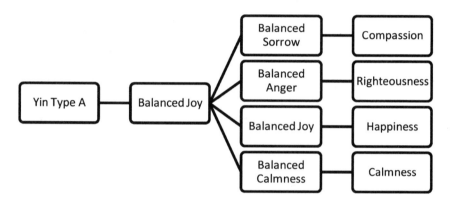

Fig 3.6. Balanced joy of the Yin Type A

than done, since her predominant emotion of sorrow is always ready to manifest, especially when others are not being straightforward and frank—behaviors that often rub her the wrong way.

THE FOUR LEVELS OF INTERACTION

Nothing exists in isolation, and according to Sasang medicine our well-being and overall health depend first and foremost on interaction. When it comes to interaction, most of us think of the relationships between friends and family members or our connection with nature and our surroundings. How about the relationship between our bodily organs? The relationship between our lungs and liver, for example, has a direct effect on our relationships with family, friends, and lovers. As we discussed above, the lungs correlate with sorrow and the liver with joy. The smooth flow of liver energy brings out joy, but when it is blocked, the sorrowful lungs may wreak havoc. The interaction between our organs is indicative of how we relate to pain, work, stress, and other aspects of life. Do you desire to escape or engage when the going gets tough? Does pain make you angry, sad, or anxious? Our organs also have a direct effect on how we interact with our environment. Sasang medicine lists four levels of interaction (see table 3.1), each depending on the balance of yin and yang flow to and from each of our organs.

TABLE 3.1. THE FOUR LEVELS OF INTERACTION

Level of Interaction	Affiliated Organ	Yin Yang Body Type Affiliation	Emphasis
Sa mu	Lung	Yang Type B	Interaction with cosmos, heaven, universe (the biggest picture)
Kyo wu	Spleen	Yang Type A	Interaction with society, strangers (the big picture)
Dang yo	Liver	Yin Type A	Interaction with groups, like-minded people (the small picture)
Ko cho	Kidneys	Yin Type B	Interaction with family and nature, intimacy (the smallest picture)

As discussed in chapter 1, each of the yin yang types is born with a stronger organ system and a weaker one. Hence each type will emphasize the level of interaction associated with their stronger system and have the tendency to avoid, ignore, disregard, or take for granted the level of interaction correlating with their weaker system. The yang types have an affiliation toward the yang levels of interaction (*sa mu* and *kyo wu*) and the yin types toward the yin levels (*dang yo* and *ko cho*). Yang Type Bs naturally engage in sa mu, which is associated with their stronger lungs, but have difficulty getting acquainted with dang yo, which belongs to their weaker liver. With a stronger liver, Yin Type As easily master dang yo but warming up to sa mu takes time and effort. Adapting to kyo wu, which correlates with the spleen, is a challenge for Yin Type Bs, but engaging with ko cho, which is associated with their stronger kidneys, comes as naturally as breathing. Kyo wu is second nature for Yang Type As thanks to their stronger spleen, but getting cozy with ko cho is another story. The stronger ko cho and dang yo get, the weaker kyo wu and sa mu become. Can yin and yang levels of interaction coexist? Sure they can! But this takes a tremendous amount of self-reflection, effort, and the ability to stay balanced in situations that otherwise would bring us down.

Sa Mu and Dang Yo

Practically all of the major religions discuss how we are connected with the divine but admit how disconnected we are capable of being. Sa mu, and the connection with the divine, is the Yang Type B's priority as it is associated with her stronger lung system. The Yang Type B focuses on the big picture, being closer to the cosmos and often harboring lofty ideas about how to administer public affairs. The Yang Type B's sorrow is born from her grief and disappointment when others lose track of this connection. Sa mu is also the priority of the lungs, which encourage the upward flow of blood and energy within the body, often at the cost of disregarding the other organs below. Sa mu is considered a yang level of interaction since yang correlates with upward movement and heaven.

The balanced Yang Type B's strong sa mu is capable of giving others a sense of purpose, drive, and enthusiasm. She is aware when others do not wish to join her quest but does not feel sorrowful or angry as a result. While engaging in dang yo, the balanced Yang Type B is able to find commonality with others, believing that they too are a reflection of the heavens. Unbalanced, the Yang Type B is easily disappointed with the current state of affairs and living in a world full of corruption and lack of connection with others and the divine. But unlike the yin types, disappointment makes the Yang Type B engage further, rather than distance herself, often turning sorrow into bursts of heat and anger, insulting and harming others. Little does the uncultivated Yang Type B know that engaging in dang yo and mingling with other like-minded folks is the only way to put an end to the misery and bring out her joy. Yet she decides to stand clear, since dang yo requires that she slow down, smell the roses, and commingle.

Associated with her weaker liver system, dang yo is rarely on the Yang

Type B's mind. When engaging in dang yo, she attempts to rock the boat, carrying out her ideas of how things should be. This doesn't go over well with the dang yo crowd, who aim at finding commonality and camaraderie. Sasang medicine holds that joy comes from engaging in dang yo. The Yang Type B's lack of joy comes from a craving for adversity and for challenging herself to the extreme—a quality found in sa mu.

The Yin Type A's strong dang yo, on the other hand, gives her an appreciation for living in the moment and relaxing with close friends and/or family. Yin Type As treasure dang yo, as they emphasize the importance of giving and sharing and are satisfied with painting a smaller picture. Balanced Yin Type As use their strong dang yo to bring joy and camaraderie to themselves and others. They don't single out only those who are like them but instead find commonality with others who, at least initially, may look and act differently. Even the slightest difference in opinion, belief, or appearance causes discomfort and suspicion when dang yo is unbalanced.

Menopause challenges the Yin Type A to reevaluate her circle of friends since friendships often transform during this phase, becoming deeper in some cases and more distant in others. The Yin Type A must sift through her relationships, weeding out individuals who soak up too much energy or steer her astray. Menopause provides the opportunity to invite into her comfort zone others with whom she may not have much in common but can still share a friendship bond, rooted in mutual respect and appreciation. Postmenopausal health depends on the Yin Type A's ability to expand her horizons by meeting new friends, creating new ideas, and focusing on the big picture—a trait that is actually associated with sa mu and her weaker lungs. Dang yo is considered a yin level of interaction, where yin correlates with downward movement, rooting the spirit and living in the moment.

Ko Cho and Kyo Wu

The *dan jeon*, meaning "elixir field" or "sea of qi," resides in the lower abdomen—an area considered to be the energetic center of the body and the residence of a "third lung." Life begins in this area, which roughly correlates with the location of the uterus. Inhaling into this area, as if it were a third lung, is traditionally believed to preserve, root, and balance bodily energy. In Sasang medicine, the uterus and dan jeon both correlate with the kidneys, the strongest organ of the Yin Type B, and the weakest of the Yang Type A. Yin Type Bs have a natural ability to root their energies, often appearing calmer than the other body types. Yang Type As, having difficulty in this regard, often feel unsettled and easily angered. The lower abdomen also correlates with ko cho, or intimacy, which goes hand in hand with calmness. Without calmness, one cannot be intimate, and without intimacy one cannot be calm. Intimacy, in this sense, is not only experienced with a partner but also with oneself and one's surroundings. Ko cho is also the kidneys' priority and is considered a yin level of interaction. Yin Type Bs prefer calmness and quiet and being alone or with those who make them feel comfortable. This encourages blood and energy to flow inward and downward, filling the sacrum, bladder, uterus, and lower extremities, occasionally at the cost of disregarding the upper body organs and emotions.

Kyo wu, which correlates with the Yang Type A's stronger spleen, is the interaction between strangers and individuals with different opinions or ideas. When the yin types meet others, they often look for common interests and desires, but the yang types couldn't care less, as long as they are respected and acknowledged. Kyo wu is driven by the Yang Type As' temperament of anger, which motivates them to seek adversity and change. Befriending others with different opinions, cultures, and backgrounds is a way to express one's anger against the normal, non-changing, or concrete aspects of human interaction—qualities associated with ko cho and their weaker kidney system.

Whereas Yin Type Bs crave intimacy, Yang Type As disregard it and instead desire formality and relationship structure, which in their eyes makes life more productive. For the Yang Type A, birthdays and anniversaries rarely mean anything, but taking out the garbage or putting food on the table gives her satisfaction and may even classify as her version of intimacy. For the Yin Type B, taking out the garbage or cooking is secondary to remembering birthdays, goodnight kisses, or other signs of tenderness. In a sense, kyo wu is more practical than ko cho, but practicality can get in the way of romance. A healthy relationship is one that balances kyo wu and ko cho, making time for intimacy but acknowledging that structure and formality are also essential.

The balanced Yin Type B's strong ko cho is capable of providing warmth and comfort to others without smothering them, giving them space to grow and live their own lives. She acknowledges the significance of kyo wu and is willing to set intimacy aside to get the job done, believing that it will always be there when her heart summons it. Relationship challenges do not cause fear for the balanced Yin Type B but instead encourage her to adapt and make appropriate changes. Even the closest of friends and family become sources of anxiety and unsettled energy for the unbalanced Yin Type B. She deeply fears kyo wu and instead hides behind the intimacy of ko cho, often descending into her own world. She may be plagued with social anxiety, choosing to stay home or be protected by a familiar environment.

The loss of a parent, an empty nest, and potential marriage issues weigh heavily on the mind of a Yin Type B, who values intimacy and often fears change. The menopausal Yin Type B may search, often in vain, for more intimacy, returning to the past, where in her dreamy mind everything was "perfect." Kyo wu and the obligations of daily life have the tendency to swallow up what is left of intimacy during menopause if she loses sight of it. If you are a Yin Type B who feels this way, then it's time to reestablish a balance between ko cho and kyo wu and reclaim your inherent power of intimacy, but also to prepare yourself for change and the need to modify your definition of intimacy.

The story is different for the Yang Type A, whose strong kyo wu gives her the courage to face relationship challenges head-on. If there's a problem, she believes in a quick fix and is ready to move on even if the issue has not been resolved yet. The unbalanced Yang Type A may feel as if her relationship has hit a brick wall despite her practical solutions. Only through balancing kyo wu with ko cho can she slow her pace down and learn to treasure those who are closest to her. Intimacy teaches her how to be patient and yielding and realize that practicality is not the only answer when human emotions are involved. The balanced Yang Type A utilizes anger to stay motivated and kyo wu to stay engaged, even if it means shifting into a lower gear. The unbalanced Yang Type A easily loses her cool, as anger and/or rage flare up when her ideas of right and wrong are challenged, and she sacrifices household affairs and intimacy for the sake of societal gain and stature.

The Yang Type A's weaker kidney system, which hosts the uterus, undergoes significant transformation during menopause. As discussed previously, this area is also associated with calmness, an emotion difficult for her to grasp. Until this point in life, she has been able to brush comfort aside in order to keep the fast-paced, cut-to-the-chase rhythm of her stronger spleen system going. Yet as she goes through menopause, a voice within her kidneys starts to whisper, "Stop living so quickly," as her knees and lower back may also join the chorus, encouraging her to slow down. The balanced Yang Type A heeds this call, taking time out for intimacy, meditation, quiet, and living in the moment. Otherwise, she will just keep rushing along, risking loss of love and further weakening the energies of her lower abdomen and uterus.

EMOTIONS AND THE FOUR BODY QUADRANTS

Sasang medicine delineates four sections of the anterior and posterior body that correlate with different emotional and physical tendencies according to each body type. The four sections of the anterior body are the chin, chest, and upper and lower abdomen. The posterior body consists of the cervical spine (neck), thoracic spine (upper back), lumbar spine (lower back), and sacral spine (buttocks region). Each of these areas hosts a positive trait that reflects our human nature and connection with divine energy. Yet they each host negative traits too, reflecting ignorance of our humanity, and these traits manifest if we do not realize and discover our connection with others and the universe and refuse to improve ourselves.

The Anterior Body

The chin, chest, and upper and lower abdomen in the anterior aspect of the body correlate with the lung, spleen, liver, and kidney systems, respectively (see table 3.2). Yang Type As often feel a burning in their chest when experiencing hot flashes because this area is the most developed aspect of their anterior body, correlating with heat. Yin Type Bs often feel a deep sense of coldness in their lower abdomen when they are not feeling well because this area is the most developed aspect of their anterior body, associated with the kidneys and cold. The Yin Type As' upper abdomen may start to protrude during the menopausal years because this area is the most developed aspect of their anterior body, associated with the liver and the process of absorption. Menopause may instigate burning and heat in the neck and chin area of the Yang Type Bs, since this is the most developed aspect of their anterior body.

TABLE 3.2. THE ANTERIOR BODY

Body Type	Strongest Anterior Section	Organ System	Possible Menopausal Changes
Yang Type B	Chin	Lungs	Heat in the neck/chin
Yang Type A	Chest	Spleen	Heat in the chest
Yin Type A	Upper abdomen	Liver	Stagnation/fat tissue accumulation in the abdomen
Yin Type B	Lower abdomen	Kidneys	Cold accumulation and stagnation in the lower abdomen*

*The kidneys are the source of cold energy within the body, making the Yin Type Bs prone to cold-induced health issues. Despite being left in the cold, the Yin Type Bs may still experience hot flashes during menopause as heat escapes to the upper body. Rarely do they feel uncomfortable when this happens, since it gives them a break from the cold.

The chin, chest, and upper and lower abdomen are associated with your *song*, or heavenly endowed nature, and host the seed of wisdom and enlightenment that you receive from this connection. Depending on your body type, energy will naturally be attracted to one of these four areas, where it accumulates and occasionally overflows. Since your song nature is a gift from the heavens, discovering and learning how to utilize it is the key to optimizing your health. Balancing your song nature is a three-step process:

1. **Recognition**—Discover your inner strengths by reflecting on how you see and react to others and how others react to and see you.

2. **Sincerity**—Reflect consistently on your actions, avoiding common emotional roadblocks, while cultivating your song nature and natural talents.

3. **Belief**—Believe in your gift, special path, and connection with others and the universe.

The Chin

The chin is associated with knowledge and the ability to calculate one's actions—a quality known as *ju chek*. When balanced, the energy of our chin portrays charisma, uprightness, and sharpness. But if we raise it too high, as the idiom "leading with one's chin" conveys, ignorance and arrogance abound. This is why Lee Je-ma said that arrogance, along with charisma, also resides in the chin. The chin resides within the lung system, which is the strongest area of the Yang Type B and the weakest of the Yin Type A. The Yang Type B's stronger chin often protrudes, and she naturally appears arrogant or, at the least, intimidating. The weaker chin of the Yin Type A often retracts, making her appear less dignified. If the need to feel powerful and dignified gets out of hand, it can transform into arrogance and haughtiness. Balancing the chin energy is more challenging for the Yin Type A than for the Yang Type B, since it is associated with the former's weakest organ system. Unlike the Yin Type A, power and authority come naturally for the Yang Type B, making it easier to control and less enticing.

The Chin

Strongest type: Yang Type B

Weakest type: Yin Type A

Associated song nature: Ju chek (*ju* = calculation, evaluation; *chek* = plan), which is the intuitive ability to evaluate one's circumstances and make sound judgments. Ju chek is also the knowledge and ability to calculate one's actions.

Unbalanced ju chek emotional effects: Haughtiness, arrogance, "holier than thou" attitude, lack of self-reflection

Unbalanced ju chek physiological effects: Facial symptoms/disorders (acne, rosacea, facial spasms, Bell's palsy, jaw pain/spasms)

Balanced ju chek emotional effects: Leadership qualities, psychic abilities, insight, power, influence

Balanced ju chek physiological effects: Reduced or absence of facial symptoms, increased flow of energy to the upper body, increased upper body strength, enhanced function of cardiovascular system

Client—Mrs. Yin Type A, age fifty-three: My husband thinks the world revolves around him, taking everything I do for granted. Well, now I'm fed up with cooking, cleaning, and "serving" his every need!

Sasang doc: Keep your chin up! The Yin Type A is very sensitive to whether or not others are arrogant or ignorant of their needs—a quality associated with dang yo—even to the point of being arrogant and ignorant themselves and blinded by feelings of revenge. This is how your husband is and likely will be for years to come. Menopause won't let you simply brush it aside anymore; something has to be done. Remember not to lead with your chin—an area associated with kyo shim (self-conceit). Instead, take a deep breath and nourish your lungs before making a decision about which direction to take. Utilize *heng gom,* your special ability to reflect and initiate change from within. Remember, it's not your husband himself but how you feel about your husband that affects your health.

The Chest

The chest is associated with our ability to govern and administer—a quality known as *kyung ryun.* When balanced, the energy of our chest emits confidence and dignity. But if the chest sticks out too much, its energy may get stuck, leading to overconfidence and extravagance. This is why Lee Je-ma said that extravagance, together with dignity and self-confidence, inhabits the chest. The chest resides within the spleen system, which is the strongest area of the Yang Type A and the weakest of the Yin Type B. It is easier for the Yang Type A to control her dignity and self-confidence than it is for the Yin Type B. The uncultivated Yin Type B may confide only in herself, shutting herself away from society, indulging in her own unrealistic dreams and desires. When the Yin Type B balances her chest energy, a profound sense of kyung ryun abounds.

During menopause, the Yin Type B has a tendency to retreat inward, cutting herself off from social interaction and external affairs. Kyung ryun comes more easily for the Yang Type A because a deeply embedded sense of anger keeps her engaged, stimulating her desire for change. If the menopausal Yang Type A controls her anger, the chest energy will flow smoothly throughout the body. This is done by releasing the notion that she is the only one worthy of respect and/or the only victim of disrespect. Once she learns not to take things so personally, her anger can be directed toward inhumanity in general rather than unleashed on this or that person.

The Chest

Strongest type: Yang Type A

Weakest type: Yin Type B

Associated song nature: Kyung ryun (*kyung* = teaching, reason, principle; *ryun* = ruling, reigning, governing), which is the ability to govern and administer affairs.

Unbalanced kyung ryun emotional effects: Isolation, depression, failed relationships, disconnection, mistrust, cowardice, social anxiety

Unbalanced kyung ryun physiological effects: Weight gain, indigestion, organ prolapse, herniation, fatigue

Balanced kyung ryun emotional effects: Social responsibility, confidence, feeling of oneness with others (despite differences in opinion, culture, and ethnicity), increased social/societal awareness

Balanced kyung ryun physiological effects: Enhanced digestive* function (reduced/resolved bloating, gas, diarrhea), increased metabolism, increased blood and energy flow to the chest

Client—shell-shocked Yin Type B, age sixty-four: I thought that retirement would reduce my stress level and make me happier, but I still feel that something major is missing from my life. It seems like one abusive relationship after another has driven me to this point.

---

*Digestion in Sasang medicine signifies the ability to adapt and absorb not just food but new experience, to face adversity, and to assimilate.

Technically, I should be fine, living on my own and surrounded by my close friends and the mountains and trees. I've always felt my best when being alone, but now I yearn for something else.

Sasang doc: Oh, how I understand! Being a Yin Type B myself, I always felt that nature brought me the comfort and quiet that my stronger kidney energy yearned for, and as a child, I spent most of my days alone with her. But even though she filled me with intense energy, it always seemed as if something was missing. Aware of this, Lee Je-ma cautioned against getting too comfortable in this mode, stating that a healthy Yin Type B motivates his/herself to interact and engage with others. As difficult as it may sound, imagine that your comfort can be carried with you everywhere in a suitcase. Remember that your stronger kidneys give you a natural source of inner strength and calmness that can be accessed no matter where you are. This gift has no value unless it is shared with others through a process called kyung ryun. Confide in yourself, without simply giving this gift away or hiding it from the world, and as you grow, so will your relationships, self-confidence, and dignity.

The Upper Abdomen

A developed abdomen makes us look relaxed, joyful, and down to earth, but when it protrudes excessively, laziness and clumsiness are conveyed. This is why Lee Je-ma said that laziness, along with joy, also resides in the upper abdomen.* The Yang Type B finds it difficult to smell the roses and kick back due to a weaker abdominal energy and a lack of joy, whereas the Yin Type A, born with this area developed, makes joy a priority, often to the point of disregarding obligations. Little does the uncultivated Yin Type A know, however, that within her abdomen exists the profound ability to reflect on her actions, or heng gom. Without reflection, the Yin Type A indulges in joy and disregards her responsibility. Balanced Yin Type As recognize when they are swimming in deep water, reflecting on their actions, and living life temperately. Heng gom doesn't come easily for Yang Type Bs since it is difficult

---

*The upper abdomen in Sasang medicine refers to the area from the base of the rib cage to the umbilicus, or navel.

for them to slow down and to reflect, and they drive themselves harder and harder, until the body can no longer persist. Disregarded heng gom is often coupled with vulgar, rough, and even violent behavior. The balanced Yang Type B recognizes this tendency and engages heng gom, despite every inclination to do otherwise. During menopause, the Yang Type B has a tendency to take on all of the world's problems, ignoring the changes occurring in her own body. By recognizing and heeding her inner voice, menopause flows much more smoothly.

The Upper Abdomen

Strongest type: Yin Type A

Weakest type: Yang Type B

Associated song nature: Heng gom (*heng* = actions, deeds, movement; *gom* = self-reflection, self-examination), which is the ability to reflect on one's actions.

Unbalanced heng gom emotional effects: Rudeness, vulgar or rough behavior, absentmindedness

Unbalanced heng gom physiological effects: Injury from lack of awareness and proprioception, exhaustion, weakness of abdominal function (sluggish bowel movement, liver congestion*)

Balanced heng gom emotional effects: Self-awareness, joy, composure

Balanced heng gom physiological effects: Enhanced energy and blood flow to the liver and small intestine, weight loss, enhanced coordination, consistent energy

Client—Not-So Reflective Yang Type B, age fifty-eight: I haven't been able to keep food down for three days. I keep on going, with or without food, because there's so much to get done and I can't stop now. But my legs frequently collapse, sending me straight to the ground. But other than that, I'm just fine. You know . . . the usual stuff. Got divorced, think I'm going to get laid off, and got fined recently for initiating and participating in a political demon-

---

*Reminder: The liver correlates with the small intestine, and since this is the weakest section of the body for Yang Type Bs, they are prone to liver and upper bowel congestion and toxicity. If Yin Type As do not tap into their liver-related heng gom, they too will experience such issues.

stration that turned violent. Lots to keep busy with, not much to be happy about. Can acupuncture or herbs help? How long do you think treatment would last? Got things to do, you know.

Sasang doc: Accupuncture and herbs could possibly help. (Doc takes her pulse.) The pulses that correlate with your lower body are very weak, while your upper body ones remain strong. Your inability to keep foods down is from pent-up sorrow, anger, and heat within the stomach and chest—a common condition for your body type. These symptoms will get worse the more you push yourself. Heng gom is the ability to slow down and reflect on your thoughts, behaviors, and actions. Once this is accomplished, a profound sense of joy and happiness abounds as energy fills the lower body. It's common for people with your body type to push themselves so hard that they don't even recognize anything is wrong until things get completely out of hand and they collapse from exhaustion.

The Lower Abdomen

The lower abdomen is the most intimate aspect of our anatomy, hosting the uterus and genitals. For most of our lives, this area is kept hidden under our clothing and often regarded by society as offensive, taboo, and so on. This is the territory of Yin Type Bs, who easily feel ashamed and unappreciated as masters of intimacy, or *do ryang*. Many women desire to be open and accepting but avoid intimacy for fear of getting hurt. The fear of intimacy among the other types makes societal interaction difficult for the Yin Type B. The uterus and genital areas were designed for intimacy and the ability to unite yin and yang energies. Hence the balanced Yin Type B has a profound ability to love, embrace, and empower, just as the uterus is capable of nurturing new life. The unbalanced Yin Type B craves intimacy but is ashamed to admit it. Her genital energy may be hidden behind an iron wall of layer upon layer of shame, shyness, and social fear, or she may submit herself to anyone who hints at intimacy, as if to say, "Thank goodness, someone finally unleashed me." The intimacy switch is difficult to toggle for the unbalanced Yin Type B, who either completely hides it or pours it out. Born with a weaker lower abdomen energy, the Yang Type A has difficulty being affectionate and intimate. Love and affection for her is often expressed outside the bedroom and through action rather than intimacy. Chapter 11, "Rocking the Boat," discusses this in detail.

Intimacy takes on new meaning in menopause, as the influence of sex hormones and desire to procreate start to wane and our ideas surrounding intimacy mature further. The menopausal Yin Type B is faced with the challenge of widening her scope of intimacy to include a larger circle of friends and family without feeling shameful or excessively self-conscious. The menopausal Yang Type A may rightfully start to question her lack of desire for intimacy, either because of a nagging spouse or simply because she has neglected it for so long.

The Lower Abdomen

Strongest type: Yin Type B

Weakest type: Yang Type A

Associated song nature: Do ryang (do = laws, regulations, manners, system, organization, consideration; ryang = considering, pondering), which is the ability to embrace and tolerate others.

Unbalanced do ryang emotional effects: Coldness, anger, fear of intimacy, mistrust, lack of affection

Unbalanced do ryang physiological effects: Decreased sexual function and/or desire, obstructed circulation in lower abdomen (scanty menstrual, urination, and bowel flow, decreased libido)

Balanced do ryang emotional effects: Loving, caring, compassionate, empowering

Balanced do ryang physiological effects: Improved sexual function and desire, smoother circulation in lower abdomen (improved menstrual, urination, and bowel flow)

Client—Judgmental Yang Type A, age forty-nine: My lower back has been killing me since yesterday. My friend at work took the day off—she's been having a difficult time lately, battling cancer and missing a lot of work—and my supervisor gave me all her work. Shortly afterward I got up to make a few copies and there it was. The pain radiates from my buttocks down the outside of my left leg and it won't let up.

Sasang doc: (Examines her lower back.) Looks like your sacroiliac joint is out of alignment. As a Yang Type A, it's likely that your sacral area pain is a result of unfettered anger stemming from your predominant emotion and a sensitivity toward being disrespected by your supervisor. The situation may have been unfair to you, but I suggest tolerating it for the sake of your friend who is ill. Tolerance actually feeds energy to your sacrum and, if accompanied by light stretching and gentle exercise, should get you back on track in no time.

The Posterior Body

Like the chin, chest, and upper and lower abdomen in the anterior body, the cervical, thoracic, lumbar, and sacral spine areas along the posterior aspect of the body also correlate with the lungs, spleen, liver, and kidney systems, respectively. The difference is that while the anterior portion of the body corresponds to how we see ourselves—that is, *song*—the posterior portion relates to how we carry ourselves, or *myung*.

The chin of the anterior correlates with ju chek (the knowledge and ability to calculate one's actions), while the cervical spine in the posterior correlate with *shik kyun* (knowing the right time to take action). It is necessary to calculate before taking action, and therefore shik kyun is carried out through ju chek. Accordingly, the energy of the chin flows to the energy of the cervical spine. The chest, associated with kyung ryun (the ability to administer affairs), encourages flow to the thoracic spine, which is related to *wi eui* (dignity/esteem). Through social interaction and responsibility we can build self-confidence and esteem.

The umbilicus, associated with heng gom (the ability to reflect), stimulates flow to the lumbar spine, which houses *jei gan* (manners and kindness). Indeed, heartfelt kindness cannot be expressed without self-reflection. Lastly, the lower abdomen, correlating with do ryang (intimacy and the ability to embrace others), sends energy to the sacral spine, which hosts *bang ryak* (tolerance). Tolerance is based on the ability to be intimate and feel profoundly connected with others. To put it simply, myung refines and ferments our raw song energies.

The spine (cervical, thoracic, lumbar, and sacrum) provides the structure and stability necessary to carry out even the minutest action. Strengthening the spine with a combination of stretching and other exercises becomes even more crucial as menopause approaches. Yet less obvious is how emotion and its energy affect the spine. Dignity and self-esteem, for example, are indeed capable of releasing upper back pain, while the ability to tolerate can dissipate sacral joint issues. It's a matter of convincing yourself that back pain isn't just about stretching or exercising but also involves reaching beyond your current limitations of thinking and believing that *you* are capable of controlling how *you* feel.

Recall how balancing our song nature is a three-step process involving the recognition of our inner strengths, a sincere effort to consistently reflect on our actions, and the belief in ourselves and our connection with others. In order to carry out our myung, or life path, we need to take the fourth step, action.

> **Action:** To carry out our life's path (or myung) by recognizing our song nature and utilizing this ability to improve our lives and those of others.

The anterior and posterior aspects of the mind and body are not isolated from one another; hence, if one is giving us trouble, eventually so will the other, if we do not address these aspects beforehand. In order to avoid or address lumbar and thoracic spine pain, it is often beneficial to strengthen the abdominal (rectus abdomens) muscles and chest (pectoralis) muscles, respectively. In order to manifest jei gan (kindness and morality of the lumbar spine) we have to master heng gom (self-reflection of the chin), and wi eui (dignity of the cervical spine) cannot manifest without kyung ryun (administrative ability of the chest). Hence, heng gom can also indirectly relieve lower back pain, and kyung ryun can relieve upper back pain.

The Cervical Spine

The Yang Type B's stronger lungs send energy to and develop the cervical spine. Thus the Yang Type B has a developed neck that often looks thicker and/or sturdier than that of the other types. Since the cervical spine is the most vulnerable part of the Yin Type A's posterior body, it is often plagued with chronic issues such as frequent shoulder and neck tightness and/or occipital headaches. The Yin Type A's stronger liver, however, contributes to a developed and robust lumbar spine, which, although subject to injury from overuse, tends to withstand more than the lumbar spine of the other types. The Yang Type B's lumbar spine, on the other hand, tends to be the weakest of the four types, giving her a chronic feeling of heaviness and weakness in the lower body and hip area.

The Cervical Spine

Strongest type: Yang Type B

Weakest type: Yin Type A

Associated song nature: Shik kyun (*shik* = recognition, knowledge, wisdom, intelligence; *kyun* = sight, vision), which is insight and knowing the right time to act.

Unbalanced shik kyun emotional effects: Lack of timing, tardiness, time-related stress

Unbalanced shik kyun physiological effects: Neck tightness, heavy-head feeling, inability to keep neck erect and/or to look upward

Balanced shik kyun emotional effects: Improved sense of time and punctuality, insight and psychic ability, feeling on top of your game

Balanced shik kyun physiological effects: Improved posture/flexibility of neck, reduction/elimination of neck tightness and weakness

---

If you experience neck pain and/or weakness, then try working on your relationship with time by following these body-type-specific guidelines:

- **Yang Type A:** The tendency toward anger may stagnate the energy of the Yang Type A's stronger spleen, interrupting the rhythm of her life. Her skills reside in the chest, where kyung ryun, the government and administration of affairs, resides. Controlling her tendency toward anger while managing and overseeing affairs will naturally bring out the ability to keep track of time and be on top of her game.

- **Yang Type B** (least difficulty managing shik kyun): The ability to manage time, or shik kyun, is the Yang Type B's specialty, since it comes from the cervical spine, the strongest area of her posterior body. Yet timing doesn't manifest on its own. Even the Yang Type B who gets lost in sorrow will find it hard to keep track of time and know when to act. Through reflection and control of her sorrowful nature, the Yang Type B opens the door to other abilities associated with the other types, like heng gom and bang ryak.

- **Yin Type A** (most difficulty managing shik kyun): Timing and connection with the universe—associated with yang—do not come naturally for the Yin Type A, who has a stronger sense of proprioception (spatial orientation) and connection with Earth, related to yin. The Yin Type A's predominant emotion of joy tends to get in the way of time, since she can easily lose track of it when enjoying and living in the moment. Tight neck muscles are often the result of time constraints and excessive responsibilities. The Yin Type A's heng gom, or ability to reflect, can snap her out of indulging in the moment, giving her a stronger sense of time.

- **Yin Type B:** Time is often the enemy of the Yin Type B, who prioritizes comfort and slowing life down—preferences associated with her stronger kidneys. The constant fear that time is passing by too quickly mixed with a desire to withdraw from her circumstances may cause chronic weakness and tightness of the Yin Type B's neck. Finding comfort, even when she is faced with deadlines and living in a fast-paced society, is the only way the Yin Type B can achieve balance and manifest do ryang.

Jessica, the Time-Trapped Yin Type A

For the life of her, Jessica, age forty-five, could not figure out why her neck kept aching day after day. After the last MRI, her doctor chuckled and said that her cervical spine was "the best-looking spine" she had ever seen. Jessica was also in the best shape she had ever been in, exercising five times a week, eating healthy foods, and feeling like she could run a marathon! Her neck pain felt as is if the muscles were being yanked from the base of her cranium, often leading to tension headaches. After discovering her yin yang body type, Jessica started to take a deeper look at her life and its patterns. She noticed that her headaches often occurred when she was under a time constraint or when she felt a situation of the past come back to haunt her. These episodes made her feel as if there was no catching up and that time was about to swallow her up! Jessica started to relax her grip on time, convincing herself that time was not the enemy and letting go of always feeling like she was going to be late. Her neck pain soon improved, especially in the mornings, when, overwhelmed with daily scheduling, she would feel at her worst.

The Thoracic Spine

The Yang Type As' stronger spleen sends energy to and develops the thoracic spine. Hence the Yang Type As have developed upper back muscles (from the base of the neck to the base of the thoracic spine), which pull their shoulders back, giving them a broad-shouldered/broad-chested appearance. Since the thoracic spine is the most vulnerable part of the Yin Type Bs' posterior body, they are prone to upper back discomfort, slouching shoulders, and tightness along the upper back. Their stronger kidneys, however, contribute to a stronger sacral spine, which, although subject to injury and overuse, tends to withstand more than the sacral spine of the other types. The Yang Type As' sacral spine, on the other hand, tends to be weaker than it is in the other types, making them prone to sacral/pelvic-related issues.

The Thoracic Spine

Strongest type: Yang Type A

Weakest type: Yin Type B

Associated song nature: Wi eui (wi = dignity, influence, force, power; eui = conduct, behavior, consideration), which is dignity and respect.

Unbalanced wi eui emotional effects: Extravagance, loftiness, frivolousness

Unbalanced wi eui physiological effects: Tightness and pain between shoulder blades, slouched posture

Balanced wi eui emotional effects: Humility/dignity,* self-respect, pride, self-esteem, self-worth

Balanced wi eui physiological effects: Improved posture/flexibility of upper back, reduction/elimination of upper back discomfort

---

*In Eastern philosophy, humility and dignity are one and the same, since without humility one cannot be dignified, and without dignity, one cannot be humble. Dignity without humility manifests as extravagance and loftiness, and humility without dignity shows up as self-injurious behavior.

If you experience upper back pain and/or weakness, then try working on your self-esteem by following these body-type-specific guidelines:

- **Yang Type A** (least difficulty managing wi eui): Anger is the engine that revs up self-esteem, providing a sense of purpose and justice. As the predominant emotion of the Yang Type A, it offers her a dignified presence. Yet even the Yang Type A can lack self-esteem when anger gets out of control, especially when she feels others are looking down on her. Excessive anger usually morphs into sadness, lack of self-worth, and tightness in the upper back.

- **Yang Type B:** As a yang type, self-esteem comes more easily for the Yang Type B, but sorrow, her predominant emotion, may get in the way. The Yang Type B may deny herself the ability to be self-confident by getting caught up in the affairs of the world, saddened by how people treat one another. Since shik kyun (knowing the right time to take action) is her specialty, the balanced Yang Type B understands that there is a time to lament and a time to move forward.

- **Yin Type A:** Dignity, humility, and self-esteem do not come easily for the Yin Type A, who is more concerned with mutual respect and the "give and take" aspect of her relationships. Aiming directly for dignity and building self-esteem can only result in arrogance for the Yin Type A. Heng gom, or the ability to self-reflect, is a powerful tool at the Yin Type A's disposal, but she can easily take it for granted. True dignity comes from the ability to reflect inward, acknowledge one's deficiencies and appreciate one's strengths.

- **Yin Type B** (most difficulty managing wi eui): Even though the Yin Type B is naturally skilled at bang ryak (embracing and tolerating others), dignity and self-esteem are a fundamental challenge. Her dignity is often contested by a shy and introverted nature. She imagines a world in which everyone is protecting one another but can easily get overwhelmed by responsibility and ticked off by others' words and actions. The balanced Yin Type B is capable of overcoming these tendencies and accepting and tolerating others despite their shortcomings.

Stacy's Delicate Balance between Dignity and Anger

Stacy, a Yang Type A, sought treatment at my clinic for upper back pain. I couldn't help but notice a tired and angry expression on her face and asked if there was anything else I could assist her with. Relieved by the opportunity, Stacy quickly expressed her disappointment about a project she had started at work a few months prior that increased production and enhanced employee morale. Yet a month later, her boss claimed that she was trying to take his job away and threatened to demote her. After exploding with anger in her boss's office, she retreated into the abyss of depression. Stacy's ability to improve work conditions and stand up for herself is an expression of wi eui (dignity), but uncontrolled anger from feeling disrespected took it away. Stacy's anger portrays the tendency to overreact and take things personally when our core strengths are challenged.

The Lumbar Spine

The Yin Type A's stronger liver sends abundant energy to the lumbar spine and abdomen. Hence the Yin Type A has a developed lower back and abdomen, giving her a relaxed and anchored appearance. Born with a weaker lumbar spine, the Yang Type B is prone to lower back weakness and discomfort. The Yin Type A's lower back pain, on the other hand, is due less to weakness and more to excessive tightness, a sign of strength. Excessive tightness of the lumbar spine may eventually transform into weakness as long-term energy and blood obstruction starve the vertebrae. This condition may also result in nerve impingement or disc degeneration as excessive pressure from surrounding tissue eventually decreases the intervertebral space. *Jei gan* (kindness and manners) resides in the lower back and is often a priority for the Yin Type A, but not for the Yang Type A, who often seems angered and/or sad. Lee Je-ma said that if the Yang Type A makes an effort to be kinder, then a profound sense of jei gan emerges, but artificial kindness simply triggers her anger.

The Lumbar Spine

Strongest type: Yin Type A

Weakest type: Yang Type B

Associated song nature: Jei gan (*jei* = ability, talent, genius, propriety, duty, consideration; *gan:* = endurance, responsibility), which is the ability to be consistent, kind, and moral to others and oneself.

Unbalanced jei gan emotional effects: Coldness, rudeness, immoral behavior, lack of self-respect/self-care

Unbalanced jei gan physiological effects: Tightness and pain in the lower back

Balanced jei gan emotional effects: Generous, giving, moral, kind to oneself and others

Balanced jei gan physiological effects: Improved posture/flexibility of lower back, reduction/elimination of lower back discomfort

---

Are you kind to yourself and/or others? Do you feel that others are being kind to you? A no answer to either of these questions may be the reason why a lower back pain issue goes unresolved. Jei gan, the seed of kindness and morality, stimulates the flow of energy and blood through the lumbar spine when balanced and impedes it when unbalanced. Kindness is achieved and received differently according to each yin yang body type.

- **Yang Type A:** "Why should I be kind when they act like that?!" the Yang Type A often asks, as her priority is mutual respect and dignity—a trait born from wi eui in the thoracic spine. When others are not practicing kindness, the Yang Type A is easily angered, often to the point of being rude and unkind herself. In order to break the spell of anger, she must let go of the idea that others have to be kind and humble first and take the initiative to practice humility without losing her self-esteem.

- **Yang Type B** (most difficulty managing jei gan): Kindness entails give and take, a trait that does not come easily for the Yang Type B, who is more concerned with the bigger picture than meddling in "petty" affairs, and who encourages others to focus ahead rather than on one another—a quality born from abundant yang energy. Simply suppressing this energy and deliberately practicing kindness will only create more pressure and anger for the Yang Type B in the end. She must first learn to accept that not everyone will heed her call for action, and to remain enthusiastic and accepting.

- **Yin Type A** (least difficulty managing jei gan): The expression of kindness comes most easily for the Yin Type A, whose stronger liver system correlates directly with jei gan, but whether or not it is based in morality can be a different story. Her concept of kindness is giving, often materially, to others in order to receive something in return. If she gives for the sake of giving, however, then the burden of expectation will be lifted, and she will have the ability to further strengthen her lumbar spine. Kindness expressed from a warm and kind-natured Yin Type A is capable of softening even the coldest of hearts.

- **Yin Type B**: Kindness comes more easily for the Yin Type B compared to the yang types, but rarely can she match the generosity of a Yin Type A. Through bang ryak, the Yin Type B prioritizes tolerance and embracing others, but this is often for the sake of security. Her kindness, although coming across as sincere, may be rooted in insecurity and fear of being ridiculed or hurt. The Yin Type B must first build courage and cultivate her calmness before attempting to be generous. Premature kindness will lead to more fear and insecurity in the end.

Laura and Her Left Turn Pain

After having lunch with her friends, Laura, a fifty-three-year-old Yang Type B, thought hard about whether she should make a dangerous left turn out of the parking lot or take the longer way back home. Always in a hurry, she decided to take a risk and choose the former option. As she was making the left turn, Laura was deeply saddened about how people drive and then suddenly felt her outward expression of anger burst forth as she thought, "Don't these people even see me coming? They don't slow down for anyone!" At that moment something peculiar happened: she noticed a sudden sharp pain in her lower back. As soon as the turn was completed and her anger subsided, however, the pain went away. Laura's experience illustrates how uncontrolled anger can stagnate the energy of the lower back and trigger pain.

The Sacrum

The Yin Type B's stronger kidneys support and send energy to the sacrum. Hence the Yin Type B has a developed sacrum and buttocks area that occasionally protrudes outward, appearing larger and further developed. A weaker sacrum tends to present chronic issues for the Yang Type B such as sacroiliac joint instability. If the Yin Type B suffers from sacral issues, it is rarely due to weakness but rather from excessive tightness, a sign of strength. It is difficult to differentiate between pain due to tightness and pain due to weakness since both may present the same symptoms, such as sciatic nerve impingement, with radiating pain down the lateral side of the leg(s) or local discomfort in the buttocks area. The knowledge of your body type can aid in discovering whether or not back pain comes from weakness or excessive strength.

The Sacral Spine

Strongest type: Yin Type B

Weakest type: Yang Type A

Associated song nature: Bang ryak (*bang* = direction, sharing, distributing; *ryak* = governing, control, regulation, surveying), which is tolerance.

Unbalanced bang ryak emotional effects: Anger toward others, intolerance

Unbalanced bang ryak physiological effects: Tightness and pain in the sacral area, lack of coordination, sciatica with possible radiation of tingling/burning/sharp pain down one or both legs

Balanced bang ryak emotional effects: Feeling of connection with others and humanity as a whole, accepting of others' shortcomings, ability to forgive

Balanced bang ryak physiological effects: Improved balance when walking and/or standing, reduction/elimination of sacral/sciatic discomfort

---

Bang ryak resides in the sacrum and is often a priority for the Yin Type B, who tends to embrace and forgive more easily than the other types. Bang ryak is rarely on the Yang Type A's priority list, as she would rather ignore or punish those who are at fault. Lee Je-ma said that if the Yang Type A refrains from excessive judgment and makes an effort to be more tolerant, then a profound sense of bang ryak emerges. Even though the Yin Type B has an affinity for bang ryak, she has a tendency to take it for granted, believing that others will naturally be as tolerant as she is. When others are not as tolerant, the Yin Type B tends to retreat and isolate herself rather than face the consequences. Tolerance expressed from a cultivated Yin Type B, however, is capable of embracing even the worst wrongdoers.

Menopause forces us to dig deeper and enhance our ability to tolerate and accept the world around us. The Yang Type B may find that living in a world where honesty and truthfulness are not always a priority gives her chronic sacral area instability and/or pain.

If you experience sacroiliac joint or chronic bladder issues, then try working on the ability to tolerate and embrace others by following these body-type-specific guidelines:

- **Yang Type A** (most difficulty managing bang ryak): Anger at herself and/or others and the belief that others are looking down on her inhibit the Yang Type A's ability to embrace others. Her skills reside in her chest, where kyung ryun (government and administration of affairs) dwells. Controlling her tendency toward sorrow and lack of trust while managing and overseeing affairs will naturally bring out the ability to embrace and tolerate others.

- **Yang Type B:** Sorrow and the feeling that others are not being truthful often stop the Yang Type B from embracing and tolerating. Eventually this will impede the energetic flow to her sacrum and bladder, resulting in lower body weakness or bladder and/or sacroiliac joint issues. Her skills reside in the chin area, where ju chek, or intuition, dwells. By trusting her intuition and gradually allowing herself to embrace and tolerate others, she will enhance the flow of energy to the sacrum and bladder.

- **Yin Type A:** Embracing others comes more easily for the yin types than it does for the yang, but the Yin Type A who loses sight of her predominant emotion of joy will find it hard to embrace others. Her skills reside in the upper abdomen, where self-reflection and kindness take refuge. Reflecting inward and getting in touch with her feelings and playful inner child will help her rediscover joy and the ability to embrace others.

- **Yin Type B** (least difficulty managing bang ryak): The ability to embrace and tolerate, or bang ryak, is the Yin Type B's specialty, since it comes from the buttocks, the strongest area of her posterior body. Yet embracing and tolerating don't manifest on their own, and the Yin Type B who loses sight of her predominant emotion of comfort will find it hard to embrace others. By staying calm and embracing and tolerating, the Yin Type B opens the door to other abilities associated with the other types, like kyung ryun and ju chek.

Diane's Shift from Comfort to Compassion

Diane made it her priority to avoid people, especially strangers. Yet the more she tried, the more people would approach her, attracted by her calm and gentle demeanor. Whenever Diane left her home, she deliberately stared at the ground just in case somebody tried to engage her in conversation. Recently, a close friend called her, crying about the loss of her mother. At first, all Diane could think was, "How can I get off the phone as soon as possible without sounding rude?" But just when she was about to make an excuse, a sudden feeling of heartfelt sympathy filled her, and instead she said, "Why don't you come over? I'll make dinner." Both Diane and her friend were surprised by the kind gesture, and at first she regretted saying it. Yet later that evening Diane felt an incredible sense of well-being and wholeness after her friend complimented her cooking and praised her ability to offer comfort. As much as the Yin Type B desires to be alone and free of social obligation, she also has a profound sense of comfort and desire for others to feel it too—a reflection of her innate bang ryak.

MOVING ONWARD

In this chapter we reviewed how each area of the physical body is connected to different aspects of emotion and psychology. Lee Je-ma firmly believed that through balancing our emotions, we can send ample energy to each area of our body. In the following chapters, I will introduce various common issues associated with menopause and interpret them from the standpoint of Sasang medicine. We will explore how each menopause-related issue has its constitutionally based emotional root. Addressing these issues with Sasang medicine requires that we reflect on our emotions and behavioral patterns and initiate the healing process by modifying our reactions and actions based on the changes that are occurring within. This approach is a sharp contrast to the "just fix it" mentality that modern medicine has proclaimed. Sure, if we are in a situation that is causing agonizing discomfort, a quick-fix approach may be momentarily called for, but reflecting on our constitutional tendencies and modifying our reaction to the world around us are the most efficient ways to optimize health.

Let's take Vicki, a fifty-three-year-old Yang Type A, for instance, whose hot flashes were driving her crazy. Her immediate reaction was frustration and anger, which eventually influenced how she interacted with everyone around her. She was miserable, and misery loves company. As her predominant emotion, anger was the one emotion that she could rely on to always be there. Most of the time, it would motivate her to do what she felt was right, but sometimes it would alienate her from even the closest of friends and family.

Finding out that anger was her predominant emotion came as no surprise to Vicki, who was actually relieved to know that it was associated with her type, which explained why it was such a strong emotion. I encouraged Vicki to take a break from constantly trying to rid herself of hot flashes and try addressing the anger itself. Vicki appreciated the idea that anger was also associated with her strong sense of vision and insight and the desire to initiate change. She revealed how her hot flashes started from the chest and worked their way upward to her face. I discussed how the Yang Type A's stronger organ, the spleen, governs this area of the body and is its main source of heat. We also talked about how the chest hosts kyung ryun, the ability to govern and administer affairs, and how do ryang (associated with her weaker lower abdomen) made her feel uncomfortable with intimacy, as she would often downplay her husband's affection. Upon hearing this, Vicki chuckled, since her hot flashes were often felt while at home with her husband by her side. She also mentioned that they occurred when she felt humiliated. I encouraged Vicki to treasure her innately powerful dignity, or wi eui, and not let it be affected when others are not dignified or do not offer the respect she seeks. Taking our conversation to heart, Vicki fine-tuned her body type strengths, stopped ignoring her weaknesses, and optimized her sense of well-being.

Addressing Nine Common Menopause-Related Challenges

By now chances are that you have discovered your body type, and if so, congratulations! If not, take your time and review the previous few chapters again before venturing onward, since there is much to learn about yourself in the process. I am more concerned about those who conclude their type right from the start than I am about those who take weeks, months, or even years. Self-knowledge is the root of healing and balance, and the more time you take to know yourself, the better you'll feel in the end.

HOW TO USE THIS PART

This part of *Yin Yang Balance for Menopause* addresses specific menopause-related issues that women may face before, during, and/or after menopause. Each of the following chapters begins with a story I've heard over the years, each portraying the challenges many women encounter during the menopausal transition. Some stories were blended, while others were altered slightly either to protect the identity of the individual or to emphasize certain aspects of menopause that otherwise may have been left out. While everybody's menopausal journey is different, most readers will identify with one or more of the women in these stories.

Each story is then followed by common Western and Eastern medical perspectives, including the latest research about each menopausal situation. Even though Sasang medicine is considered Eastern medicine, it has a slightly different emphasis from its Chinese medicine counterparts, focusing primarily on body type rather than external factors. This contrast will become more evident as I compare both approaches side-by-side in each chapter.

Menopause is an intricate phase of life, presenting itself in various ways according to the individual and her response to the environment. There are obviously more than just nine challenges that come with menopause, but those mentioned in the following chapters are the most common and most trying. The awareness of your body type and its emotional/physiological tendencies does not eliminate the challenges

110

that menopause may still present but instead provides the tools to guide you through. Even if you don't suffer from any of the issues listed in this part of the book, reading through each chapter will prepare you should they occur, or simply provide deeper insight into how they may influence others with your body type.

A symptom is simply the body's way of letting us know that a particular area needs attention, and as you'll see in the following chapters, each type has its own reason for the issues that arise due to menopause. The following chapters go beyond the mainstream symptomatic approach while encouraging you to envision how each menopause-related issue flows within your body, recognizing that a hot flash is not just a hot flash, and insomnia is not just insomnia. Instead, they are nonstatic and dynamic energetic movements that result from an imbalance within our stronger and weaker organ systems. Hot flashes for the yin types are the result of weakened yang energy escaping upward and away from overpowering yin, and for the yang types, they arise from excessive and rebellious yang energy overwhelming the body's yin energy. On the surface, hot flashes for the yin and yang types might appear identical, but they are addressed with completely different strategies. No matter how much fresh water a plant is given, growth is limited without fresh soil to nourish its roots. Each body type has its own hot flash root system that doesn't respond to simply moistening the leaves.

AN INTRODUCTION TO SASANG HERBAL MEDICINE

Although it can take many forms, Sasang medicine is primarily an herbal approach to restoring health. Written in 1891, Lee Je-ma's original text included hundreds of herbal formulas, with dozens borrowed from doctors of the Song, Ming, and Yuan dynasties of China. Lee Je-ma either modified these formulas or created his own to address the requirements of each body type. He believed that the primary function of each herb is to balance emotion and encourage energy flow from our stronger to weaker organ systems. Lee Je-ma himself stated that even the most effective treatment won't work without the cultivation of one's mind. He often educated his patients about balancing their body-type-specific tendencies while ingesting herbs. Occasionally he'd lament about how, despite ingesting herbs, a patient's condition deteriorated after he or she overlooked this important principle.

Sasang-based herbal remedies for each yin yang body type are included in the last section of each of the following chapters. Lee Je-ma classifies them as either lung, spleen, liver, or kidney herbs. The lung herbs encourage energy flow to the weaker lungs of the Yin Type A, spleen herbs do the same thing for the weaker spleen of the Yin Type B, liver herbs for the weaker liver of the Yang Type B, and kidney herbs for the weaker kidneys of the Yang Type A. As soon as a particular Sasang herb passes through the digestive tract, its constituents immediately proceed to its affiliated organ. In some cases, they may travel there from the stronger organs, and in others, they go directly to the weaker ones. The former situation encourages the flow of energy from the stronger to weaker organs and hence throughout the entire body in conditions of stagnant or blocked energy. The latter supports the weaker organ directly, bypassing the stronger organs to directly nourish and support their function.

Sasang herbs support not only the function of the stronger and weaker organ systems but also the emotions associated with them. According to Sasang medicine, all illnesses have both emotional and physical components, and hence each herb addresses both mind and body. For instance, for the Yang Type A, who has trouble balancing her anger, herbs such as coptis root or Japanese honeysuckle, which cool heat from her stronger spleen, could help do the trick and in the meantime clear excessive heat issues!

The following chapters include remedies for each body type with preparation and dosage instructions (when applicable). Ordering information is also provided for difficult-to-find herbs. This information is not intended to promote the business of these manufacturers but to provide you with the most direct and easily accessible sources that I could find. You can always put your favorite search engine to work in exploring other sources.

Each of the remedies provided in the following chapters may have other properties beyond the condition they are listed under. Be sure to check out the subsection titled "Common Uses" for each herb to find out other hidden benefits. You may also find it helpful to look up each symptom by name and body type in the index. When using this method, make sure to avoid herbs that do not match your body type or situation. Familiarize yourself with each herb and its associated body type by reading through the whole chapter rather than basing your choice on its symptomatic function. Sasang medicine emphasizes the body-type-specific energetic function of each herb. Some herbs help the energy flow upward to strengthen the upper body; others help it flow downward to bolster lower body function. An herb used for headaches may also be used in some cases for neck and shoulder pain, based on its energetic function. Once you are familiar with the energetic function of each herb, it is easier to apply it properly.

The "Herbal Friend" sections introduce herbs that are commonly used together to enhance healing. Also known as "pair herbs" in Eastern medicine, herbal friends either complement or counteract each other's function. Pair herbs that complement each other mutually augment their respective properties. Pair herbs that counteract each other moderate unwanted side effects from their partner, making them safer for ingestion. In the Eastern medicine clinic, it is common to have several pair herbs mixed together in a single formula. Sasang medical formulas consist of ten to fifteen different herbs, with each herb having both unique and combined (paired) functions. While single herbs are helpful for certain conditions, they rarely do the whole job on their own. The use of pair herbs in Eastern medicine coincides with its philosophical emphasis on symbiosis and the premise that a sum is even more powerful and effective than the totality of its parts.

If a remedy appeals to you but is listed under another body type, you should avoid it altogether. Ingesting herbs for body types other than your own could lead to uncomfortable and possibly health-damaging side effects. If you experience indigestion after consuming any of the herbs listed in this section, discontinue the herb immediately. Herbs that match your body type should be easily digested and assimilated. If symptoms such as bloating, excess gas, lack of or excessive appetite, and/or bowel movement issues follow ingestion of an herb, chances are that it isn't compatible with your body type.

Finally, be sure to read any "Caution" sections to avoid interactions with other medications and herbal side effects. Herbs without a caution section are, to the best of my knowledge, relatively safe to ingest. Yet even if the herb is deemed safe, it should not be consumed in excess. The dosage section provides information on appropriate dose ranges. Also, be aware that most extracts and tinctures contain traces of alcohol and if you are sensitive to even small amounts, avoid extracts or tinctures made with alcohol. Luckily, not all extracts contain alcohol, so read product labels carefully before purchasing any herb, herbal extract, or tincture. Non-alcohol-based tinctures often have glycerin among their ingredients; these are included in this book whenever possible.

Although you may be familiar with specific herbs in the following chapters, their less widely known Sasang-related functions may have escaped your knowledge. Sasang-based herbal functions may occasionally contrast with common interpretations, making it difficult for those with previous herbal knowledge to accept or comply with them. If you have any specific questions regarding the use of the herbs in this section, visit my website at sasangmedicine.com and click the "Contact Us" icon.

4

Fire Aboard

Hot Flashes

Mary's hot flashes add pleasant warmth to her otherwise freezing body, while Denise's overheat her already hot system. Donna is capable of ignoring her hot flashes, while Jeannie is stopped in her tracks by them. Justine's hot flashes are worse when she feels stressed or embarrassed, while Vicky's wake her up in the middle of the night. Marsha's hot flashes leave her feeling drenched, as sweat pours from every inch of her body, while Michelle stays as dry as a bone. Heat triggers Renée's hot flashes, yet Barbara could stand naked in the snow and still get them. Wendy breezed through menopause without a single hot flash, while Elaine experienced one every day. Terry's hysterectomy at age forty-three was followed by three years of intense hot flashes. Amy, who underwent a hysterectomy at the same age, never felt a hot flash. Pat felt a tingling sensation through her body before a hot flash occurred, but Cindy's came without warning. Heather could feel heat rising from her stomach to her head, while Kelly's hot flashes felt like someone had lit her whole body on fire. Cathy's hot flashes worsened with moderate exercise; Nancy's, though, went away after she began a new workout routine.

These experiences amount to only a small fraction of the feedback I have received from my patients. To make matters worse, not only would these hot flash symptoms differ from patient to patient, but they also varied from day to day. Even though Mary experienced a pleasant hot flash on Monday, come Thursday it was flaming as hell! Marsha's hot flash on Tuesday left her drenched, but after the one on Friday, not a drop of sweat emerged from her skin. If apples are apples and oranges are oranges, why can't a hot flash be a hot flash? Why is the hot flash experience so different from one individual to another? Of course, estrogen and progesterone levels may play a role, but not a single study out there could verify a direct correlation between levels of hormone deficiency and hot flash intensity. Many postmenopausal women, with only a fraction of the hormones they once had, are hot flash free. Clearly, there is more to hot flashes than just hormones and other physiological changes that come with menopause. We each respond to the external (work, family, friends, and so on) and internal (fluctuating hormone levels) environments in different ways based on our past experience, health state, and, perhaps most influential of all, body type. Hence the hot flash experience also fluctuates according to the individual and how she reacts to the environment, which is influenced but not dictated by hormonal changes.

Hot flashes, also referred to as "hot flushes" or "vasomotor symptoms," are among the most commonly reported menopause-related symptoms, occurring in seven out of ten menopausal women in the United States.[1] Hot flashes are usually marked by a sudden feeling of warmth that is most intense over the face, neck, and chest but can be felt throughout the body. These episodes are often followed by sweating as the body attempts to adjust the internal thermostat and cool the surface of the body. Sweating may be mild or completely absent during a hot flash in some women, and if it does occur, it is mostly experienced at night, interfering with sleep.

THE HOT FLASH EXPERIENCE

Many women are able to sense when a hot flash is about to happen by feeling an uncomfortably warm sensation in their abdomen, a headache accompanied by heart palpitations, a tingling sensation on their skin, and/or a general sense of discomfort, irritability, or hypersensitivity to stress. The hot flash sensation is usually due to a rise of temperature only at the skin level as the cutaneous vessels dilate and warm blood rushes outward to the surface. Finger temperature rises, offering researchers a valid objective tool to record the frequency and intensity of hot flashes. The pulse rate also increases an average of nine beats per minute, often triggering anxiousness and/or irritability.

While hot flash symptoms are easily detectable, their etiology is not well understood in modern medicine. One theory involves the effect of declining levels of estrogen, which elevate other hormones such as follicle-stimulating hormone (FSH) and luteinizing hormone (LH), produced in the pituitary gland, situated directly below the hypothalamus. Increased levels of FSH and LH signal the hypothalamus to dilate the blood vessels, causing a rush of blood toward the skin and decreasing the core body temperature. Other explanations involve the estrogenic influence of hormones such as epinephrine and norepinephrine, which also control vasodilation, resulting in the sensation of heat at the skin level. While these theories may hold merit, scavenging the body for a single hot flash source has led us to the discovery of yet further potential scenarios. The more we discover about human biology, the more hot flash explanations we'll find. Within each person exists a universe of infinitely integrated, constantly interacting components that cannot be singled out and accused of causing a hot flash single-handedly. We will soon discover how in Sasang medicine, our stronger and weaker organ systems and their correlating emotions play an integrative role in avoiding or instigating a hot flash.

What Is the Difference between Hot Flashes and Night Sweats?

Basically, just the name. Both are episodes of sudden flushing, heat, and potential sweat. The only difference is that hot flashes occur during the day, and night sweats happen at night, mostly between the hours of 3:00 and 5:00 a.m. Night sweats, however, often produce more sweat than hot flashes do. In Eastern medicine, this is thought to be due to the difference between yin and yang, where yin correlates with the evening and moisture, and yang with daytime and dryness. Yet there can still be ample sweating with hot flashes and reduced sweating with night sweats since no rule is ever set in stone and other factors, such as our yin yang body type, have a role to play. The term hot flash is often used to describe both daytime and nighttime flushes of heat.

Hot flashes are not exclusive to menopause, since certain types of chemotherapy, radiation, and androgen treatment for breast and/or prostate cancer may also spark them. They may occur at different times throughout one's lifetime or be exacerbated by an imbalance of the monthly cycle, hot weather, stress, anxiety, smoking, and/or caffeine. The hot flash experience varies across different ethnicities, cultures, climates, lifestyles, diets, attitudes, and genetics, making some prone to symptoms and others symptom-free. African Americans tend to suffer more from hot flashes than most other ethnicities in America,[2] while Japanese Americans report having fewer hot flashes than those of European descent.[3]

WESTERN AND EASTERN PERSPECTIVES ON HOT FLASHES

Estrogen replacement is the most efficient Western medical approach to decreasing hot flashes, boasting a success rate of up to 90 percent in eliminating them altogether.[4] Other approaches include the use of antidepressants and blood pressure and/or anti-seizure medication. Venlafaxine, an antidepressant, reduced hot flash symptoms in up to 60 percent of those who were tested.[5] With these statistics, most women who deal with consistent hot flashes would likely leap for joy at the possibility of relief, yet fewer and fewer doctors are prescribing these medications, encouraging their patients to seek alternatives.

According to the Women's Health Initiative (WHI)—a comprehensive study performed in 2004 that included over five thousand participants—the risk of breast cancer increases significantly in women from ages fifty to seventy-nine who have not had a hysterectomy and who take estrogen and progesterone together. Another study, including over ten thousand women who underwent hysterectomies and were taking estrogen, was terminated early because of the significantly higher occurrence of stroke during the trial. Before these studies, both estrogen and progesterone were viewed as relatively safe and prescribed freely; they were even compared to a fountain of youth by some doctors. Shock waves over these studies can still be felt, leaving both doctors and patients wary of hormone therapy following menopause.

Another issue with estrogen, not dealt with in the above trials, is that when treatment is ceased, there is an over 50 percent chance that hot flashes will return, often worse than before estrogen withdrawal.[6] Hence many women who experience symptom relief are advised by their doctor to keep taking estrogen, years after their last hot flash.

The above trials do not paint the whole picture of hormone replacement treatment, nor do antidepressants always cause side effects. In her book *The Wisdom of Menopause*, Dr. Christiane Northrup points out that beginning hormonal treatment in lower doses soon after or during perimenopause would have likely reduced the risks of cancer and/or stroke among participants in the aforementioned trials. She is also a proponent of bioidentical soy- and yam-based estrogens, such as 17-beta-estradiol, estrone, and estriol, designed to match the structure of human hormones. Dr. Northrup also holds that side effects can be reduced by adjusting the dosage according to the individual through obtaining bioidentical hormones from a compounding pharmacy capable of acutely adjusting dosages and hormone ratios. This approach contrasts with the standard approach to hormone therapy, which uses estrogens that are not as compatible with the human body, such as Prempro, which is derived from pregnant mare urine.

The use of antidepressants for hot flashes has increased within the past few years, perhaps in response to WHI trial hormone-related fears. The exact reason why antidepressants reduce hot flashes in some women is still not clearly understood, but it may have to do with the suggestion that emotions have a role to play in hot flashes—a premise of the Sasang medical view. Menopausal women often report experiencing hot flashes when they are feeling stressed, nervous, excited, or aroused. The use of antidepressants to control emotion, however, frequently presents side effects such as nausea, weight gain, loss of sex drive, fatigue, drowsiness, and/or insomnia. Not knowing how or why antidepressants affect hot flashes even in women who are not depressed, coupled with a high risk of side effects, is enough to steer many women clear of this option. Still others may find that the lowest possible dose of antidepressants helps reduce acute hot flashes and can be tapered off slowly once things are under control. If you decide to take the antidepressant and/or hormone therapy approach, I recommend concurrently engaging in alternative methods such as diet, herbal therapy, acupuncture, exercise, and emotional balancing. Doing so will likely enhance the effects of hormone replacement therapy and/or antidepressants and potentially allow you to reduce medication dosages through time.

In Eastern medicine, hot flashes are referred to as "rebellious heat," which rises from one or more organs within the body. Sasang medicine focuses on releasing this heat from each body type's stronger organ system through foods, herbs, exercises, and, most important of all, emotional balance. The approach to addressing hot flashes varies significantly according to where the heat originates from. The Yang Type A's heat accumulates within the spleen, the original source of bodily heat, resulting in a "fire feeding fire" scenario. Hence the Yang Type A's hot flashes are often the hottest of all four body types. The Yin Type B's heat accumulates in her stronger kidneys, the body's original source of cool energy, making her hot flashes the least uncomfortable of the four body types. In some cases, the Yin Type B may actually look forward to getting a hot flash because it gives her long-awaited feelings of warmth!

Even though many women feel as if their body has turned into a furnace when suffering from a hot flash, body temperature does not actually increase. Instead heat is displaced and pushed out to the exterior. The monthly cycle is an opportunity to release this energy from the body and start anew. If a cycle is skipped or nonexistent—as in menopause—the body has to release heat in other ways. If there is significant heat accumulation within the body, hot flashes are sometimes the only option it has. Menopause is a time when women come face-to-face with the rebellious child within, who has reluctantly waited decades for the opportunity to grab their attention. It's time to become a rebel and stretch the strict rules by which emotional and biological processes were bound. The uterus is no longer a compartment where the heat of excessive emotion can be stored and released during the monthly cycle. It is time to *become* the person you are completely capable of *being*, whether or not it is the "correct" thing to do. As discussed earlier, heat is yang, and yang is the spark that ignites passion, growth, and change.

Night Sweats

Hot flashes tend to be more intense at night than during the day, stirring up extreme heat and abundant sweat, often interrupting sleep.

At first a woman may find the heat so unbearable that she throws off the covers, only to feel extremely cold from being drenched in sweat moments later. There has been great speculation over why hot flashes mostly take place between 3:00 and 5:00 in the morning, and why they are so powerful within this time frame. Modern medicine falls short of answering these questions, simply explaining how night sweats are due to an impairment of the sympathetic nervous system and its inability to regulate internal temperature. Yes, an imbalance of the sympathetic nervous system may indeed be involved, but that doesn't explain why this system, involved in the fight-or-flight response, kicks in when we are asleep and supposedly most relaxed.

In Eastern medicine, bodily energy is said to flow from one organ to another every two hours, completing a full cycle between 1:30 and 3:30 in the morning, when energy flows from the liver, the last organ of the cycle, to the lungs, the first. Most of us are usually sound asleep during this time, with our conscious thoughts out of the way, giving our body the chance to recycle its energies efficiently without disruption. Yet the liver doesn't always want to give up its place in the spotlight, especially if it's constitutionally the strongest organ, as with Yin Type As, who either choose to stay up late or wake up easily during this time. In order for us to renew our energies, something must give, and training our strongest organs to loosen the reins is easier said than done. Menopause itself is a time for women to renew their energies, but they can only be balanced through weeding out unnecessary and unhelpful thoughts, acquaintances, activities, and material belongings. Table 4.1 on page 122 provides the various pathways our body's energy takes in the course of a day.

The reason hot flashes are more intense in the evening is different according to each of the body types. As discussed earlier, night correlates with yin, and yin with cold. If night is associated with cold, then why would hot flashes worsen? For the yin-deficient yang types, the evening may give yang energy the opportunity to dance wildly about, without constraint, as we feebly seek sleep. For the yin types, abundant evening yin energy may smother and irritate yang to the point that it escapes upward and outward, bringing heat and sweat along with it.

TABLE 4.1. PATH OF ORGAN ENERGIES THROUGHOUT A TWENTY-FOUR-HOUR CYCLE

Time	Organ
11:01 p.m.–1:00 a.m.	Gallbladder
1:01–3:00 a.m.	Liver
3:01–5:00 a.m.	Lungs
5:01–7:00 a.m.	Large intestine
7:01–9:00 a.m.	Stomach
9:01–11:00 a.m.	Spleen/pancreas
11:01 a.m.–1:00 p.m.	Kidneys
1:01–3:00 p.m.	Urinary bladder
3:01–5:00 p.m.	Small intestine
5:01–7:00 p.m.	Heart
7:01–9:00 p.m.	Pericardium
9:01–11:00 p.m.	Lymph system

THE YIN AND YANG OF HOT FLASHES

Yang energy, associated with progesterone and testosterone, causes heat to rise up from deep within the body, and yin energy, associated with estrogen, cools it and sends it back down. It is easier to imagine how excessive yang energy bullying its way through our bodies can bring about hot flashes, but how can this happen when yin gets out of hand? Let's take a closer look at the hot flash process to find the answer.

Sasang and Chinese medicines differ slightly with regard to hot flashes. The latter associates them with a deficiency of yin, which gradually wanes as we age. You may recall from chapter 1 that yin and yang go through significant changes within the female body every seven years. During the seventh of the seven-year cycles, a woman experiences the most intense change in which her kidneys, the source of yin energy, begin to decline, making it difficult to root yang, which jumps at the opportunity to ascend. Hence treatment for hot flashes in Chinese medicine primarily involves supporting yin and restraining yang energy. The Chinese medical practitioner often prescribes herbs that are yin-natured, cooling, and cloying in order to accomplish this.

This method is often successful when addressing the hot flashes due to yin weakness and yang abundance, but not everyone fits this profile. Hence patients who still have sufficient yin energy may find such herbs too cooling, heavy, and difficult to digest. Worse yet, some individuals may experience even more hot flashes after taking these herbs because, according to Sasang medicine, excessive yin is capable of clamping down on and squeezing yang to the point that it oozes and retreats upward, bringing a flash of heat with it. Hence even though a loss of estrogen, correlating to a decrease in yin, is believed to be the primary hot flash trigger, excessive amounts may also lead to the same symptoms. During perimenopause, for example, there are times when estrogen levels spike and are deemed to be the culprit behind intense, sweaty hot flashes. This coincides with the Eastern medical theory that yin at its extreme transforms into yang and vice versa. Does this mean that estrogen alone is to blame for hot flashes? While a loss of estrogen is the most obvious hormonal indication of menopausal onset, and hence gets the most attention, in actuality, any hormone that acts out or lags behind the others can cause menopausal symptoms. Menopausal bliss depends on a balance between yin and yang and between estrogen, progesterone, and testosterone.

Before diving into body-type-specific approaches to hot flashes, let's look at six general tips that anyone experiencing them may find useful.

Tip #1: Reduce Stress

A study conducted in 2011 that included 110 pre- and recently post-menopausal women revealed how a meditation known as Mindfulness-Based Stress Reduction (MBSR) significantly reduced the discomfort associated with hot flashes. Interestingly, participants didn't record any changes in hot flash intensity, but they were less affected by them. These results compared promisingly with other medications that have been known to reduce hot flashes[7] and show how meditation can change how we perceive hot flashes even if they still occur.

How we perceive hot flashes makes all the difference. Someone who is new to hot flash symptoms may be frightened, feeling as if the doom and gloom of menopause is about to swallow her whole. Others who have suffered from flashes of heat in the past may not even recognize the onset of a menopause-related hot flash. Acceptance is an essential component of the healing process. To accept does not mean to give up your faith that things will get better. Instead, it is the acknowledgment that hot flashes have arrived, and rather than curse, moan, and complain, one can have faith that when the time is ripe, they too will pass. But meanwhile, it is time to adjust, take action, rediscover yourself, and realize that hot flashes are not to be "defeated." Listen to your hot flashes and get accustomed to their occurrence without becoming possessed by them.

It is easy to fall into the trap of expecting hot flashes to occur and then, once they do, feeling as if they will never go away. Many women begin to identify themselves and their lives with hot flashes, finding it difficult to imagine life without them. Stop yourself before letting the feeling of defeat settle in and try following these simple but effective steps:

1. Accept that you are having a hot flash instead of denying it, or worse, fighting it.
2. Throw away thoughts of defeat, anguish, or other negative ideas that hot flashes may conjure up. Hot flashes can be the perfect excuse to lash out at others, think unpleasant thoughts, and feel hopeless if you choose to.
3. Breathe and center yourself. (Follow the steps in Tip 5.)
4. Let go. Whether it was an intense or a mild hot flash, once it is gone, it's time to move on. It is easy to get stuck in the healing process as we overanalyze why this or that symptom occurred, thinking that we have to solve it here and now. The onset of a hot flash in some cases may be obvious, such as an explosive argument with a spouse. The reason why a hot flash occurs in others may not be so obvious, though, leaving a feeling of cluelessness. Actually, all that needs to be done in such situations is to keep the channel of further discovery open, and eventually wisdom and balance will flow in. You may never find an answer as to why

your hot flashes occurred and be pleasantly surprised when they no longer do! What could possibly have resolved such flaming intensity? Often it is nothing but time, resilience, patience, and the wisdom that you have accumulated throughout the process.

5. Record when the hot flash occurred. Did it occur upon awakening? At work? Before bed? While sleeping? Hot flashes that occur first thing in the morning may indicate the feeling of being overwhelmed with daily responsibility. Hot flashes before bed or while sleeping may act as a relief valve, letting out the steam of daily stress. If your hot flashes occur at specific times during the day or night, or after particular situations, then prepare beforehand with deep breathing and calming your mind.

Tip #2: Exercise

Moderate exercise can reduce hot flashes, but strenuous exercise can induce them. Not even the most skilled trainer or doctor could tell you exactly how much exercise is too much or not enough. Listen to your body during and after exercise and expand and/or cut back on your routine accordingly. An exercise that triggered a hot flash last week might be doable this week. Determining exactly which exercise triggers your hot flashes and how much exercise will help moderate them is an ongoing challenge that changes according to not only the person but also to her age and the time. It also takes a considerable amount of effort and self-reflection. If you are starting an exercise routine or have difficulty figuring out which one is best for you, try following these practical steps:

1. Start simple, increasing your workout time and intensity slowly but surely. While there are many potentially supportive training methods, many of my patients have had the most success with interval training—enhancing and decreasing the intensity of a workout at regular intervals within a training session. This method contrasts with the idea of pushing beyond one's limits without giving the body a chance to recharge.

2. Stay consistent, convincing yourself to do at least some form of exercise five days a week.

3. Exercise primarily to stay healthy and balance your energies, rather than simply to lose weight, gain muscle, and so forth.

4. Pace your breathing. When engaging in cardiovascular exercise, maximize your lung capacity by inhaling and exhaling as deeply as possible. I recommend counting to the highest number you can while inhaling and repeating the same amount while exhaling. Try pacing your breaths with each repetition, so that if you are bicycling, for example, each cycle, whether initiated by the left or right foot, may count as one pace. Then it is up to you to determine how many paces per breath—five paces breathing in, five out . . . six paces in, six out, and so on. As your workout becomes more intense, it will naturally be difficult to keep the same breathing rhythm, so be sure to adjust it accordingly, so you don't have to gasp for air.

Tip #3: Balance Food Intake

Hot flashes almost always originate from heat stagnation and accumulation in one or more digestive organs. For the yang types excessive heat is often generated from the esophagus and stomach, and for the yin types, the liver and kidneys are often its source. Sasang medicine emphasizes the importance of eating according to your body type. I suggest referring to the appendix in this book or to my other book, *Your Yin Yang Body Type,* for extensive body-type-specific dietary suggestions. Here are a few general guidelines.

What to Eat

In general, avoiding excessively spicy, fatty, sour, sweet, and salty foods is of fundamental importance in avoiding hot flashes. Each flavor has its own energy that, in turn, affects different areas of the body. Excessive intake of any of these flavors may overstimulate, stagnate, and congest their correlating body areas. Moreover, consuming foods that are not compatible for your type may also instigate the onset of hot flashes.

How Much to Eat

Too much of any type of food, even if it is compatible with your body type, may irritate the stomach and potentially instigate a hot flash. Also, the consistent churning of heavy, difficult-to-digest foods often gives rise to excessive heat from friction within the stomach and intestines. Insufficient food intake, on the contrary, may stir up stomach acid, giving rise to excessive heat in the upper body. Only you have the ultimate ability to determine how much is too much/too little food intake. Listen closely to what your stomach is telling you and try not to ignore the signal of hunger or contentment. The road to optimum health begins within, by developing the ability to hear what your body is telling you without ignoring or overreacting to its message.

When to Eat

As mentioned earlier in this chapter, every organ of the body has its own active and latent period throughout a twenty-four-hour cycle. The stomach is most active and ready to perform between the hours of 7:00 and 9:00 a.m. Our ability to digest food efficiently starts to wane as we get farther away from this time period. Stomach time is an opportunity to ingest our heartiest meal of the day, lessening the chance of feeling fatigued, bloated, or heavy after eating. Some of us may find a cup of coffee and piece of toast in the morning adequate, but this habit may leave us fatigued and in need of more caffeine to keep us going as the day progresses. As a light eater myself, I recall being overwhelmed when my Taiwanese friend offered me a breakfast the size of a dinner, explaining that it is customary to do so in his home country! After giving this method a whirl, I began to feel more energized through the day. Now I routinely consume at least 30 percent of my daily caloric intake during stomach time.

Eating a larger meal in the morning isn't for everyone. Those who are active throughout the day need the extra calories in the morning to charge their batteries, while others who are more stationary may notice feeling/looking heavier and bloated after eating a substantially sized breakfast.

Eating dinner after 7:00 p.m., when our yang (metabolic) energy retires and yin (resting) dominates, may result in unsettled digestive energy and hence a hot flash. If you digest foods rapidly, then not eating for three or more hours before bedtime, in itself, could trigger a hot flash as the stomach juices swoosh about wildly, begging for more food. Nibbling on a rice cracker or drinking a warm cup of almond/rice/goat's milk an hour or so before bed may suffice. Keep in mind that drinking a substantial amount of fluid directly before sleeping may trigger the need to wake up and urinate.

How to Eat

Eating in a rush or while stressed, forgetting to chew your food slowly, or focusing on something other than food while eating can also initiate hot flashes. Relaxing the mind, as if meditating, enhances the process of digestion, whereas a cluttered and unsettled mind simply disrupts it.

Tip #4: Try Acupuncture and Acupressure

A study performed at Stanford University demonstrated how nine sessions of acupuncture over a seven-week period greatly reduced the intensity of hot flashes.[8] Along with assisting the flow of energy throughout the body, acupuncture needle insertion is also a way to release excessive heat. Patients who receive acupuncture for hot flashes often feel a chill throughout the body during the treatment as the body attempts to adjust its internal thermostat.

I often utilize the points shown below to relieve hot flashes, since they have effectively provided relief for my patients over the years. These points correlate with different organs of the body that may absorb heat and have difficulty letting it go. They can be compared to relief valves that let out excessive steam from an engine, which in the human body can be done via energy meridians flowing from each organ to the surface of the body. These points are most effective if they are addressed daily, even when hot flashes are not present.

Please note that you do not need to insert a needle at these points for the treatment to be helpful. Using acupressure, or applying pressure to each point, often yields significant results. Applying significant pressure to each point until it feels tender often yields better results than a light touch. Avoid using sharp metal objects that could penetrate your skin or applying excessive pressure.

☯ LIV2 (SECOND POINT ON THE LIVER MERIDIAN): "MOVING BETWEEN"

This acupressure point is the second from the tip of the foot along the liver meridian, located between the first and second toes (see fig. 4.1 on the next page). There is often a short crease that continues from the inner side of the big toe downward to the upper part of your foot. LIV2 is located at the point where this crease terminates. LIV2 releases heat from the liver, where hot flash heat often originates.

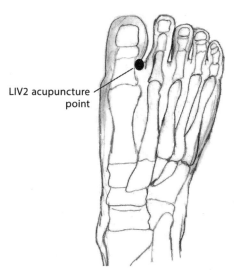

LIV2 acupuncture point

Fig. 4.1. LIV2, second point on the liver meridian

✳ Use your index finger to apply direct pressure to LIV2 while counting to ten and breathing slowly.

✳ Gently release and then switch to the other foot.

✳ Repeat this process up to five times.

🌀 ST44 (FORTY-FOURTH POINT ON THE STOMACH MERIDIAN): "INNER COURT"

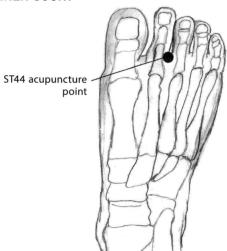

ST44 acupuncture point

Fig. 4.2. ST44, forty-fourth point on the stomach meridian

This acupressure point is the second from the tip of the foot along the stomach meridian and is located between the second and third toes (see fig. 4.2 above). There is often a short crease from the outer side of the second toe downward to the upper part of your foot. ST44 is located where this crease terminates. This point is indicated for the release of heat from the stomach, where heat tends to accumulate before a hot flash.

* Use your index finger to apply direct pressure to ST44 while counting to ten and breathing slowly.
* Gently release and then switch to the other foot.
* Repeat this process up to five times.

☯ HT9 (NINTH POINT ON THE HEART MERIDIAN): "LESSER SURGE"

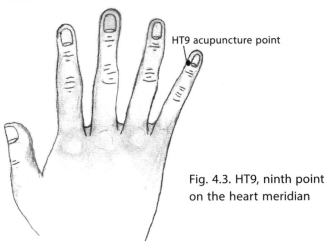

HT9 acupuncture point

Fig. 4.3. HT9, ninth point on the heart meridian

Imagine two lines, one from the tip of your pinky nail, located on the side facing the ring finger and extending straight downward, and another across the bottom of the nail perpendicular to the first line. HT9 is located where these two lines intersect (see fig. 4.3 above). I often utilize this point to promote calmness and release excessive heat from the heart, our emotional center.

* Use your fingernail, a toothpick, or a pen to apply pressure to HT9 while counting to ten and breathing slowly.
* Gently release and then switch to the other hand.
* Repeat this process up to five times.

Tip #5: Breathe

A study conducted in 1996 demonstrated how three weeks of consistent slow and deep breathing significantly reduced hot flash symptoms.[9]

Several of my patients have reported that they can prevent the onset of a hot flash by breathing deeply as soon as they feel it coming. Breathing is the first and last thing we do as humans and in my opinion is the most convenient balancing tool we have, since it can be done right away, wherever we are.

There are numerous breathing techniques, most of them developed from the ancient yogic practice of pranayama. A Chinese technique, referred to as *dan tian* breathing, has shown promising effects in reducing hot flashes among many of my patients.

DAN TIAN BREATHING

* Lie down with your hands resting on your lower abdomen.
* Slowly inhale while gently pushing your lower abdomen outward, letting the ingoing air fill it up. Try to avoid filling your chest with air, focusing only on your lower abdomen.
* Exhale, simply releasing the air from your abdomen, letting it flow back upward. At the very end you may want to gently squeeze your abdomen to ensure that all of the air has been released.
* Repeat these steps every day for at least five minutes before getting out of bed in the morning and before going to sleep. Imagine that you are bringing energy and heat downward from your head to your feet when inhaling and then releasing all the tension in your body when exhaling.

Tip #6: Consume Hot-Flash-Reducing Foods and Vitamins

The internet is saturated with hot flash remedies, often accompanied by exaggerated claims. While many of these approaches are somewhat effective in relieving hot flashes, they do not work for everyone or in every situation and aren't always backed by substantial research and/ or literature. Table 4.2 on page 132 provides a list of six common hot-flash-relieving foods/supplements and the body type they are most compatible with. In the latter half of this chapter, I will present several herbal hot flash remedies in detail for each body type. The combination of eating according to your yin yang body type and supplementing with body-type-specific herbal hot flash remedies doubles your chances of reestablishing balance.

TABLE 4.2. HOT-FLASH-REDUCING FOODS AND SUPPLEMENTS

Supplement/Food	Yang Type Compatibility	Yin Type Compatibility	Common Sources	Effect
Vitamin E*	Very compatible	Supplement with lowest recommended dosage	Wheat germ oil, canola oil, sunflower oil	Nourishes yin and anchors yang heat
Flaxseed[†]	Supplement with lowest recommended dosage	Supplement with lowest recommended dosage	Original form	Nourishes and supports the function of the liver, lungs, and large intestines
Soybeans[‡]	Very compatible	Not compatible	Original form or in tofu, tempeh, soy-based yogurt	Nourishes yin and has cooling energy
Magnesium[§]	Supplement with lowest recommended dosage	Tolerable in food but not recommended as a supplement	Dark leafy greens, pumpkin seeds, sesame seeds, sunflower seeds, cashews, almonds, seafood, beans, whole grains, avocados, yogurt, bananas	Promotes the downward flow of energy, roots the mind and spirit
Sage[¶]	Not compatible	Very compatible	Original form or as a supplement	Promotes harmonious flow of yang heat throughout the body
Wild (Chinese) yam[‖]	Tolerable but not recommended	Very compatible	Original form (can be found in Asian food markets or as a supplement)	Supports and nurtures yang energy, and to a lesser degree yin energy

*Ziaei et al., "Effect of Vitamin E."

[†]Ghazanfarpour et al., "Effects of Flaxseed and *Hypericum perforatum*."

[‡]Taku et al., "Extracted or Synthesized Soybean Isoflavones."

[§]Park et al., "Pilot Phase II Trial of Magnesium Supplements."

[¶]Bommer et al., "First Time Proof of Sage's Tolerability and Efficacy."

[‖]Wu et al., "Estrogenic Effect of Yam Ingestion."

HOT FLASHES AND
THE YIN YANG BODY TYPES

Hot flashes induced by excessive yin and weakened yang are more common among the yin types, while those arising from abundant yang and weakened yin are experienced more frequently among the yang types. From the Sasang point of view, the seventh cycle of the seven-year cycles in women is associated with not only a weakening of yin but also a fluctuation of yang energy. During this cycle, each yin yang body type must cultivate herself further in her own way by getting in touch with and balancing her innate physiological and psychological inclinations. If an individual is constitutionally more yin-natured, then she will be prone to yin symptoms such as hot flashes with cold spells, sluggish digestion, diarrhea, and/or depression, but if she is yang-natured, then yang symptoms such as frequent heat spells, skin dryness, and/or anger abound.

Hot Flashes and Emotion

In research, hot flash testing is usually separated into two categories: subjective and objective. The former category relies on the patient's subjective recording of hot flashes, and the latter on measurements such as core body temperature, heart rate, and finger blood flow. A study conducted in 2005 demonstrated how women who reported being joyful and calm exhibited significantly fewer subjective hot flashes than those who were angry, frustrated, and/or stressed. This study also revealed how anger, frustration, and/or stress resulted in higher levels of subjectively recorded hot flashes even without increases in body-surface temperature, heart rate, or finger blood flow. Hence unbalanced emotions can trigger the feeling of a hot flash even if there are no objective findings to back them up! If you think that's interesting, here's the real punch: Even though the joyful and calm group reported fewer subjective hot flashes, both groups averaged the same amount of objective ones. Hence even if estrogen and the hypothalamus are going absolutely bonkers, joyfulness and calmness may be enough to keep them from fazing us!*

*Thurston et al., "Emotional Antecedents of Hot Flashes."

Sasang medicine holds that how we feel emotionally determines whether or not we have a smooth or rough menopausal transition. This may be hard to swallow, since it is easier to imagine that hot flashes influence how we feel emotionally than it is to convince ourselves that our emotions can induce and aggravate menopausal symptoms like hot flashes. Each emotion has its own temperature: anger, for instance, is hot, and calmness is cold. These emotional inclinations make certain body types more prone to hot flashes than others, depending on the setting of their internal thermostat. The yang types tend to express hotter emotions, and the yin types cooler ones. Yet all four of the yin yang body types may experience hot flashes, since hot emotions are not exclusive to the yang types. Actually, the yin types may occasionally find it more challenging to deal with hot flashes than the yang types since they have less experience dealing with pronounced heat and hot-natured emotions.

Let's take a look at how to address hot flashes according to the unique requirements of each yin yang body type.

YANG TYPE A

Even when she is not experiencing a hot flash, the Yang Type A is prone to overheating thanks to her stronger spleen—the body's source of heat. Her angry temperament, which triggers the release of heat from the spleen, can easily generate hot flashes. Comfort, on the other hand, which is associated with her weaker kidneys and the element of water, produces cold energy. The Yang Type A's menopause-related issues and the stresses of daily life may take her past the boiling point, turning anger into rage and water into fire. Herbal treatment for the Yang Type A is aimed at cooling the spleen and supporting the kidneys.

The Yang Type A with hot flashes is not always a raging bull. Actually, she may present herself as joyful, gentle, or even calm! But this is often an attempt to conceal her true nature and avoid offending or disappointing others. Until this point in her life, the Yang Type A may have been able to suppress and conceal her anger, or at least keep it from exploding. Yet menopause creates an entirely different dynamic for her: as the energies shift within her body, so do emotions, demanding her attention. Sure, the Yang Type A is able to feel joyful and calm, but only through getting in touch with and balancing her anger. If something rubs her the wrong way, she is not able to simply brush it aside like the yin types, since anger will rapidly build up. Yet responding with excessive anger only fans the flames of rage. Anger does not have to be expressed with one's fist; it can be a motivational force that leads to positive and effective action.

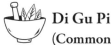 ## Di Gu Pi
(Common: Lycium Bark; Latin: *Lycium chinense*)
In Eastern medicine, Di Gu Pi, or lycium bark, is used to treat steaming bone syndrome, a condition in which excessive heat radiates outward from the depths of the body—a common hot flash dynamic. As a cold-natured herb, lycium bark doesn't only cool the body, it also nourishes the Yang Type A's deficient kidney yin. It focuses primarily on cooling the stomach, clearing heat stagnation, and enhancing digestion. Lycium bark also clears heat from the skin, where it accumulates during a hot flash. The Yang Type A may notice an uncomfortable or painful skin sensation preceding or during the onset of a hot flash. This, also addressed with lycium bark, comes from trapped heat as it gets pushed outward from the depths of the body.

Common Uses
Lycium bark relieves hot flashes, excessive sweating, dry/painful skin, and indigestion (due to heat stagnation).

Sources
A tincture of Di Gu Pi can be purchased from the Hawaii Pharm website.

Preparation and Dosage
Please follow the manufacturer's suggestions.

Herbal Friend: Zhi Mu
(Common: Anemarrhena;
Latin: *Anemarrhena asphodeloides*)

Zhi Mu (meaning "mother's wisdom"), or anemarrhena, is an herb that truly lives up to its name. While most cold-natured herbs have a tendency to be drying, this herb has the remarkable ability to moisten the bodily organs while efficiently clearing heat. This can be likened to a mother's ability to nourish and calm a fussy infant. Zhi Mu and Di Gu Pi work together to nourish yin and clear heat, calming those fussy hot flashes. Zhi Mu can also be purchased as a tincture from the Hawaii Pharm website. Both herbs can be ingested together in equal doses. Please see the manufacturer's dosage suggestions for further details.

YANG TYPE B

As mentioned above, both yang types tend to overheat since they lack yin cold energy. Yet the Yang Type B is not as prone to excessive heat-related issues as the Yang Type A. The former needs the cool energy of the liver to balance her warm lung energy, while the latter needs the ice-cold energy of the kidneys to douse the flames of her hot spleen energy. The Yang Type B is by no means incapable of experiencing acute hot flashes since sorrow, correlating with her stronger lungs, can easily morph into the heat of anger, associated with the spleen, and then into scorching hot flashes.

As with any of the other types, a hot flash can appear out of nowhere, making it difficult to trace or connect with our emotions. It is easier to hold hormones accountable for these otherwise spontaneous aggravations. Yet Sasang medicine holds that even these situations can be tied to our predominant emotions, which often hide below layers of coping skills. If the Yang Type B controls her tendency toward sorrow and distrust of others—a tendency related to her weaker liver—then her hot flashes will naturally lose their impetus as time goes by.

Balancing one's predominant emotion is a process that takes a tremendous amount of sincerity, patience, and self-reflection. It is often difficult to get in touch with one's inner feelings, since day-to-day emotions can conceal them. Even when they are discovered, there is no certainty that balance and harmony will naturally unfold. The Yang Type B may choose to avoid and/or suppress her sorrow, which simply makes her more sorrowful and angry. Sorrow brings about love and compassion when it is channeled in the right direction.

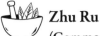 **Zhu Ru**
(Common: Bamboo Shavings; Latin: *Bambusa* supp.)

Bamboo plays an important role in Eastern philosophy because of its well-developed root structure and flexible stem, which give it the ability to bend without breaking. A person who is rooted, flexible, and capable of yielding to the winds of change without collapsing is often likened to the bamboo tree. As an herb, bamboo shavings clear uprooted heat from the chest, neck, and head. Anxiety and irritability are often a result of unsettled energy and excessive heat in the upper body. Hence bamboo is often prescribed for chronic anxiety and stress. It also quenches thirst by clearing heat from the stomach, where the yang types store plenty of hot yang energy. As an added benefit, a study performed in 2005 showed that bamboo has significant cholesterol-reducing effects.[10] Another study, conducted in 2013, demonstrated how it is also capable of reducing inflammation and acting as an antioxidant.[11]

Common Uses
Bamboo shavings relieve hot flashes, stomach acid, vomiting, nausea, gastroesophageal reflux, excessive sweating and/or thirst, irritability, and anxiety.

Sources
A tincture of Zhu Ru can be purchased from the Hawaii Pharm website.

Preparation and Dosage
Please follow the manufacturer's suggestions.

Herbal Friend: Lu Gen
(Common: Common Reed; Latin: *Phragmites communis*)

Lu Gen, also known as common reed, is often spotted close to rivers, streams, and marshes because of its strong affiliation with water. With a hollow stalk, common reed slurps up water as one does with a straw. As a medicine, it transports moisture to the upper body and moderates yang heat. It is often used to tame the excessive lung energy of the Yang Type B by transporting yin cool energy upward, while draining excess yang heat energy in the upper body. Hence common reed addresses upper body heat-related issues such as hot flashes, acid regurgitation, heartburn, and vomiting. A tincture of Lu Gen can be purchased from the Hawaii Pharm website. Equal doses of Lu Gen and Zhu Ru can be taken together in one serving to clear heat and address hot flashes.

YIN TYPE A

Even though she has more yin cold energy than the yang types, the Yin Type A is not immune to hot flashes. Actually, most of my clients who receive treatment for hot flashes are Yin Type As, in part because they have difficulty adjusting to unprecedented bursts of heat. The yang types easily overheat in general and are therefore less inclined to do anything about hot flashes. The Yin Type A's liver is responsible for hot flashes despite being associated with cool bodily energy. How can the body's source of cool energy produce so much heat? The stronger liver of the Yin Type A often bites off more than it can chew, absorbing excessive toxins from incompatible foods and uncomfortable experiences. Just as heat is produced by the microbial breakdown of a compost pile, the accumulation of toxins within the liver also yields warmth, and if substantial enough, even hot flashes.

The liver is stimulated and nourished by joy, an emotion so enticing that it's hard to let go of, especially for the Yin Type A. What brings joy on one occasion, however, doesn't always bring it on another. As life shifts gears during menopause, the Yin Type A's definition of joy often transforms too, as she asks herself, "Is this what I really want out of _____ (life, relationships work, etc.)?" She may feel something unexplainable brewing inside, leading to bouts of irritability, frustration, or unprecedented desires. Since joy is what makes or breaks the Yin Type A's emotional and physical health, it is essential that she recognize and work with these feelings rather than simply suppress them.

The Yin Type A believes firmly in "give and take" and is capable of being the most generous of the four body types. By the time menopause kicks in, she has probably devoted every ounce of effort toward rearing children and taking care of other household duties, trusting that she will always, or at least eventually, receive something in return. Perhaps someday her children will thank her or her husband will start to cook and clean or give her foot massages. While these outcomes may come true in the future, menopause is a time when liver joy can no longer be placed on hold. The body is our greatest teacher, and through chronic hot flashes, pain, or fatigue, it tries to get our attention. We all have an alarm somewhere in our body that informs us when things are out of sync. Our first instinct is to fear it, fight it, or even try to ignore it rather than simply listen, learn, and find harmony here and now. This is a time for the Yin Type A to give to herself and receive the benefits of wellness and inner joy.

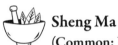 ## Sheng Ma
(Common: Black Cohosh; Latin: *Actaea racemosa*)
Sheng Ma, or black cohosh, is highly regarded in both Native American and Chinese medicines as an herb of many uses, and it has a wide reputation for addressing menopausal issues. Research has shown that black cohosh can alleviate hot-flash-related[12] and postmenopausal insomnia.[13] In Sasang medicine, black cohosh is prescribed for its ability to clear congestion and heat from the Yin Type A's hyperactive liver. Flaring heat and unsettled energy in the upper body make it difficult to sleep, possibly contributing to skin flushing, tinnitus, nausea, excessive stomach acid, acne, and fever. Black cohosh is also used to treat sore throat, coughing, and sinus congestion, which are instigated by the Yin Type A's stronger liver, as it takes advantage of her weaker lung system.

Common Uses
Black cohosh relieves hot flashes, headaches, throat issues (sore or swollen throat, tonsillitis, swollen glands), coughing, acid stomach, acne, tinnitus, nausea, and sinus congestion (with heat signs, such as fever, sore throat, etc.).

Sources
With its common use for hot flashes and postmenopausal symptoms, black cohosh is readily available on the Nature's Way and Planetary Herbals websites.

Preparation and Dosage

Please follow the manufacturer's suggestions.

Caution

Black cohosh is a cold-natured herb. If you cannot drink cold fluids without getting a stomachache, diarrhea, indigestion, or sneezing, then black cohosh may not be suitable for you. These symptoms will occur after ingesting black cohosh if there is not enough heat in the body. Very high doses may cause a slower heart rate, lower abdominal cramps, dizziness, tremors, or joint pain.

Herbal Friend: Huang Qin
(Common: Skullcap Root; Latin: *Scutellaria baicalensis*)

In Sasang medicine, Huang Qin, or skullcap root, is prized for its ability to resolve a variety of heat-related issues in the body, which can manifest as inflammation, hot flashes, anger, excessive appetite, or infection. Black cohosh and skullcap root enhance each other's ability to clear heat and address these symptoms. Skullcap root extract is available from manufacturers such as New Chapter and Nature's Way. Follow the manufacturer's suggestions for appropriate dosage and ingest skullcap root and black cohosh together for optimum results.

YIN TYPE B

Among the four yin yang body types, the Yin Type B is the least prone to hot flashes, or to be precise, she is less concerned and affected by them. Since the Yin Type B's stronger kidneys provide plenty of cold energy, heat is rarely an issue for her. Actually, an occasional hot flash could offer her relief, especially on a cold wintry day. Yet hot flashes aren't always fun even for the Yin Type B, since in her case, a deficiency, rather than excess, of yang energy is to blame. During a hot flash, the Yin Type B's excessive yin cold energy from her kidneys chases yang heat away from the lower body, pushing it upward. As yang heat rises from the kidneys, it stifles the heart, making anxiety and nervousness a common hot flash companion.

The Yin Type B's hot flashes are rarely preceded by the sensation of heat in the abdomen—signaling yang heat accumulation—that is common among the other types. During a hot flash, the abdomen of the yang-heat-deficient Yin Type B is as cold as ice while her upper body feels hot and stuffy. Copious sweating for the Yin Type B is also different than it is for the other types, since it leaves her feeling drained and exhausted as abundant cold chases yang heat outward through the skin pores. I've met several Yin Type Bs who, after sweating excessively, were on the verge of collapsing. Clammy sweating throughout the body is an ominous sign for this type, often indicating other acute health issues and collapsing yang energy. Lee Je-ma says this can be avoided if the Yin Type B calms her tendency to overreact and become anxious over petty things. This is easier said than done because there's a constant battle between her desire to be comfortable and her need to achieve lofty goals. This feeling is exacerbated during menopause, as the Yin Type B often feels as if the clock of life is ticking away, and her dream of the perfect life she once imagined is fading.

 ## An Xi Xiang
(Common: Benzoin Oil; Latin: *Styrax benzoin*)

In Eastern medicine, An Xi Xiang (meaning "peaceful rest fragrance"), or benzoin oil, is often used as incense or as an ingredient in tea that includes other herbs to raise the spirit, uplift the mood, and promote balance and harmony of the emotions. Lee Je-ma credits An Xi Xiang with the ability to clear the body of pathogens and toxins, while balancing the heart and mind. Along with other Yin Type B herbs, this one also supports the digestive system, making it easier for the Yin Type B to digest not only food but life's challenges, transforming them into a source of strength and well-being.

Common Uses
Benzoin calms anxiety, uplifts emotions, relieves indigestion, addresses pain in the chest/abdomen from food stagnation, and alleviates coughing.

Sources
Bulk Apothecary offers an essential oil of benzoin on its website.

Preparation and Dosage

I recommend dabbing a tiny bit of this essential oil under the nose with a cotton swab or ball. It may also be applied to the wrists or to armpits to prevent body odor. Several drops may be burned with a diffuser or oil burner. Benzoin can be applied topically several times a day to retain fragrance.

Caution

Although benzoin is used as an ingredient in medicinal teas, it is usually ingested only under the care of a professional. Most sources warn against ingesting it and recommend it for topical use only. Yet even topically, this potent medicinal has plenty of healing power. The application of essential oils directly onto the skin may produce localized skin sensitivity, such as rashes or redness. Try diluting the first few applications of benzoin with small amounts of water until your skin gets used to it. If your skin is not irritated, then try applying it directly.

Herbal Friend: Rou Gui
(Common: Cinnamon; Latin: *Cinnamomum cassia*)

Rou Gui (*gui* means "to restore"), or cinnamon, replenishes the body's yuan (source) energy, which is produced in the kidneys. It also warms up and enlivens the Yin Type B's kidneys, which have a tendency to stagnate and freeze the energies of the body. Excessive kidney-induced cold may clamp down on the Yin Type B's weaker yang energy, pushing it upward. Hence cinnamon helps restore kidney yang energy, preventing it from bombarding the upper body and alleviating the Yin Type B's hot flashes and headaches. Together with the warmth of An Xi Xiang, cinnamon strongly reinforces the Yin Type B's yang energy to improve digestion and harness escaping heat. Raw cinnamon bark can be purchased from most supermarkets and natural food stores. Suppliers such as Nature's Answer, Solaray, and Gaia offer an extract of cinnamon in capsule form on their websites.

Raw cinnamon bark is prepared by boiling three (two- to three-inch) bark slices with two cups of water. Let simmer over low heat for fifteen minutes and drink it while it's still warm. The exact amount of cinnamon may vary, depending on your taste preference. For capsules, refer to the manufacturer for dosage guidelines.

5

Sealing the Portholes

Osteoporosis

At age forty-seven, two years after her hysterectomy, Wendy tripped over a tree branch and fractured her hip bone. She remembers thinking right after her fall that it was just a little thump, yet she couldn't figure out why it was so difficult to get up again! Frightened by this experience, she visited her doctor. He diagnosed her with Stage 3 osteoporosis and prescribed 1,500 milligrams of calcium per day.

At age fifty-three, she was told by her doctor that her osteoporosis had worsened despite decades of supplementing with calcium and vitamin D. He discussed how our bones do not absorb calcium without exercise and asked if she had an exercise routine. "Of course I exercise!" she responded. "I get up, rush to work, run around the office doing this and that errand, and clean the house." Her doctor chuckled and asked again if she set the time aside for exercise. Wendy fell silent, wondering how on earth she would ever find the time. Her doctor continued, "It's the rhythm and consistency of brisk walking outside or on a treadmill, bicycling, or other cardiovascular activity that encourages our bones to regenerate." Wendy reluctantly began a daily walking routine and reduced her calcium intake to 750 milligrams, and her follow-up bone density test results at age sixty-seven were astonishing! Not only had her bone density increased, but Wendy felt overall healthier too.

The importance of calcium intake after menopause and/or hysterectomy cannot be understated, but as with other supplements, it is often ingested in excessive amounts because many of us subscribe to the idea that more is better. Excessive intake of calcium may lead to hypercalcemia, a condition that has been linked to a higher risk of heart and kidney disease. Some sources argue that excess calcium supplementation may result in calcium deposits, in the form of calcium carbonate stones, within the arteries and kidneys.[1]

While declining levels of estrogen after menopause might sound like a sure path to osteoporosis, this is not always the case. Loss of bone mass can be delayed or prevented, and bone mass can even be increased, by taking care of your bones as early as possible. Calcium intake coupled with vitamin D and exercise are indispensable ways to maintain and potentially increase bone mass. With that said, consuming higher than recommended levels of calcium won't necessarily add further benefit. The current recommended dietary intake of calcium established by the Food and Nutritional Board (2010) for postmenopausal women is 1,200 milligrams/day, and for vitamin D, it's 500 international units/day, which increases to 800 after age seventy. Yet a recent study demonstrated that 750 milligrams of calcium a day is sufficient, and anything more doesn't decrease the risk of bone fracture further.[2]

Estrogen also has an important role to play in bone growth and sustainability, although the exact mechanism behind this relationship is still unknown. We know that bones have estrogen receptors, but what role they play in stimulating healing and increasing absorption of calcium still remains a mystery. The fact that bone density often decreases from lack of estrogen after menopause is convincing enough to confirm that a strong relationship nevertheless exists. Studies show us that bone mass reaches its peak in females at ages twenty-five through forty and then slowly declines until menopause. From age fifty-two to age sixty— the period of time when estrogen levels sharply decline—the body experiences its greatest reduction of bone mass. Yet from age sixty-five onward, the decline in bone mass slows to a crawl, as the body adjusts and finds alternative methods (other than estrogen) to maintain it.

Since the body's natural estrogen has a direct effect on bone mass, wouldn't estrogen replacement be the best option after menopause? While some studies suggest that low levels of estrogen replacement may decrease the risk of fracture by 20 to 35 percent,[3] potential side effects such as vaginal bleeding, breast tenderness, risk of myocardial infarction, and ovarian cancer may outweigh the benefits.[4] Although these side effects may be mediated by closely regulating the dose and type of estrogen, conflicting evidence regarding its ability to address osteoporosis portrays how there's no absolute one-size-fits-all approach. Moreover, there are several factors that influence the effects of estrogen such as age, extent of osteoporosis, health history, and so on.

With the estrogen debate still lingering, doctors have turned to other methods to prevent and treat osteoporosis. Bisphosphonates, for example, are currently the most frequently prescribed medication. This medication group, consisting of brand names like Fosamax and Actonel, inhibit osteoclast cell activity to prevent the breakdown of bone cells. A review of available research conducted in 2002 showed that bisphosphonates are capable of preventing bone fracture in an average of 27 to 49 percent of all trial participants.[5] Despite boasting this ability, bisphosphonates aren't easily absorbed through the stomach and tend to result in indigestion. Other side effects may include flu-like symptoms, bone pain, and/or low blood-calcium levels.

The World Health Organization recommends that women with a bone density loss of −2.5 or greater should consider taking pharmaceutical medication to prevent bone fracture.[6] If your bone density test scored in this range, then I'd suggest discussing the above options with your medical doctor. Regardless of your T-score results, I believe you'll find the methods in this book, either in combination with a pharmaceutical approach or by themselves, to be of significant benefit.

THERE'S MORE TO OSTEOPOROSIS THAN CALCIUM AND ESTROGEN

At age thirty-eight, osteoporosis was the last thing on Jill's mind. Sure, she wondered why her mom had fractured her hip twice at the age of forty, but never did she think it would happen to her. Jill's first fracture, which happened when she was helping a friend move a file cabinet, came as a complete surprise. Jill always had a robust upper body, making her the go-to woman when her friends needed a helping hand. She was so proud of it that she never told anyone how weak her lower body felt most of the time. After her first fracture, it all slowly but surely started to make sense: she and her mom both looked stronger than most of their acquaintances, but only in areas that others could see. Hidden underneath was a weaker foundation that was prone to cracking.

Studies show that genetics may also contribute to the onset and extent of osteoporosis,[7] and as we will soon discover, so does your yin yang body type. A genetic tendency toward osteoporosis doesn't mean that it will inevitably become an issue. Bone mass improvement relies on three basic factors: having the *intention* of enhancing health, holding the *belief* that it is possible, and taking the appropriate *action* based on the unique requirements of your body type.

Did You Know?

Osteoporotic fractures often do not produce significant pain. Hairline fractures are common among individuals with osteoporosis. This type of fracture forms an extremely thin line across the bone, is difficult to detect in X-rays, produces minimal to no pain, and often goes undiagnosed. Hairline fractures commonly occur at the femoral (hip) joints and facet joints (between the vertebrae) in serious cases. With Stage 4 osteoporosis, hairline fractures may occur with light injury or simply from everyday bone stress.

Osteopenia is considered a lighter form of bone mass reduction than osteoporosis, though it still describes a significant loss of bone mass with a higher risk of fracture. One in ten sixty-year-old women and one in five seventy-year-old women have osteoporosis. Forearm fractures are the most common type of osteoporotic fracture, followed by hip, shoulder, and spine fractures. Once an osteoporotic fracture occurs, there is an **86 percent** increased chance of another fracture occurring in the same location.[8] So be very careful!

Taking action doesn't mean excessive exercise. Instead it requires that you develop the ability to know what constitutes too much and too little activity. Strike a balance with your body, compromising at times and pushing along when necessary. If you feel pain or excess strain, then stop or at least slow down. If you walk daily, don't forget to take into consideration the distance back home. Challenge yourself to exercise every day, or at least every other day, within your limits. Emotional and physical health is in your hands. But remember, before you step on the gas pedal and drive, you have to know your vehicle. The amount of pressure you apply depends on whether it is a race car or a lemon. Even a lemon can get you from place to place, although it may take longer. Knowing your body's limits and capabilities is the first step toward maximizing your bone health. Slow down when slowing down is called for and don't be ashamed or blame it on getting older. There is a time to slow down and a time to speed up. Listen to and be aware of what your body is telling you and steer clear of an overenthusiastic mind.

WESTERN AND EASTERN PERSPECTIVES ON OSTEOPOROSIS

Whereas in the West, loss of bone mass during and after menopause is associated with fluctuations in estrogen and progesterone, in Eastern medicine, it is associated with a deficiency of kidney function, which is responsible for producing and sending bodily essence, or *ek gi* (in Korean), to the bones, storing it in the form of marrow. Modern medicine also associates the kidneys with bone health, crediting a hormone called erythropoietin that stimulates the production of marrow, which, in turn, produces white and red blood cells within the bones. Erythropoietin deficiency contributes to a loss of bone marrow and bone cell (osteoclast/osteoblast) production. The kidneys are also said to activate vitamin D within the body.

Even though modern medicine acknowledges the association between the kidneys and bone health, treatment of osteoporosis is primarily focused on the bone itself by administering drugs that delay the process of bone degeneration. In traditional Eastern medicines, strengthening and supporting the kidney function is a priority. As we will soon discover, each body type has its own approach depending on its inherent organ-related strengths and weaknesses.

THE YIN AND YANG OF OSTEOPOROSIS

In Eastern medicine, the kidneys are said to be the source of yin energy—the mother of all fluid and essence within the body. An abundance of yin may sound like an ideal condition for nourishing our blood, skin, muscles, and bones, but actually, it's not all that simple. Excessive yin production will naturally weaken opposing yang energy, causing the stagnation of blood and energy within the body and inhibiting the flow of essence from the kidneys to the bones. Yang energy is responsible for pushing yin from one place to another. Yin is not always fond of yang's pushy behavior, but without a little nudge, yin will stay put and eventually cause health issues. Simply stated, even though they oppose one another, yin and yang depend on each other for all body functions. Although bone health is primarily a yin-dominated process, without yang, it is useless.

Try the following tips to enhance your bone strength no matter what body type you are. Check each one off the list to make sure you are covering all the bases before jumping into the specific suggestions for your body type.

Tip #1: Take Vitamin D

Without vitamin D, calcium cannot find its way to your bones. This precious substance also protects us from numerous illnesses such as breast, prostate, and colon cancers, depression, insomnia, and an unbalanced immune system.[9] Supplementing with vitamin D (with calcium) may suffice, but keep in mind that your body produces it naturally when exposed to sunlight. If you do not get enough time out in the sun, start thinking about doing so. The Vitamin D Council recommends approximately fifteen minutes of bare skin exposure to the sun for fair-skinned individuals, and at least twenty minutes for those with darker skin.[10] Your skin cannot produce Vitamin D from indirect sunlight, so sitting in front of a window won't do the trick. If you are a fair-skinned sun worshipper, remember that the sun's rays can also be damaging, and intense sun exposure for more than twenty minutes can easily burn your skin.

In my neck of the woods—the Pacific Northwest—a condition called SAD (seasonal affective disorder), which is caused by a lack of sunlight, affects up to 9.9 percent of the population. Especially in the winter, many of my patients suffer from SAD, which makes them feel drowsy, depressed, and unmotivated. From my experience, acupuncture and exercise along with vitamin D supplementation are effective in treating this condition. If you do not get enough sun exposure or have low levels, then eating foods or consuming supplements with vitamin D (see tables 5.1 and 5.2) is the way to go. The recommended daily intake of vitamin D for women ages fifty-one to seventy is 600 international units, and after the age of seventy it increases to 800 international units.

TABLE 5.1. YANG-TYPE-COMPATIBLE FOODS RICH IN VITAMIN D

Food/Drink	Serving Size	Percentage of Daily Recommended Value
Whole milk	1 cup	24%
Mushrooms (maitake)	1 cup (diced)	196%
Halibut	3 oz	233%
Cod liver oil	1 oz	700%

TABLE 5.2. YIN-TYPE-COMPATIBLE FOODS RICH IN VITAMIN D

Food/Drink	Serving Size	Percentage of Daily Recommended Value
Sardines	12 g	5%
Almond milk†	100 g	10%
Sockeye salmon*	3 oz	111%
Herring	1 oz	115%

*Although rich in omega-3 and omega-5 fatty acids, salmon *oil* has very little to no vitamin D content.
†Vitamin D–fortified almond milk is also available on the market.

The use of artificial UV sunlight is becoming increasingly popular in the Pacific Northwest, offering promising results. A study performed in 2010 demonstrated how exposure to UV light for ten to fifteen minutes, five times a week for eight weeks, significantly enhances vitamin D levels in patients who suffer from malabsorption.[11] Before you go out and buy a sunlamp, there are a few factors to keep in mind: Most sunlamps on the market do not emit UV light and therefore cannot facilitate the production of vitamin D inside your skin. Second, UV lamps are often used for tanning, and excessive exposure may cause serious skin burning. UV light exposure should be done in short spurts (as the study above suggests) and with the use of UV protective eyewear. I couldn't find the UV light brand, Sperti Del Sol, mentioned in the above study, but others, like Sperti Fiji and Sperti Vitamin D, can easily be found online.

Tip #2: Exercise to Strengthen Your Bones

Even though emotional stress can lead to illness, physical stress on our bones makes them stronger. Actually, without stress, our bones cannot grow at all! The pulling and prying of tendons and ligaments on our bones is what elongates and gives them shape. Hence a sedentary lifestyle after menopause will more than likely contribute to the onset and/or exacerbation of osteoporosis. How much is enough? First, it depends on the type of cardiovascular exercise. Running may do wonders for cardiovascular health but can cause damage to the knees and soft tissue of someone forty years or older. If you are a runner, try to limit running time, combining it with walking and other cardiovascular activities such as bicycling, elliptical, swimming, aerobics, and so forth. If you were diagnosed with osteoporosis or arthritis in your lower extremities, eliminating running altogether and sticking to the latter exercises is the way to go. Are you an avid walker/hiker? These are excellent methods to encourage your bones to absorb more calcium. For the postmenopausal individual, I suggest using walking poles to prevent fractures from slipping. Tai Chi is another form of exercise that helps promote balance and build bone mass through a series of slow and fluid movements. A study performed by S. L. Wolf and colleagues showed how a group of women with a mean age of eighty who performed fifteen minutes of Tai Chi a day over four months had a 47 percent lower risk of falling compared to a control group.[12] Another study showed how daily performance of Tai Chi significantly reduced the loss of bone mass in postmenopausal women.[13]

Excessive twisting, such as swinging a golf club, or high-impact loading from lifting excessive weight can increase chances of fracture. Occasionally something as simple as bending forward to lift an object may also cause fractures in individuals with osteoporosis. Eliciting the help of a cane, chair, or other sturdy piece of furniture may suffice, but if necessary, bend both knees to pick up the object to avoid placing too much stress on your lumbar spine.

Tip #3: Consume Calcium-Rich Foods

To prevent kidney issues and encourage efficient absorption, I suggest getting most if not all of your calcium intake from body-type-specific foods (see tables 5.3, below, and 5.4, page 152) and supplementing only when necessary. The menopausal yang types need higher dosages of calcium (up to 1,200 milligrams/day) than the yin types (up to 750 milligrams/day) because of their tendency to lose bone mass more quickly.

TABLE 5.3. YANG-TYPE-COMPATIBLE CALCIUM-RICH FOODS

Food/Drink	Serving Size	Estimated Calcium
Shrimp	3 oz	125 mg
Kale	8 oz	180 mg
Black-eyed peas	½ cup	185 mg
Adzuki beans	1 cup	197 mg
Broccoli	8 oz	200 mg
Tofu (prepared with calcium)	4 oz	205 mg
Milk (skim, low-fat, whole)	8 oz	300 mg
Soy milk	8 oz	300 mg
Sardines	3 oz	325 mg
Collard greens	8 oz	360 mg

TABLE 5.4. YIN-TYPE-COMPATIBLE CALCIUM-RICH FOODS

Food/Drink	Serving Size	Estimated Amount of Calcium
Oranges	1 whole	55 mg
Figs	2 figs	65 mg
Almonds (dry roasted)	¼ cup	72 mg
Dandelion greens	1 cup chopped	103 mg
Bok choy	8 oz	160 mg
Salmon	3 oz	180 mg
Beans (white)	1 cup	191 mg
Lentils	1 cup	198 mg
Yogurt (Greek)	6 oz	200 mg
Almond milk, rice milk	8 oz	300 mg

Note: Most vegetables are cold-natured and may freeze up the digestive system of yin types, but they are not necessarily off limits for them. Flash steaming or cooking yang type vegetables transforms cold nature into warm nature, making it easier for the yin types to ingest them.

Tip #4: Consume Isoflavone-Rich Foods

As we have discussed above, estrogen is an important component of bone health. Isoflavones are food components that resemble the structure of estrogen and are treated as such within the human body, where they mimic estrogen's actions. Soybeans are by far the richest isoflavone food, boasting 128 milligrams per 100-gram intake. For the yang type, pretty much any soy-based product will do, but for the yin types, fermented soy-based foods such as tofu, tempeh, and miso soup are a bit easier to digest than soy milk, which often causes them digestive upset. Although not as rich in isoflavones as soy, other foods such as red clover sprouts, chickpeas, lentils, flaxseed, and lima beans may be easier on the digestive system of the yin types (refer to the discussion of phytoestrogens in the appendix for more details).

Tip #5: Watch Your Sodium Consumption

Sodium, according to Eastern medicine, guides energy to the kidneys and supports bone health, but excessively salty foods overwhelm the kidneys and eventually weaken them. So how much is too much? The problem is that the typical modern diet already contains too much sodium. Most sources recommend a maximum of 1,500 to 2,300 milligrams a day. The weaker kidneys of the Yang Type A benefit from ingesting closer to the higher end of this spectrum, while the stronger kidneys of the Yin Type B appreciate no more than 800 milligrams. Accordingly, foods that are naturally salty, like seafood, shellfish, and seaweed, are more compatible for the Yang Type A than for the Yin Type B. So how about the Yang Type B and Yin Type A? I'd recommend no more than 2,000 milligrams for the Yang Type B and up to 1,500 milligrams for the Yin Type A. If you are diabetic or suffer from high blood pressure, then further limiting your salt intake is advisable. As a general rule, consuming foods that naturally contain salt is a healthier option than ingesting it from sodium chloride (table salt), MSG, and other chemically derived sources.

OSTEOPOROSIS AND THE YIN YANG BODY TYPES

Osteoporosis does not favor a particular body type, since nobody, yin or yang, can avoid the process of aging. Yet the yin types in general have an advantage over the yang types because bone health relies on the kidneys, which are yin organs. If the kidney-strong Yin Type B takes care of herself, she is likely to have the strongest bones of all four types. Because of all their yin energy, the kidneys are also responsible for cooling the body. Born with weaker kidneys and abundant heat, the Yang Type A's bones are always looking for attention and are prone to osteoarthritis. Still, unless Yin Type Bs cultivate their yang heat energy through exercise and yang (warm or hot) foods, their bones may never get to see their fame and glory.

Sasang medicine holds that an essential bond exists between what we eat and the health of our skin, muscles, tendons and bones. The bones are produced by *ek* (essence), originating from the breakdown of food in the large intestine. This process requires the cold and congealing energy of the kidney system, where the large intestines reside. The digestion of food in the stomach, on the other hand, relies on the warmth of the spleen system, where the stomach resides. The warmth of the esophagus and cool nature of the small intestines also play a significant role in transforming food into essential body tissues. Please see table 5.5 for further details.

TABLE 5.5. ORGANS, TEMPERATURES, AND BODY FLUIDS

Digestive Organ	Temperature	Product Created from Food	Body Part Nourished and Transformed
Esophagus	Warm	*Jin* (clear fluids)	Skin/hair
Stomach	Hot	*Go* (thick fluids)	Tendons
Small intestines	Cool	*Yu* (oily fluids)	Muscles
Large intestines	Cold	*Ek* (extract/essence)	Bones

Each of the four body types sends energy from their stronger organ to the kidneys in order to maintain bone health—a process that depends on balancing our emotions and eating habits and sticking to a consistent exercise routine. The Yang Type A's bones benefit from "cooling" the anger produced from an inherently stronger spleen and choosing foods and exercises that don't overheat her system. The Yang Type B could always work on slowing down to avoid overburdening her aging joints and refraining from ingesting foods and drinks that are too stimulating. The Yin Type A, on the other hand, may have to fight the natural urge to relax and motivate herself to exercise regularly. The Yin Type B's stronger kidneys may freeze up, making her bones brittle, if she doesn't stay warm and interact with others, especially during the colder months.

Now let's explore how osteoporosis relates to each of the four body types in more detail.

YANG TYPE A

As we've discussed above, Yang Type As are most prone to bone-mass loss owing to their weaker kidneys. Yet not all Yang Type As experience significant bone loss after menopause. Above all else, the Yang Type A's bone health depends on how grounded her kidney energy is. Excessive uprooted anger from a stronger spleen pushes her energy upward and away from the kidneys, while rooted anger is capable of nourishing them. So what does it mean to "root" anger? Anger is a vital part of the Yang Type A's psyche, and it's behind everything she says and does. For her, the challenge isn't to suppress anger but to know how to express it without offending or injuring herself or others. Her sudden bursts of excessive anger are often a result of having too many irons in the fire and feeling as if she has to do all the dirty work. From a scientific perspective, this triggers the release of excessive amounts of cortisol into the bloodstream, which in turn inhibits the production of osteoclasts (bone cells). If any of the four Sasang predominant emotions of sadness, anger, joy, and calmness are given free rein, they can easily injure our weaker organs. Health depends on balancing the yang and yin emotions, anger with calmness and sadness with joy. The balanced Yang Type A reflects inward, taking a deep breath and calming her mind before getting angry, but unbalanced, she lashes outward.

If the Yang Type A experiences chronic hip or lower back pain, light rather than excessive exercise may be the answer. The sacroiliac joint, which connects the pelvis to the sacrum, is often the first joint of the back to dislocate. Going to a chiropractor, osteopath, and/or acupuncturist to monitor and address this situation could potentially avoid further issues down the line. I once met a seventy-five-year-old Yang Type A who kept herself in excellent shape and was admired by her neighbors as she walked and exercised in the park every morning. A few years back she experienced hip pain and decided that she would address it by exercising harder. As the weeks went by she was in even better shape, but her hips continued to hurt even more. Her X-rays showed severe degeneration of her hip bones, to the point of no return. Unfortunately, only a few weeks later, she was unable to walk without severe pain and became housebound.

Impulsiveness is one of the Yang Type A's strongest traits. She often acts before thinking, always ready for the next move before finishing her last one. This way of thinking sometimes comes in handy, especially when accompanying yin folks, who often think too much before taking action. The yin types may continually question whether or not they are making the right decision, while the Yang Type As "think" with their body. There is no time for the Yang Type A to dwell or fret about this or that issue. As the Yang Type A ages, however, her body has trouble catching up. Menopause is a time for Yang Type As to reflect on their actions, health, and well-being. While they do not have to aspire to be as slow-moving and slow-thinking as the Yin Type B in order to stay healthy, since this would be counterintuitive, they can "borrow" certain Yin Type B traits, such as do ryang—the ability to plan and strategize.

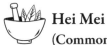 ## Hei Mei
(Common: Blackberries; Latin: *Rubus fruticosus*)

In my home state of Oregon, many of us are all too familiar with blackberries. This fruit, which was introduced from Europe to the eastern United States in the early 1800s, traveled rapidly toward the Pacific Northwest, taking over fields and roadsides along the way! Most Oregonians view blackberries as a menace rather than a medicine. However, blackberries are an invaluable medicine for Yang Type As because they strengthen the kidneys, their weakest organ. Since the kidneys support the lower back and legs, this herb addresses chronic lower back pain. Blackberries, which target the hips, knees, ankles, and toes, are very rich in nutrients, such as dietary fiber, vitamins C and K, folic acid, and manganese. They are ranked one of the best antioxidant foods by the National Institutes of Health. Antioxidants eliminate free radicals and help the body fight off infection.[14] The tiny seeds in blackberries are high in omega-3 and omega-5 fatty acids and protein. Lastly, blackberries are highly concentrated with phytoestrogens, a natural source of estrogen that plays a major role in keeping the bones strong and the tendons flexible after menopause.

Common Uses
Blackberries alleviate joint pain (e.g., hips, knees, ankles, and toes), bone pain, postmenopausal issues (osteoporosis, osteopenia), and frozen shoulder.

Sources
Blackberries are seasonally available fresh or frozen at most supermarkets. Off-season (winter) supplies are sometimes available in

supermarkets on the West Coast. Dried blackberries are available all year round from Nuts.com. Freeze-dried blackberries, which can be easily dissolved in water, are available from the Z Natural Foods website.

Preparation and Dosage

A handful of fresh or dried blackberries a day can provide plenty of energy to the Yang Type A's kidneys. Three cups of blackberry tea a day can help prevent bone-related issues. Blackberry tea is prepared by boiling a handful of dried blackberries in two to three cups of water. Let the tea simmer for fifteen minutes and drink it cool or warm, depending on your preference. Blackberries also make a yummy ingredient or garnish in salads, oatmeal, or yogurt.

Herbal Friend: Sheng Di Huang
(Common: Rehmannia or Chinese Foxglove;
Latin: *Rehmannia glutinosa*)

Sheng Di Huang, or rehmannia, is commonly used for Yang Type As because it supports their weaker kidneys in several ways. First, it is one of the strongest herbs to nourish the kidneys. Second, it is commonly used for nourishing the blood, which is considered the "mother" of yin. Third, it strengthens the lower back, knees, and ankles—areas that are particularly vulnerable to bone-related issues among the Yang Type As. Rehmannia is also capable of preventing bone-mass loss—a property that is believed to be the result of its effect on estrogen.[15] Modern science is still not sure how and why rehmannia supports bone function even though, for thousands of years, Chinese medicine has been aware of its yin- and bone-nourishing qualities. Together, rehmannia and blackberry nourish bone marrow, strengthen the bones, and nourish the blood.

Rehmannia can be purchased as a tincture on the Herb Pharm website. The Sasang-based formula Dokhwal Jihwang Tang, which contains rehmannia and several other herbs to help nourish and support the reproductive organs, is available on sasangmedicine .com: Click "Sasang Store" from the main menu and then the "Add to Cart" icon beneath "Herbal Pills." Type "Dokhwal Jihwang Tang" under "Ordering Instructions."

YANG TYPE B

Deficient yin, which correlates with the lower body, often makes Yang Type Bs appear clumsy, as they experience difficulty stabilizing their weaker legs. An abundant upper body energy with a wobbly foundation gives them a robust and occasionally monstrous appearance, despite being inwardly feeble. Yang Type Bs' weaker lower body is due to weaker lower body organs (liver and kidneys) that have trouble feeding their bones. In general, Yang Type Bs have less risk of osteoporotic bone fracture compared to Yang Type As, since their kidneys are not their weakest organ. Yet to avoid the risk of fracture, they also have to be extra careful not to lose their balance, being mindful of their lower body and rooting their energies.

The connection with heaven, or *chon shi*, comes from the Yang Type B's stronger lungs. This trait gives her a profound sense of connection with the cosmos. Once she gets a taste of it, the Yang Type B may lose her connection with the earth, disregarding the needs of her own flesh and bones. If her head is in the clouds, she may also be completely unaware of obstacles in the way, tripping over things left and right.

The feeling of oneness with the cosmos sounds pretty awesome, right? This feeling is so important to the Yang Type B that she will do anything in her power to sustain it. Those who have had such an experience know how difficult it is to return to earth. The Yang Type B transforms this feeling into her everyday reality. The other types may also get a glimpse of it by achieving something great, taking psychedelic drugs, or engaging in a spiritual practice. For the Yang Type B, it's there no matter what, and if she doesn't take action to sustain and tame it, she'll get ill. Internally, this trait shifts her energies upward, toward the head and away from the lower extremities. Hence arthritis and bone density loss in the lower extremities are a common issue for the Yang Type B. When balanced, she is capable of feeling at home within her own body, while simultaneously reaching up to the heavens.

Song Jie
(Common: Chinese Red Pine/Masson Pine; Latin: *Pinus massoniana*)

In winter, deciduous tree branches become brittle while the leaves wither away, but conifers like the Masson pine retain their leaves and branches and stay flexible and nourished all year round—a sign of incredible structural integrity! Just about every part of the pine tree can benefit the health of a Yang Type B. Its pollen stimulates blood movement, its bark helps with skin abrasions and tendon and muscle pain, and its nodes assist with joint and bone issues. The bark and nodes of the Masson pine tree contain a healing flavonoid that can be found in Pycnogenol, a trademarked formula that has anti-inflammatory, antioxidant, immune-supporting properties and helps strengthen blood vessel walls. A study performed in 2012 showed that Pycnogenol also has positive effects on bone strength and mineral density.[16]

Common Uses
Masson pine supports bone health and alleviates allergies, common colds, water retention, joint pain, and muscle and/or tendon pain.

Sources
Masson pine bark extract is available from the Planetary Herbals and Puritan's Pride websites. Be careful! Even though there are several other sources of pine bark extract, they are often mixed with ingredients not suitable for Yang Type Bs.

Preparation and Dosage
Follow the manufacturer's instructions for dosage.

Herbal Friend: Wu Jia Pi
(Common: Devil's Club; Latin: *Oplopanax horridus*)

In Sasang medicine, Masson pine bark is often mixed with devil's club to treat allergies and common colds by supporting the immune system and assisting with the flow of lung energy. They are also combined to strengthen the liver and kidneys of the Yang Type B, thus assisting with bone health and rehabilitation. Use two parts devil's club to one part pine bark extract. Follow the manufacturer's instructions to determine the recommended dosage range for each supplement. Devil's club is available from manufacturers such as Herb Pharm and HerbalRemedies.com.

YIN TYPE A

Generally speaking, Yin Type As inherit stronger bones than the yang types, making it relatively easy for them to maintain bone mass after menopause thanks to a stronger liver, which feeds the muscles, sending them energy and blood. Muscles increase bone mass by pulling and increasing pressure on the surface of each bone, stimulating the absorption of calcium. Also with a stronger liver comes the tendency to absorb excessive fat and by-products from food, contributing to weight gain. While not all Yin Type As are heavyset, those who do pack on a few extra pounds put even more pressure on their bones, stimulating bone growth. While I do not suggest gaining excessive weight, it's a fact that lighter postmenopausal women are more prone to osteoporosis compared to those who are heavyset. Excessive weight gain over a shorter period of time, however, may increase the risk of fracture. Moreover, significant body weight forces the tendons to pull excessively on the bones, causing them to thicken and become arthritic.

Did You Know?

Were you ever diagnosed with arthritis? If so, welcome to the club. Most of us show at least some sign of arthritis after the age of thirty. Yet it's not until we experience joint pain that the A-word becomes a concern. Arthritis (osteoarthritis) isn't a disease or the beginning of the end of one's youth. Actually, it's nothing but another word for "bone growth." The pulling of our tendons and ligaments on the bones is what increases height, but when our bones stop growing vertically, they start extending horizontally. That's right! We keep growing (laterally) and experience growing pains throughout our entire lifetime.

The Yin Type As' temperament of joy gives them a profound ability to live in the moment, relax, and chill out. If they take this ability to the extreme, then inactivity and idleness become the norm. A lack of physical activity leads to an impaired neuromuscular function and an increased fracture risk. Hence it is essential that the Yin Type A challenge herself to stay active. Her stronger liver is also paired with skill and talent, a trait brought out through heng gom, or self-reflection. In short, if the Yin Type A reflects on her actions, her liver will radiate with joy and share energy with the rest of her body. Without self-reflection, it will hoard the body's energies, crave joy only for itself, and disregard the ability to express profound talent. The tendons of an unbalanced and unreflective Yin Type A lose their flexibility, constantly yank away at the bones, and bring about arthritis and/or osteoporosis. The Sasang medicine association between liver health and bone density might seem a bit far-fetched, but modern research is beginning to recognize this connection. Recent studies have linked liver disease with a 40 percent increase in bone fractures.[17] As science advances, such findings reveal just how integrated and mutually dependent the different components of our body are. The Sasang medicine model stretches things even further by emphasizing the influence of our thinking on organ and bone health.

Wouldn't it be great to feel joyful all the time? Who, in their right mind, would rather be angry? Joy is an emotion that just about everyone defines as a positive one. The Yang Type A's anger, on the other hand, is almost always interpreted as negative. Sasang medicine does not label emotions as good or bad, since each one has its place. Joy, if taken to the extreme, can breed stagnation, while anger embraced with calmness could be motivating and stimulating. The Yin Type A balances her joy by accepting other emotions like anger and sorrow, without feeling that joy has left her in the dust. Balanced joy from the liver sends energy downward to the kidneys, which then send energy to the bones, lower back, and extremities. The Yin Type A who lacks joy, or desperately holds on to it, often experiences lower back pain and weakness. So spread the word that balanced joy can enhance your bone density! But remember that joy without sorrow is like having a liver without lungs. We need both emotions and organs to stay alive and function. If you look hard enough, you'll find joy within anger and sorrow, and anger and sorrow within joy.

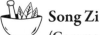 **Song Zi**
(Common: Pine Nuts; Latin: *Pinus* spp.)

Pine nuts are ingested to strengthen the bones, making them a suitable remedy for osteopenia or osteoporosis. Pine nuts are especially beneficial for the lower body skeleton, such as the lower back, hips, knees, ankles, and/or toe joints. Each pine nut has up to 35 percent of its weight in protein, therefore making it a great source of cellular energy. In Sasang medicine, pine nuts, like many other Yin Type A herbs, have the added benefit of nourishing and protecting the lungs from infection and boosting the immune system.

Common Uses

Pine nuts ease lower-body joint pain (e.g., toes, ankles, knees, and hips), osteoporosis, osteopenia, tooth decay, tooth pain, skin dryness, and menstrual issues.

Sources

Several varieties of pine nuts are available. European pine nuts, also called stone nuts, are slender and longer than the Asian variety. Despite a difference in shape, the two varieties are equally beneficial for the bones. Less expensive pine nuts can be purchased in bulk from Nuts.com. Organic pine nuts are available on the Woodstock Foods website and at Trader Joe's natural food stores.

Preparation and Dosage

Pine nuts make a good snack and can also serve as a valuable ingredient in numerous delicious recipes. In Korea, pine nuts are often sprinkled into teas to add a pleasant nutty taste. Try it with your favorite tea!

Herbal Friend: Li Zi
(Common: Chestnuts; Latin: *Castanea* spp.)

Eating roasted chestnuts beside an open fire at Christmas may be the only time we pay any attention to them in the West. In the Sasang medicine clinic, however, they are prescribed for bone-related issues such as osteoporosis, osteopenia, and lower-body joint issues because of their significant potassium and magnesium content. Chestnuts are also prescribed for indigestion caused by cold accumulation in the body, which is signaled by a sensitivity to cold, a lack of appetite, and watery dark brown/tarry stools. Chestnuts make an excellent nutritious snack because they are high in minerals, vitamins, and phytonutrients, while still keeping a low-calorie/low-fat profile. They are also gluten-free, making them a good option for those with gluten sensitivities. Roasted, dried, and powdered chestnuts can be purchased by the pound from Nuts.com.

Chestnuts are commonly peeled and ingested directly from the shell. Chestnut powder (also known as chestnut flour) can be used as a gluten-free white-flour alternative for baking. After being soaked and peeled, dried chestnuts also become a yummy ingredient for a variety of healthy dishes. A tea made of dried chestnuts is prepared by combining four raw and peeled chestnuts with two cups of water; bring to a boil and then simmer over low heat for thirty minutes. Drink two to three warm cups per day to relieve diarrhea and indigestion. Chestnuts and pine nuts can be ingested together for added bone benefit along with immune and digestive support.

YIN TYPE B

While Yin Type Bs are less prone to osteoporosis than the other types, they are not completely immune to it. It all depends on whether or not they preserved their health through the premenopausal years. Even our strongest organs may suffer the consequences of a poor diet, lack of emotional balance, or both. As we have discussed previously, the kidneys feed energy to and nourish the bones via the ek, or bodily essence. Calmness, the emotion associated with the kidneys, facilitates this process, so the calmer we are in general, the more essence we produce. But if the Yin Type Bs' calmness gets out of hand, locking them into their own little world and lacking interaction, then the bones will not have enough opportunity to develop. On the contrary, active Yin Type Bs tend to suffer less from fractures than the other types. The trick is to stay calm and active at the same time!

With a weaker spleen group, which is in charge of food metabolism, the Yin Type B's digestive system tends to lag behind the rest of her body, often producing fatigue and grogginess. The spleen group also correlates with our tendons, giving the Yin Type B a fragile stooped-over appearance. Our bones rely on the constant pull of the tendons in order to grow and rebuild. So a healthy digestive system is essential for bone health. If the Yin Type B does not focus on keeping her digestive system healthy, then no matter how strong her kidneys are, she will not be able to produce enough essence to maintain bone integrity. How does the Yin Type B know if she has a healthy digestive system? The answer is simply whether or not she has a good appetite and can ingest cold water without indigestion. Both scenarios indicate that she has enough yang energy to metabolize food and keep her body warm.

The Yin Type B can experience remarkable improvements in her health if she stays active most of the time, while the opposite is true for the Yang Type A, who mostly benefits from slowing down. With strong kidneys, also associated with basal energy, the Yin Type B can keep going, slowly but surely like the Energizer Bunny, whereas the Yang Type A, with weaker kidneys, tends to burn out easily. From the outside the Yin Type B often looks weaker and more fragile than the Yang Type A, her energetic opposite, because bone strength is less impressive than muscle. So keep it moving, Yin Type Bs, even if the mirror doesn't appreciate it as much as your bones do.

If you are a Yin Type B who somewhere along the way swayed off the path of well-being, then it may be necessary to turn over a new leaf while giving your kidneys a little boost with Sasang medicine herbs. It may be tempting to take this or that over-the-counter remedy promising to increase your bone mass, but most will overstimulate the Yin Type B's already vibrant kidneys, instigating digestive issues. Below you'll find herbs that enhance bone health by cultivating the yang of her weaker digestive system.

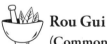

Rou Gui
(Common: Cinnamon; Latin: *Cinnamomum cassia*)
Rou Gui, or cinnamon, has the dual function of supporting the digestive system and strengthening the bones. The latter function stems from its

ability to reinforce the kidneys, which are in charge of bone and joint health. Cinnamon has high levels of manganese, essential for building bone and other connective tissue. It is also rich in fiber, calcium, and iron, all of which help strengthen the bones. In a Copenhagen University Hospital study, 200 patients with arthritis pain were given half a teaspoon of cinnamon powder with one tablespoon of honey—another Yin Type B friend—every morning. Most patients showed significant relief of knee pain after one week. After one month, 75 of the 200 participants who had been immobile before the study were able to walk without any pain at all.[18]

Common Uses
Cinnamon relieves headaches, circulatory issues (numbness, tingling, and/or coldness of the extremities), joint and muscle inflammation, lower back and knee pain, and sensitivity to cold.

Sources
Cinnamon bark can be purchased from most supermarkets throughout the United States. Suppliers such as Nature's Answer, Solaray, and Gaia offer a capsulated extract form of cinnamon on their websites.

Preparation and Dosage
Raw cinnamon bark is prepared by boiling three two- to three-inch slices of bark in two cups of water. Let the tea simmer over low heat for fifteen minutes. More or less cinnamon can be added depending on your taste preference. If you're using capsules, refer to the manufacturer's dosage guidelines. Cinnamon can also be added in powder form to protein drinks.

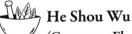 **He Shou Wu**

(Common: Fleeceflower Root; Latin: *Polygonum multiflorum*)

This herb is called He Shou Wu, meaning "Mr. Black Hair," because it is believed to delay the graying of hair thanks to its essence-nourishing properties. It is also known as fleeceflower root and has been used for thousands of years in Eastern medicine for nourishing and supporting the essence, or ek, of the body, which is produced in the kidneys and resides within the bones, where it builds and nourishes the blood. A study performed in 2004 showed that fleeceflower root can prevent bone calcium loss.[19]

Common Uses
He Shou Wu strengthens the kidneys, benefits the bones, nourishes the blood, and is often used in formulas to address premature graying of the hair, lower back and knee soreness/pain, and nocturnal emissions.

Sources
He Shou Wu, also known as Fo Ti, can be purchased in capsule form on the Nature's Way website by typing "Fo Ti" in the search bar. It can also be purchased in tincture form from Nature's Answer on the Swanson Health Products website.

Preparation and Dosage
Follow the manufacturer's dosage recommendations. Both fleeceflower root and cinnamon can be taken together in one sitting.

6

Woman Overboard

The Depths of Depression

Rebecca had everything going for her: a successful career, loving husband, and two children in college. For years she would leap out of bed, make breakfast for her husband and children, and rush off to work as a family counselor. Day after day, Rebecca reminded other women of how to reclaim their lives and renew their energies when menopause showed up at their door. Yet there she was, tissue in hand, staring at the floor in her living room. "What's the matter, honey?" her husband asked. As she struggled for an answer, all Rebecca could say was, "I dunno, something's not right." Little did she know that deep inside her mind and body, a battle had been brewing for years. In the past, she had brushed these feelings aside by keeping herself busy with work and household chores. Now they were surfacing, and no matter how much she tried, Rebecca could no longer ignore them. Something was indeed not right, and even Rebecca did not have a clear answer as to why she felt this way; neither was she to blame. On the surface everything was perfect, but underneath, the foundation was cracking away. Between work and family, Rebecca had somehow lost sight of her inner self along the way, and now that she was on the path toward menopause, her body and mind were giving Rebecca an ultimatum: "Heed our call or else!"

It is estimated that 8 to 15 percent of all women are faced with depression at one time or another as they go through menopause. Close to nine million women nationwide are plagued with depression at some point in their lives. Even though depression is affected by hormonal changes and genetic factors, it is not dictated by them. Despite fluctuations in hormone levels and the existence of genetic precursors, many women go through menopause without becoming depressed. The issue is whether or not women allow these factors to take over and define who they are.

Even if you aren't genetically or hormonally prone to depression, factors such as being a member of the sandwich generation, feeling a loss of youthfulness, or missing your child(ren) after they leave the house all contribute to the emotional issues associated with menopause. The rapid fluctuation of hormones and other biological changes simply add more fuel to the fire. Women who are prone to depression before the onset of perimenopause or menopause may experience increased depression around this time.

Depression is actually more than just feeling sad and can manifest in a variety of ways depending on the individual and situation. The *Diagnostic and Statistical Manual of Mental Disorders* (DSM) includes three general criteria in the diagnosis of depression:

1. Depressed mood
2. Loss of interest and enjoyment in usual activities
3. Reduced energy and decreased activity

The DSM also states that major depressive disorder is a more serious form of depression that includes the above criteria with the addition of at least five of the nine symptoms listed below occurring on a daily basis:[1]

1. Depressed mood most of the day
2. Diminished interest or pleasure in all or most activities
3. Significant unintentional weight loss or gain
4. Insomnia or sleeping too much
5. Agitation or psychomotor retardation noticed by others
6. Fatigue or loss of energy
7. Feelings of worthlessness or excessive guilt
8. Diminished ability to think or concentrate, or indecisiveness
9. Recurrent thoughts of death

Many, if not most, people experience depression at least once in their lifetime; hence the diagnosis of clinical depression is not as easy as it may seem. The DSM distinguishes between depressive episodes and major depressive disorder: The former is often relatively easier to address through making lifestyle changes such as eating and exercising right for your body type and avoiding certain emotional traps with the help of a friend, family member, or counselor. Major depressive disorder, on the other hand, usually requires the assistance of a trained professional.

When to See a Professional about Depression

- If you are having suicidal thoughts
- If depression is interfering with your everyday life
- If it is causing you to constantly shut others out of your life
- If it lingers no matter what you do

WESTERN AND EASTERN PERSPECTIVES ON DEPRESSION

Before we dive in, let's discuss depression from the standpoint of modern medicine and science and then from an Eastern medicine view. Depression is thought to be a result of a lack of serotonin in the brain, a loss that specific drugs, such as selective serotonin reuptake inhibitors (SSRIs), can prevent. It is also believed that estrogen and serotonin have a close relationship, where the increase/decrease in one causes an increase/decrease in the other. Hence as estrogen levels decrease during and after the menopausal transition, so does serotonin, making women prone to depression. As we saw in chapter 1, progesterone and estrogen regulate one another, so higher progesterone results in lower estrogen levels, also contributing to depression. Progesterone is dominant during the latter half of the monthly cycle, during and directly after pregnancy, and periodically throughout perimenopause. Hence women often report feeling depressed during these phases. Yet the jury is still out over whether or not depression is caused by an estrogen, progesterone, and/or serotonin imbalance, since a reduction in estrogen levels or a lack of serotonin in the brain does not always lead to depression.

In its search for a physiological source of depression, modern medicine has identified several possible perpetrators, but no prime suspects. Will there ever be a final verdict? I've met numerous people who hop from one medication to another as their doctors follow new trends in research or as symptoms come and go, but the end result is often the same: lingering depression. Perhaps modern research is looking for depression in all the wrong places.

The use of SSRIs and/or estrogen to treat depression may sound tempting since most of us would love to rid ourselves of depression by simply controlling the chemical processes within the body. Yet side effects from such medication often include nausea, nervousness, dizziness, reduced sexual desire, drowsiness, and weight gain. Whereas some individuals may benefit from these and other antidepressant and hormone-based medications, others find that the benefits do not outweigh the risks. Antidepressants act as a buffer between our mind and emotions. Yes, if there is a raging battle within us, then perhaps a buffer may be the first step toward resolution. Yet inevitably both sides must come to terms with one another if there is to be lasting peace. In some cases, the advice of a specialist may be necessary to determine the best medical approach.

Eastern medicine views depression not as a chemical or neurological issue but as a lack of harmony and balance of organ-related energies within the body. Each emotion is associated with a particular organ, and when the two are in balance, they promote organ energy flow, but when they aren't, energy becomes stagnant. Each organ in the body can be compared to a member of an immediate family. If the sister liver gets along with the brother lungs by exchanging ample amounts of energy, then their correlating emotions of sorrow and joy will be also be in harmony, benefitting mother heart, daddy kidney, and so on. Maintaining balance in an immediate family can be quite a challenge, let alone among our internal organs! Yet in a family supported by a strong bond of love, even if children misbehave or parents argue from time to time, there is no long-term negative effect. The same goes for the relationship between our organs, since liver joy and lung sorrow are destined to argue once in a while. Yet as we saw in Rebecca's situation, liver joy was the predominant emotion for most of her life, and she slammed the door in sorrow's face every time it came knocking. It was simply a matter of time before lung sorrow busted through.

THE YIN AND YANG OF DEPRESSION

In Sasang medicine, depression is seen as a combination of several emotions, contrary to the common Western idea, which defines it as a feeling of despondency. The cause of depression differs according the body types and their predominant emotions. For example, the Yin Type A's hyperdeveloped liver, associated with joy, may be the underlying source of depression. How could joy be the root of depression? If the Yin Type A feels entitled to joy and things don't flow well, then depression can easily take over. Other predominant emotions, such as comfort and anger, can also instigate depression. Table 6.1 provides a list of predominant emotions and their effects for the four body types.

TABLE 6.1. PREDOMINANT EMOTIONS AND BODY TYPES

Body Type	Strongest Organ	Predominant Emotion	Behavior when Balanced	Origin of Imbalance
Yang Type A	Spleen	Anger	Standing up for oneself and others	Others looking down on them or treating them unjustly
Yang Type B	Lungs	Sorrow	Speaking the truth	Others keeping secrets
Yin Type A	Liver	Joy	Helping others	Others not helping them
Yin Type B	Kidneys	Calmness	Protecting others/giving them a sense of security	Feeling insecure or unprotected

Before we get into specific discussions of depression and each body type, let's consider the following tips for handling depression regardless of your type.

Tip #1: Don't Ignore Your Feelings

Depression doesn't randomly show up without reason; an underlying component usually needs to be addressed. If you feel stagnant, locked, or unable to move forward in life, then take a deep look within and sift through the possible causes. Most of the time, these feelings are a result of unaddressed emotions, desires, and feelings that are asking for your attention. It might be helpful to consult a therapist or friend who would listen and discuss effective ways to address unresolved emotional issues, especially if they are interfering significantly with your life.

Tip #2: Keep on Flowing

No matter how hard it may seem when you are feeling depressed, getting out of the house and staying active is essential to keep you out of the abyss. If you prefer to be alone, then try going for a walk alone, and if you need to talk with someone, have him/her accompany you. The home is where we settle our energies and slow them down. Since depression often causes stagnation and blockage of our energies, simply getting out of the house can be energetically uplifting.

Tip #3: Exercise; It's Medicine

Exercise is one of the best medicines for depression. The rhythmic movement of your body coupled with sweating and stronger breathing encourage the flow of energy throughout the body and the release of endorphins and dopamine—our happy hormones. One study showed that two hours of exercise twice a week for ten weeks significantly reduced levels of depression compared to a no-exercise control group.[2] You don't have to push yourself too hard in order to feel better emotionally and physically. The point is to exercise within your limits and eventually to the point of working up a sweat. According to Sasang medicine, sweating releases stagnant emotion and energy from the body through the skin pores.

Tip #4: Try Acupuncture and Acupressure

Acupressure is an effective method for promoting energy flow throughout the body. Each acupressure point on the body acts as a flow controller, enhancing flow where it is needed and slowing it down when it is out of control. Acupuncture and acupressure utilize the same points on the body, and both have been used for thousands of years to address emotional and physical imbalances.

PC8 (EIGHTH POINT ON THE PERICARDIUM MERIDIAN): "LABOR PALACE"

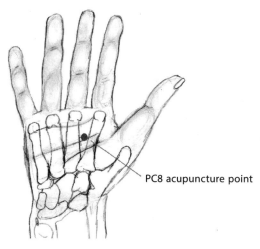

PC8 acupuncture point

Fig. 6.1. PC8, eighth point on the pericardium meridian

This point is located between the tendons of the pointer and middle fingers along—or directly below in some people—the second highest horizontal crease of the palm (see fig. 6.1 above). When a tight fist is made, the point is where the tip of the middle finger touches the palm of the hand. Similar to its cousin HT8 (see page 201), PC8 calms the heart and facilitates emotional processing. The name of this point, "Labor Palace," comes from its ability to provide a safe haven for labored thoughts and emotions. Applying significant pressure until the area feels tender often yields better results than a light touch.

✻ Apply direct pressure to PC8 with the tip of your index finger while counting to ten and breathing slowly.

✻ Gently release and then switch to the other hand.

✻ Repeat this process up to five times.

DEPRESSION AND THE YIN YANG BODY TYPES

Depression affects each yin yang body type in different ways depending on their constitutionally unique energies. Generally speaking, for yang types, it often involves situations that get in the way of their determined yang energy, while for yin types, it is often a result of placing their own yin-related joy/calmness on the back burner for too long, or clinging to it with all their might. Sure, the yin types may experience depressive episodes when something/someone gets in their way, and the yang types when joy or comfort is neglected, but these situations rarely manifest as major depressive disorders. Balancing our body type's predominant emotion is an essential step to avoiding and overcoming depression.

We all have a unique path in life that, if traveled, brings out the best in us. Yet no path is ever forged for us, and we may have to bush-whack our way through unchartered wilderness when our navigation equipment fails. Depression is an emotional state that all of the body types are capable of experiencing when they feel stuck along this path. The menopausal transition is often a time when life gives us a wake-up call, forcing us to take a good look at where we've been and where we're going. It is a time when our focus shifts from birthing and rear-ing children to rebirthing and re-rearing ourselves. As I mentioned in the introduction, orcas are the only other mammal that experiences menopause. Whale studies show that the postmenopausal orca has a central role to play in the survival of her family. Orcas enter menopause around the age of forty and have been known to survive until the age of ninety.[3] Whether we are human or whale, the fact is that there is life beyond procreation, and with the knowledge of your body type, the path toward abundant emotional and physical health unfolds.

Let's take a closer look at how depression may affect each of the body types.

YANG TYPE A

As mentioned above, when the yin yang body types fall into depression, it is usually because of an imbalance of their own unique predominant emo-tion. Hence if the Yang Type A has difficulty controlling her predomi-nant emotion of anger, depression will often ensue. This process usually kicks in as a result of feeling belittled or disrespected, initially making her extremely angry but eventually leading her to exhaustion. The Yang Type A's sensitivity to oppression is due to an affiliation with wi eui, or showing mutual respect and dignity, which is associated with her stronger spleen. Lack of inherent kidney energy, correlated with calmness and comfort, also contributes to the Yang Type A's propensity toward anger.

Ann, the Agitated Yang Type A

Ann, a forty-six-year-old Yang Type A with a chip on her shoulder, sought treatment for lower back pain. She asked, "So can you fix it?" After I inquired about when her lower back pain had started, she told me that it came on suddenly after she had watched the news the previous night. Not having yet determined her body type, I assumed that an uncomfortable chair or couch had led to the discomfort, but she maintained that it was a reaction to "those condescending idiots in Washington D.C." The feeling of being directly assaulted by arrogance made Ann furious at first, but then she felt distraught, depressed, and helpless—a common pitfall of the Yang Type A. During her treatment, I inserted several acupuncture needles to cool excessive heat radiating from her hyperdeveloped spleen—the source of her anger. Not only did Ann feel more relaxed afterward, but her back pain also significantly diminished.

During the menopausal transition, the Yang Type A may become hypersensitive to injustice. Bursts of anger may emerge seemingly from nowhere when she is stressed or uncomfortable. Things get even worse when the Yang Type A feels she has been disrespected or belittled. Menopause is the Yang Type A's invitation to stand up for herself and others and make a difference but also to distance herself from issues over which she has little or no control. For the Yang Type A, the first step toward preventing and addressing depression is to avoid getting angry over minor issues.

The menopausal Yang Type A often has an aversion to calmness as her spleen yang energy spends most of its time in the upper body and away from the deep-seated and dark yin energy of the lower body. Calmness for her means giving up or falling behind a rigorous daily schedule. "I must keep busy!" she says, abhorring the thought of being lazy and irresponsible. In her haste, she often overlooks and takes for granted family relationships and personal health. Her tolerance of those who are more laid back and easygoing also decreases. Situations that used to be easily brushed aside, like returning home to find her yin-type hubby on the couch casually munching away on a snack while watching football, may start to aggravate her beyond belief. But little does she realize that her own self-comfort is the only path to postmenopausal health. The balanced Yang Type A sets time aside to slow down, breathe deeply, and pamper herself. She realizes that "being" is more important than "doing," and that the rest of her life depends on the ability to shift into a lower gear.

Herbs can also help curb the Yang Type A's anger by cooling her throbbing spleen and encouraging the downward flow of rebellious yang energy to the kidneys. The herbs below are commonly prescribed in the Sasang clinic for the Yang Type A who is struggling with uncontrolled anger and/or depression.

 Zhu Ye
(Common: Bamboo Leaves; Latin: *Lophatherum gracile*)
As we've seen with Zhu Ru (bamboo shavings) in the "Fire Aboard" chapter, bamboo is often praised in Asia for its resilience and ability to bend in strong wind without toppling over, and it is often used in Eastern medicine to promote resilience of the spirit. The Yang Type A's virtue of humility is like that of bamboo, bending and yielding to others without belittling herself. Although her humility cannot be matched by the other types, getting there is a significant challenge because anger often gets in the way. Bamboo leaves help curb the anger of the Yang Type A by strongly rooting her anger while lifting up her wounded spirit. With their ability to cool and root energy, bamboo leaves also encourage the smooth flow of urine in cases where there is a lack of or a difficult flow due to heat accumulation.

Common Uses
Zhu Ye calms the mind and spirit, promotes a smooth urine stream by draining excess yang and heat from the upper body, and treats mouth sores, swollen gums, and thirst due to heat rising upward from the stomach.

Source

A tincture of bamboo leaves can be purchased from Hawaii Pharm; look for Dan Zhu Ye tincture on their website.

Preparation and Dosage

Refer to the manufacturer for standard dosage and a Sasang specialist (see "Continuing the Voyage," page 335) for modified dosage.

 Bo He

(Common: Field Mint; Latin: *Mentha arvensis*)

Bo He, or field mint, soothes and cools the stomach energy of Yang Type As and also has a calming effect on the mind, alleviating stress and anger and promoting sleep. Field mint is also beneficial for Yang Type A headaches. Chilled field mint tea makes for a refreshing drink in the summer or whenever you need to cool down. Mint also contains a significant amount of iron and vitamin D, which can help counteract SAD, a form of depression brought on by a lack of sun exposure. Field mint may also help pick up your mood on a gloomy day.

Common Uses

Field mint relieves headaches, throat disorders (swollen and sore throat, tonsillitis, and/or swollen glands), stress, anxiety, insomnia, and depression.

Sources

The term *mint* is an umbrella term that includes spearmint and peppermint, and they all have similar characteristics and health effects. While mint/spearmint/peppermint tea is sold at most supermarkets, keep in mind that tea bag sources routinely combine mint with ingredients that may or may not agree with your body type. For an extensive list of body-type-compatible foods and herbs, please refer to my book *Your Yin Yang Body Type*. Mint is also available in tincture, extract, and capsule forms. While mint itself is readily available, field mint, also known as wild mint, is not as easy to find. In our clinic, we import field mint directly from China. Field mint grows wild in open fields throughout the United States and Canada. While field mint may have the strongest effect, other types of mint can be substituted.

Preparation and Dosage

Insert a tea bag into a mug of hot water and let steep for two minutes. If field mint leaves are available, boil 9 grams per two cups of water and let simmer for fifteen minutes over low heat. Strain out the leaves before drinking. Up to four cups of mint tea can be consumed per day. For the best cooling effect, drink it chilled. Field mint tea goes well with a bamboo leaf tincture. You can mix the tincture directly into the field mint tea or take the two separately.

Can't Other Body Types Get Irritable during Menopause Too?

Other body types can get irritable as well, but the reasons irritability manifests is different for each type. The Yang Type B's irritability is usually because she does not feel respected or appreciated. For the Yin Type A, it's a result of feeling betrayed or unacknowledged. The Yin Type B's menopause-related irritability may be the result of a desire to escape rather than face life's every-so-often harsh reality.

YANG TYPE B

Yang Type Bs are no strangers to sadness, as it is their predominant emotion. One might think that sadness would make them appear grumpy and seem to be sulking all the time. Actually, sadness doesn't bring them down like it might the yin types; instead, it cranks them up, often to the point of anger. If Yang Type Bs are not careful, sadness can get out of control and morph into extreme anger or rage because of their affiliation with sa mu, or sense of societal duty. They can easily take the gift of sa mu too far and feel as if they always have to be in charge, believing that others must heed their advice. When an imbalanced Yang Type B believes that someone is keeping a secret, sadness will get out of control. Yet it's rage rather than sadness that gives the Yang Type B a reputation for often being authoritarian and stern.

During the menopausal transition, the Yang Type B's stronger sorrow-filled lungs often get stronger while her weaker sacral and lumbar areas, which correlate with comfort and joy, get weaker. If she has not experienced much comfort and joy before menopause, then it will be even more challenging for her to embrace the transition. Dishonesty and betrayal are major obstacles to the Yang Type B's joy. During menopause she becomes hypersensitive to others' faults and imperfections. By making a sincere effort to trust herself even if others may not be trustworthy, she sends energy to her liver, and slowly but surely joy unfolds. Herbal medicine can also be helpful here, since plant energy can encourage the smooth flow of yin and yang energy within the body. The herbs below gently help the excess yang energy descend and transport it from the lungs to the liver.

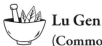 ## Lu Gen
(Common: Common Reed; Latin: *Phragmites communis*)

With its strong affiliation for moisture and its hollow stalk, Lu Gen, or common reed, is often spotted close to rivers, streams, and marshes, slurping up water like a straw. After ingestion, common reed transports moisture to the upper body and moderates yang heat. In Sasang medicine, it is often used to tame the excessive lung energy of the Yang Type B by sending cool yin energy to the lungs and encouraging the descent of excess upper body yang heat energy. By softening the flow of upper body energy, this herb also assists with stomach issues such as acid regurgitation, heartburn, and vomiting.

Common Uses
Common reed addresses anxiety, worry, indigestion (stomach acid, heartburn, and/or vomiting), shortness of breath, and dry heaves.

Sources
A tincture of Lu Gen can be purchased on the Hawaii Pharm website.

Preparation and Dosage
Refer to the manufacturer for standard dosage and a Sasang specialist (see "Continuing the Voyage," page 335) for modified dosage.

Caution
Consult with a specialist before administering to children or during pregnancy.

Food Friends: Buckwheat and Persimmon

While balancing your mood with Lu Gen, how about eating more buckwheat and persimmons? Both of these Yang Type B foods act as mood boosters in their own right. In Sasang medicine, buckwheat is used to detoxify and stimulate energy flow, especially to the Yang Type B's weaker liver and intestines. It has high levels of tryptophan, which is known to stimulate the release of serotonin, a neurotransmitter that makes us feel happy and relaxed. Lee Je-ma credited persimmons with the ability to nourish the heart and lungs, while uplifting the spirit. With their astringent nature, persimmons are also used in Sasang medicine to quench thirst and address diarrhea.

Can't Sadness Bring Down Other Body Types Too?

Other body types can also experience sadness, but the reasons sadness manifests differs according to the type. The Yang Type A's sadness is usually the side effect of excessive bursts of anger. For the Yin Type A, it's a result of lacking joy and a reason to smile. The Yin Type B's menopause-related sadness may be from not having enough quiet time to relax and recoup.

YIN TYPE A

Rebecca, introduced at the beginning of this chapter, is a Yin Type A born with a stronger liver, which correlates with the emotion of joy. It is difficult to imagine that joy can result in depression, but it is often the most dubious yet likely suspect. Do you recall how all things have aspects of both yin and yang? Depression is no exception, since within depression is joy and within joy lurks depression. Stated in another way, we wouldn't feel depressed if we never knew what joy felt like, and we wouldn't feel truly joyful if we never felt depressed! The Yin Type A's stronger liver always seeks joy, and if it does not find it, sadness abounds. A person with this body type is often the most joyful, and even when she is sad or depressed, periodic traces of joy can still occur, as if her inner joy needed to come up for air, sometimes resulting in a manic-depressive state. The Yin Type A has a strong sense of dang yo, or group orientation, from which she draws energy and establishes her footing. Being with others and sharing ideas, gifts, food, and so forth is what brings joy to the Yin Type A.

The lungs, which correlate with sorrow, are the weakest organ of the Yin Type A, and hence sorrow is a trap that easily catches her when she's off guard. It's easy for the Yang Type A to fill her lungs with self-worth and reliance, but the Yin Type A depends on the physical presence of others and reciprocal give-and-take relationships to keep her fulfilled and joyful.

If the Yin Type A doesn't consistently invite enough joy into her life, she can easily become ill. The menopausal Yin Type A is prone to questioning her sense of dang yo and wonders if certain friends or lover(s) are being genuine. She often thinks twice about her relationships, questioning whether or not they are true sources of joy. During menopause, a woman's inner voice becomes stronger, letting her know when it needs her attention. If it is time for more joy, then cleaning out the closet of unhelpful relationships might be necessary. It may also be time to reflect on what it is she is really seeking from others and to ask herself if it can be found within instead.

Can't the Other Body Types Feel a Lack of Joy during Menopause?

Other body types can certainly feel a lack of joy, but the reasons for it differ according to the type. The Yang Type As' lack of joy is a reaction to their sense that they, or others around them, are not being treated fairly. For Yang Type Bs, it's a result of feeling as if no one is following their advice and direction. The Yin Type Bs' menopausal lack of joy may come from either isolation or taking on overwhelming responsibilities.

Since yang correlates with the upper body and yin with the lower body, it's challenging for the yin types to get an objective bird's-eye view of their life. Actually, shik kyun—the ability to distinguish, filter, and decipher—comes from the lungs, the Yin Type A's weaker organ. Depression kicks in when the Yin Type A has lost a sense of where she is going and where she has been as she staggers through the darkness. Her stronger spongy liver can easily make matters worse as it clings to everything in reach. The depressed Yin Type A is no stranger to thoughts like "I know he's not a nice man, but I still need to be with him!" or "This job will eventually kill me, but I have to stick with it." If the yang types aren't happy, everyone around them will feel the heat even if they try to conceal their emotions. The yin types do a better job of masking their feelings even if they are suffering within. By strengthening her lungs, the balanced Yin Type A distinguishes between friend and foe, profit and loss, harmony and disharmony, and makes tough decisions, trusting her inner voice.

Without first releasing the excess worry, stress, insecurity, toxins, and so on of a Yin Type A's liver, it would be unfeasible to send energy to her lungs. Be patient with yourself because it takes years (some may argue lifetimes) to unravel the knots of excess within our organs. Yet with each step along the way another flower within you blooms, and before you know it, a beautiful garden begins to emerge. Sasang medicine utilizes hundreds of herbs to release liver excess, promote the flow of energy to the lungs, and uplift the spirit. Here are a few of the top contenders.

 ## Suan Zao Ren
(Common: Sour Jujube Seed; Latin: *Ziziphus spinosa*)

Suan Zao Ren, or sour jujube seed, is commonly used in Eastern medicine to calm and soothe the heart and mind. These little red seeds nourish and support the function of the heart and lungs—a task that effectively chips away at the Yin Type A's depression. Sour jujube is used in a variety of herbal formulas for these reasons. Its seeds contain substantial amounts of flavonoids, alkaloids, and saponins, the combination of which likely contributes to their calming effects.

Common Uses
Sour jujube seed relieves insomnia, anemia, depression, anxiety, nervousness, stress, night sweats, thirst, and palpitations.

Sources
Even though sour jujube is readily available in China and Korea, it is difficult to obtain raw in the United States. It is, however, part of a popular and easy-to-obtain formula, Suan Zao Ren Tang (sour jujube decoction), which helps with sleep and can be purchased from the Chinese Herbs Direct and Vita Living websites.

Preparation and Dosage
Follow the manufacturer's recommended dosage instructions.

Caution
If you are taking medications for insomnia, consult a professional before trying sour jujube. When combined with other sleep medications, it may cause excessive drowsiness.

 Long Yan Rou
(Common: Longan Fruit; Latin: *Euphoria longan*)
Long Yan Rou, or longan fruit, is used in Sasang medicine mainly to calm the spirit and mind and support brain function. Long Yan translates as "dragon eyes," and accordingly, this herb is also used to assist with age-related eye disorders, such as cataracts. Dried longan fruit is also rich in copper; a 3.5-ounce serving accounts for 90 percent of the recommended daily allowance. Deficiency in minerals such as copper contributes to the development of osteoporosis in women as they age. The Yin Type A's stronger liver has a tendency saturate and congest itself with minerals, causing deficiency of copper, magnesium, and potassium in other areas of the body. Long Yan Rou helps circulate liver energy and distribute minerals along the way.

Common Uses
Long Yan Rou assists with insomnia, forgetfulness, anxiety, fear, lack of focus, headaches, sadness, and depression.

Sources
Organic Traditions offers a 3.5-ounce bag of organic dried longan fruit that is available on the LuckyVitamin website, and an 8-ounce bag of the nonorganic variety can be found on the Dragon Herbs website.

Preparation and Dosage

Consume up to ten dried fruits a day, or ingest via Suan Zao Ren Tang (sour jujube decoction).

Herbal Friend: Yuan Zhi
(Common: Seneca Snakeroot;
Latin: *Polygala senega*)

Yuan Zhi (meaning "enhance willpower"), or snakeroot, encourages the flow of energy to the Yin Type A's lungs and brain, stimulating mood and memory. In Sasang medicine it is said to "awaken the true qi of the lungs." Alcohol-based and nonalcoholic tinctures are available on the Hawaii Pharm website; search for "polygala." Yuan Zhi arouses and inspires, while Long Yan Rou nourishes and supports the mind and spirit. For best results take both herbs together. Please follow the manufacturer's guidelines for the applicable dosage.

Jeannie, the (Not So) Joyful Yin Type A

"How can you stay so happy all the time?!" Jeannie's friends would often ask while, unbeknownst to them, she was falling deeper into the abyss of depression. Jeannie was indeed a joyful-natured person, always encouraging others with her radiant smile. She didn't recognize when depression kicked in and couldn't explain why she started oversleeping, sobbing when alone, and drinking excessively. Sorrow is difficult to distinguish and process for Yin Type As because it is associated with their hypodeveloped and energetically deprived lungs. Instead of addressing her depression, Jeannie simply brushed it aside, hoping that her joy would return. It was only when she realized that joy and sadness can coexist, expressing themselves when appropriate, that her condition began to improve. Instead of ignoring or eradicating sadness, she decided to slowly get in touch with it and gave herself permission to cry on her friend's shoulder and watch sad movies, each time feeding her thirsty lungs with more energy.

YIN TYPE B

The Yin Type B's strong sense of ko cho, or household affairs, gives her a passionate desire for intimacy at home with family and/or simply being alone. This trait is coupled with intense willpower, giving her an unprecedented drive. A lack of intimacy or inability to achieve what she set out for can leave the Yin Type B with a deep sense of despair and insecurity. If the Yin Type B weren't so introverted, the advice of others might have put an end to this misery. Yet she often chooses to go through it alone, hiding her feelings. While this may work in some situations, it does not necessarily work in others. Menopause is an opportunity for the Yin Type B to stand tall and face her fears one by one.

Being around others for too long can easily exhaust the menopausal Yin Type B, causing her deficient yang energy to escape upward and outward as if to say, "Beam me up, Scotty. It's getting too hectic down here!" This feeling is often enhanced when lofty goals of the past have not been met. The Yin Type B is a dreamer who sets and plans goals that often require cracking the shell of intimacy and exposing herself to the world, which may send her crawling right back inside. Menopause gives the Yin Type B permission to let go of her lofty goals and reevaluate her relationships with others and work. It is a time when a quiet home suddenly loses its appeal; with children off to college, the world outside becomes more attractive to her.

If the Yin Type B could build a cocoon around her stronger kidneys and isolate them from the hustle and bustle of the lungs and spleen (both yang organs), she'd do so in a heartbeat. It's when the stronger areas of our body isolate themselves and disregard the weaker ones that we get off-kilter. The Yin Type B's kidneys cannot remain comfortable without integrating the heat of the spleen. Spleen energy gives us the ability to speak our mind and cut to the chase—a quality born from kyo wu. Oh, how the Yin Type B wishes that others would just keep to themselves! Little does the uncultivated Yin Type B realize that it is only through the ability to express herself in the face of adversity that she is capable of finding comfort and avoiding the abyss of depression. As appealing a path though it may sound, isolating herself further during and after menopause will only result in more discomfort and loneliness. Yet if she loses her sense of comfort along the way, it's back to square one. Warmth is the answer to her despair and steamy baths, cardiovascular exercises, and hot-natured foods can help do the repair. Her cold kidney home may seem like a place to chill and feel secure, but it actually hinders her growth in the long run. The blazing spleen possesses an endless supply of heat waiting to be tapped.

Can't the Other Body Types, Get Cold Easily and Feel Insecure?

Other body types can also get cold and feel insecure, but the reasons why differ according to the type. The Yang Type A's cold and insecurity come from a tendency to burn herself out with anger and over-reaction. For the Yang Type B, these feelings are the result of burning up too much yang heat and feeling belittled. The Yin Type A's cold and insecurity come from losing someone or something important to her.

Below are some herbs that stimulate the Yin Type B's deficient spleen and assist with depression.

 ### An Xi Xiang
(Common: Benzoin Oil; Latin: *Styrax benzoin*)

As we've seen in the "Fire Aboard" chapter, benzoin is prized for its ability to calm the Yin Type B's spirit and promote digestion of food and experience (see page 141). An Xi Xiang's warmth and strong aroma lift the clouds that easily encroach and darken the Yin Type B's hyper-sensitive mind.

Common Uses
Benzoin calms anxiety, uplifts emotions, relieves indigestion, addresses pain in the chest and abdomen from food stagnation, and alleviates coughing.

Source
Bulk Apothecary offers essential oil of benzoin on its website.

Preparation and Dosage

I recommend dabbing a tiny bit of benzoin oil underneath the nose or onto the wrists with a cotton swab or ball. It can be reapplied topically several times a day to refresh the fragrance. You can also burn a few drops in a diffuser or oil burner.

Caution

Although benzoin is used as an ingredient in medicinal teas, it is usually ingested only under the care of a professional. Most sources warn against ingesting this herb and recommend it for topical use only. Applying essential oils directly onto the skin may produce rashes or redness. Try diluting the first few applications of benzoin with water until your skin gets used to it. If your skin is not irritated, then try applying it directly.

 ## Huo Xiang
(Common: Patchouli Oil; Latin: *Pogostemon cablin*)

In Eastern medicine, patchouli is used as a tea to clear the sinuses, support the digestive system, and balance the flow of energy throughout the body. Its aromatic fragrance can be inhaled to stimulate the function of the Yin Type B's weaker spleen and pick up her mood, enhance memory, and clear away cluttered thoughts. Yin Type Bs in particular benefit from patchouli because its warm nature helps the stomach break down and assimilate foods, and it treats allergies, colds, and other respiratory issues. Patchouli has also been used for decades in the West as a fragrance and essential oil. Remember that strong, recognizable smell from the hippie era?

Common Uses

Patchouli alleviates indigestion, allergies, common colds, congestion, coughing, shortness of breath, lack of appetite, depression, and brain fog.

Sources

Patchouli oil is available from manufacturers such as NOW Foods and Plantlife.

Preparation and Dosage

A few drops of patchouli oil may be dabbed onto a cotton ball and rubbed under the nostrils to clear the sinuses or onto the abdomen to promote digestion up to three times a day. I suggest alternating daily between applications of benzoin and patchouli oils for the best effect.

Caution

Please see caution for benzoin on previous page.

7

No Wake Zone

Improving Your Sleep

E lena's friends used to make fun of how she could sleep anywhere, any time. Her husband envied how she could fall right asleep while he tossed and turned the night away. It wasn't until she reached the age of forty-eight that Elena experienced her first sleepless night. She woke up the next morning feeling groggy and discovered that her husband was sleeping on the couch. "What happened to you last night? Why are you sleeping on the couch?" she asked in amazement. He described how she kept swishing this way and that, occasionally smacking him in the face with her arm. Elena couldn't believe her ears, since until then she had slept without moving a muscle. Brushing the whole experience aside, Elena and her husband hit the sheets the following evening without thinking anything of the previous night. Two hours later Elena whispered in her husband's ear, "Honey, are you awake?" All she received was a grunt, then a snuffle, and finally a "Go back to sleep, honey." Days turned into weeks and weeks into months of insomnia, and Elena, along with her husband, began to look and feel like a zombie. Elena couldn't figure out what was going on, since she was not ill, there were no added stressors in her life, and now she had the entire bed to herself. Sometimes she would fall asleep quickly, only to wake up again around 3:00 a.m. with a hot flash followed by intense sweating or an urge to urinate, or for no reason whatsoever! Elena noticed her heart racing and a feeling of anxiousness whenever she had

189

trouble getting to sleep or upon awakening in the middle of the night.

What Is Insomnia?

Insomnia is basically a lack of sleep, and those who suffer from it know exactly how energy-depriving a condition it can be. But according to the DSM-IV , the criteria for diagnosing insomnia are as follows:[1]

- The primary complaint is difficulty getting to sleep and staying asleep and/or feeling rested from sleep for more than one month.
- It takes thirty minutes or longer to fall asleep three or more nights a week.
- Sleep disturbance isn't related to other issues such as apnea, narcolepsy, or circadian rhythm disorder.
- Sleep disturbance doesn't occur exclusively during the course of another mental disorder.
- Lack of sleep is interfering with social, occupational, or other important daily functions.

Elena arrived at my clinic looking frail and upset, desperate for a solution and hoping that acupuncture would do the trick. "I don't want to take medication," she said, "so is there anything you can do to help me?" I reassured her that the only thing standing between her and a deep, nourishing sleep is an imbalance of energy, and that if she followed my tips and body-type-specific suggestions, chances were that things would improve immensely. I explained how sleep depends on the nightly descent of bodily energy from the heart to the kidneys, but that excessive activity, stress, excitement, or other stimulants may interfere with this process. As I went on to discuss the Eastern view of menopause, and how it is seen as the seventh of the seven-year cycles of life—a time when accumulated life experience and body energy culminate and rise to the upper body—Elena's eyes suddenly widened as she recalled that her sleeplessness began after she skipped her monthly cycle for the first time at age forty-eight.

According to the National Sleep Foundation, insomnia is experienced by approximately 50 percent of all menopausal women. Yet meno-pause is not the only perpetrator, since one in four Americans resort to some kind of sleep aid. It shouldn't come as a surprise that so many people suffer from insomnia given that most of the industrialized world runs its engines both day and night. Most of us avoid slowing down because it is equated with failure and lack of productivity. Even if we desire to slow down after a busy and stressful day, a revved-up mind may have other intentions. Lack of sleep is an issue that can equally affect all of the four body types.

Chronic lack of sleep is often the source of so many other, often obscure, and seemingly unrelated symptoms like chronic unrelenting headaches, chronic migrating pain, fibromyalgia, anxiety, irritability, poor memory, immune deficiency, weight gain/loss, and so forth. Sleep replenishes our life force, and without it we simply cannot function. We will soon discover how each of the yin yang body types contributes to and is affected by insomnia in slightly different ways.

While stress is the most frequent sleep reducer, other not-so-obvious factors may also play their part. The energy of an unsettled digestive system, for instance, can rebel upward against the heart, bringing about anxiety and/or insomnia. Consistent pain or the urge to urinate may also interrupt a night's sleep. The sympathetic dog or cat owner may also miss out on sleep if they give their pet bed privileges. The same goes for a partner who snores! Aside from getting rid of your partner or pets, there are other successful ways of approaching the issue.

Despite the various reasons for disrupted sleep, hot flashes are the most common reason for waking up in the middle of the night for peri-menopausal women. This chapter will review the reasons why hot flashes and other menopause-related factors have a profound effect on sleep and will offer both general and body-type-specific methods for improvement.

ONE THING LEADS TO ANOTHER

A fifty-four-year-old female patient visited my clinic complaining of severe dizziness, spasms throughout her body, and a number of other unusual symptoms, such as eyelid twitching, blurry vision, floaters, and a pounding headache above her left ear. She had been to various doctors who diagnosed her over the years with different syndromes such as fibromyalgia, polymyalgia, psychosis, and so on. Yet even with treatment, her symptoms continued to worsen. I noticed that she looked exhausted, so I asked her about sleep. Tears started pouring down her cheeks as she recalled how each night sleep had become a daunting chore since the onset of her perimenopause. I gave her several ideas about how to improve her sleep and a body-type-specific herbal formula consisting of ten herbs to address anxiety and insomnia. Soon afterward her sleep improved and so did her unusual symptoms.

FATIGUE AND SLEEP

Fatigue is often associated with insufficient sleep, but even with less sleep, it's possible to feel energized and replenished if sleep quality is maintained. Chronic fatigue can frequently be traced to insufficient *deep* sleep, although an underlying illness may also be a source. Patients who suffer frequently from insomnia say they get plenty of sleep but still feel tired throughout the day. A good night's sleep requires that we spend 20 to 25 percent of it in the rapid eye movement (REM) phase. During this phase of sleep the body recharges its batteries, slowing down all functions and focusing inward. Getting to bed around the same time each night enhances our ability to enter REM sleep. Sleep schedule fluctuations may trigger fatigue since they throw off our body's natural rhythm.

Studies show that stimulants such as caffeine directly interfere with deep sleep. Occasionally I'll encounter patients who, when asked about their energy level, say they have tons of it. Yet when it comes to pulse checking—a diagnostic method used in Eastern medicine to assess energy levels—it is surprisingly deep and weak, indicating fatigue. My next question is usually about whether or not they drink coffee, to which the answer is often "just a few cups a day." Coffee and other stimulants may temporarily boost energy, but in excess, they'll eventually destroy it.

DO YOU REMEMBER YOUR DREAMS?

Contrary to popular belief, remembering dreams doesn't indicate a healthy sleep. Actually, in most cases, if we remember our dreams, it's a sign that we've resurfaced from REM sleep prematurely. Without adequate REM sleep, we cannot replenish our energies, making it difficult to get the following day started. If you remember your dreams, it doesn't necessarily mean that you are sleep-deprived; those who attempt to remember their dreams as soon as they wake up may be able to do so without compromising REM.

Are you REM deficient or just someone who remembers their dreams? A sleep study can provide a definitive answer, but simply reflecting on your energy level may suffice. If you remember your dreams and wake up tired, groggy, dizzy, and/or out of sync, it's likely that you are missing out on REM sleep. If you remember your dreams but still feel energized and ready to leave the house in the morning without the help of caffeine or other stimulants, then REM may not be an issue.

WESTERN PERSPECTIVES ON INSOMNIA

From the standpoint of Western medicine, insomnia during or after menopause is due to age-related changes that occur in the ovaries and their regulation of hormone levels within the body. Surging estrogen and progesterone production within the ovaries makes it challenging for menopausal women to get sufficient REM sleep, frequently bringing about fatigue and grogginess upon awakening. Estrogen replacement has been found to improve REM in menopausal women, but the mechanism behind this effect is still unknown. One study found that estrogen replacement improved sleep by reducing or eliminating hot flashes, hinting that an improvement in sleep might be simply a result of enhanced comfort more than anything else.[2]

In Western medicine, estrogen therapy is the most effective method of treating menopause-related hot flashes and insomnia, but, as mentioned in our discussion of hot flashes in chapter 4, it doesn't come without risks, and as we will soon discover, alternative approaches often work just as well, if not better than hormones. If you have tried everything else and are at your wit's end, then a discussion with your doctor about using plant-based estrogens (also known as phytoestrogens), or a small dose of bioidentical estrogen, may be an option. Yet before you take this route, I suggest tapping into the powerful source of your own internal healing energy by trying the natural methods below, especially if you know that you are prone to estrogen-fed cancers or other hormone-related sensitivities.

Antidepressants are also routinely prescribed by doctors for insomnia on the belief that depression and insomnia go hand in hand. Lack of sleep may eventually induce depression, while depression might lead to a lack of sleep. SSRIs, such as Zoloft, Prozac, and Celexa, are the most commonly prescribed antidepressants for insomnia, followed by tricyclics, such as Pamelor, Elavil, and Silenor, which are not as strong as the former and have a mild sedative effect. Interestingly, even though SSRIs are prescribed for insomnia, they have also been known to interfere with sleep, attesting to their unpredictable effects on the nervous system.

Both SSRIs and tricyclics have other considerable side effects, such as high blood pressure (tricyclics only), sexual malfunction, weight gain, dry mouth and throat, racing pulse, and confusion. As if this weren't enough, Paxil has been known to cause birth defects. Yes, many of us would try absolutely anything if we lose night after night, day after day, and week after week of sleep, but with these risks, such drugs should be taken as a last resort.

For some of us, insomnia may feel like an uncontrollable beast, and for others, it may be somewhat more tamable. Remember that, ultimately, you are the master of your own mind and body, although it may not seem so at times. Most Western medications alter the chemistry within the body, either limiting it or forcing it to function in a particular way. Manipulation isn't synonymous with harmony, since the former has to do with artificial control and the latter with natural balance and equilibrium. Our bodies constantly strive to achieve balance but often get thwarted along the way. Occasionally, we may have to trick or manipulate the body to avoid getting stuck in an unhealthy pattern, but inevitably we will have to work *with* it, forming a symbiotic and mutually enhancing relationship.

EASTERN PERSPECTIVES ON INSOMNIA

In Eastern medicine, quality of sleep is related to the state of yin and yang within the body. When yin and yang are balanced, the body nat-

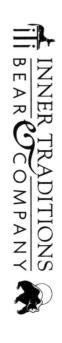

INNER TRADITIONS & COMPANY

Inner Traditions • Bear & Company
P.O. Box 388
Rochester, VT 05767-0388
U.S.A.

PLEASE SEND US THIS CARD TO RECEIVE OUR LATEST CATALOG FREE OF CHARGE.

Book in which this card was found _____

☐ Check here to receive our catalog via e-mail.

| Company |
| ☐ Send me wholesale information |

Name _____

Address _____ Phone _____

City _____ State _____ Zip _____ Country _____

E-mail address _____

Please check area(s) of interest to receive related announcements via e-mail:

☐ Health   ☐ Self-help   ☐ Science/Nature   ☐ Shamanism
☐ Ancient Mysteries ☐ New Age/Spirituality ☐ Visionary Plants   ☐ Martial Arts
☐ Spanish Language ☐ Sexuality/Tantra   ☐ Family and Youth   ☐ Religion/Philosophy

Please send a catalog to my friend:

Name _____ Company _____

Address _____ Phone _____

City _____ State _____ Zip _____ Country _____

Order at 1-800-246-8648 • Fax (802) 767-3726

E-mail: customerservice@InnerTraditions.com • Web site: www.InnerTraditions.com

urally sinks into a deep sleep. The body and mind slow down when yin energy accumulates in the evening and speed up when yang energy ascends in the morning. Emotional stress, dietary imbalance, and a lack of exercise all contribute to an imbalance of yin and yang, and in turn, insomnia. Difficulty getting to sleep is due to yang imbalance; difficulty staying asleep arises from yin imbalance. Some of us may have difficulty with both getting to sleep and staying there, indicating an imbalance of both yang and yin.

Difficulty Getting to Sleep

An imbalance of yang energy is often marked by tossing and turning with thoughts churning wildly. This imbalance is stirred up by excessive activity before bed, several cups of coffee (especially when consumed in the afternoon or evening), stress, anxiety, or even joy! With so much yang energy pushing upward to sustain a demanding daily schedule, yin descent in the evening is practically impossible. Just when you thought things couldn't get worse, the liver energy kicks in at 11:00 p.m., shoving even more energy upward, joining the party of vibrating energy inside the head and adding to the challenge of unwinding.

Difficult Staying Asleep

Yin energy is responsible for rooting and softening yang energy within the body. Without yin, yang would run wild and drive away sleep. In order to get a deep sleep, yin and yang need to strike a balance. Yet when it comes to brute strength, yang always has the advantage, and a tendency to ignore yin. In Oregon, we have large trees that occasionally plummet to the ground when pushed by even a relatively light wind. I am often surprised when I see how undeveloped their roots are—a small, unsophisticated bundle, barely hanging from the bottom of a fallen giant. Humans also have a tendency to focus on action and movement, forgetting the importance of quiet and nonaction, making it difficult for yin to keep us asleep at night. Difficulty staying asleep is due to an imbalance of yin energy, which ideally is capable of nourishing, caressing, and rooting the energy of the heart and other organs at night.

Most menopausal women with insomnia awaken between the hours of 1:00 and 3:00 a.m., often feeling hot and/or sweaty. Modern science explains that waking up around this time has to do with a circadian rhythm within the body, and its slow release of cortisol throughout a twenty-four-hour cycle. Excessive physical and/or emotional stress during the day interferes with this cycle, causing it to spike later in the evening rather than during the day when we can use the extra energy. Higher stress levels correlate with higher levels of cortisol release from the adrenal glands. Most of us are familiar with the adrenal glands and how they produce adrenaline, the fight-or-flight hormone, which is excreted when we are under a lot of pressure or in a dangerous, life-or-death situation. When cortisol levels become exhausted, the adrenal glands will start to excrete more adrenaline, leaving us feeling wired, anxious, irritated, and exhausted all at the same time.

In Eastern medicine, each of the organs is stimulated at different times of the day as the ebb and flow of yin and yang energy make their way through the body. The cycle renews itself between 1:30 and 3:30 a.m., a period when energy shifts from the last organ of the energy cycle, the liver, to the first organ, the lungs. Most of those who have difficulty staying asleep at night, or with releasing stress, wake up at this time since recycling requires letting go of one cycle before starting another. The relationship between the liver and the lungs is often one of obligation and remorse rather than mutual admiration and support. The stronger liver often absorbs excess energy from the lungs, while the stouter lungs often take it away from the liver. Their disdain for one another stems from having fundamentally different energies. The Hun, or ethereal spirit, residing within the liver, desires to be free of obligation, material influence, and physical form, whereas the Po, or material spirit of the lungs, craves them. Hence a battle is waged between the desire to be free of life's challenges and the feeling of obligation and attachment.

THE YIN AND YANG OF INSOMNIA

In Eastern medicine, the shift of yin and yang energy within the body during the menopausal phase is thought to be the basis of insomnia. How we travel through the corridor of menopause greatly depends on how balanced or imbalanced our energies are before entering it.

Suppressed yang energy is no longer containable once we reach the corridor. Until this point in life, we may have brushed aside specific emotions and desires for the sake of pleasing others, staying out of trouble, or simply getting through the day. The more we suppress this energy, the stronger it eventually becomes. During menopause, the lid that seals these emotions slowly, and in some cases abruptly, opens, unleashing anger, irritability, grief, and unsettled emotions—all wreaking havoc on a night's sleep. For some of us, insomnia is a result of yin weakness; our yin is incapable of rooting upward-bearing yang. For others, it is due to an abundance of yin that, over the years, suppresses yang to the breaking point, which then rebels upward day after day, night after night.

Before we dive into body-type-specific methods for overcoming insomnia, let's take a look at a few time-tested, general tips for improving your sleep.

Tip #1: Keep Your Routine

The body is a creature of habit, preferring to eat, exercise, go to the bathroom, and sleep around the same time every day. A shift in routine can easily confuse the body and interrupt its rhythm. Sleeping an hour or so later than usual may trick the body into believing that we don't have to sleep at all. This holds true for other bodily processes, like eating and bowel movement. Eating dinner an hour or more later than we usually do may make it harder to digest, since the stomach prepares itself for food around the same time every day. If we ignore the urge to go to the bathroom, the signal eventually fades and constipation ensues.

Tip #2: Hit the Sheets before 11:00 p.m.

According to Eastern medicine, the energy of the body shifts from organ to organ every two hours. From 11:00 p.m. to 1:00 a.m., the body's energy gathers around the liver, which is responsible for creative thinking and focus. If you are suffering from a lack of sleep, then the onset of creative thinking and focus right before going to bed can only make matters worse. For others, this period may actually be a great time for creative thinking, writing, studying, or catching up on unfinished business. Yet if staying up past 11:00 p.m. becomes a habit, fatigue and lethargy will eventually manifest during the day. Getting to bed before creative thoughts fill our mind contributes to a deeper sleep and more energy the following day.

Tip #3: A Bed Is for Sleeping!

Some of us love to use our bed for doing absolutely everything aside from sleeping. However, the more active you are in bed, the less your body associates the bed with sleep. If you are having trouble with sleep and like to read, jump up and down on your bed, have pillow fights, or play hide-and-go-seek under the covers, try reserving these activities for another comfortable place in your home. Reserving your bed simply for rest—and of course making love*—can often help improve sleep.

Tip #4: Focus on Your Breath

Counting sheep may work for some people, but others may just keep on counting until they have accounted for every sheep on the planet. Instead, try to focus on the feeling and sound of slowly inhaling and exhaling while you lie in bed. Your breath helps not only to relax the body but also to clear your mind of accumulated daily clutter, and focusing on it in a meditative state could actually produce the same brain waves achieved during healthy sleep.

Tip #5: Repeat the "Just Let Go" Mantra

If you are one of those people who can't shut down their minds before bed, then this tip is for you. While in bed, try repeating the word *relax* as you inhale and the words *just let go* when you exhale, over and over again. Every time a thought knocks on the door of your consciousness, continue to repeat, "Relax . . . just let go."

Tip #6: Darken Your Room

Darkness has a profound effect on the mind and body, explaining why many of us feel drowsy after sunset. Have you ever tried studying, working, or writing in candlelight? I couldn't last twenty minutes without yawning and dozing off. Darkness signals the body to slow down, whereas light encourages it to rev up. Hence eliminating any trace of light from your bedroom increases the chances of getting a deeper sleep.

---

*Having an orgasm directly beforehand has been known to facilitate a deep sleep.

Melatonin is a naturally occurring substance within the body that responds to darkness, helping us relax, especially at night. In the modern world, most of us spend too much time in artificial light even into the depths of the evening, and this interferes with the release of melatonin within the body. A higher rate of insomnia among fair-skinned individuals is likely due to lower levels of melatonin within the body. If you feel wired at night, then melatonin supplementation may be the answer. Those of us who feel more secure leaving a light on at night when sleeping may also find this supplement helpful in reducing photosensitivity. Dr. Weil, known for his sound advice regarding natural supplements, recommends an as-needed 2.5-milligram dose of sublingual melatonin tablets before bed, or 0.25 to 0.3 milligram if taken regularly.

Tip #7: Avoid Exercise Directly before Bed

Exercise motivates the movement of yang energy throughout the body, while sleep is the process of settling it down. Intense exercise within two hours of sleeping may overstimulate the organ energies, making it difficult to sink into sleep. Intensive earlier exercise or lighter evening exercise/stretching doesn't have this effect and could actually benefit sleep by clearing the mind of daily stress and tiring the body.

Tip #8: Avoid Foods and Fluids Directly before Bed

Do you have to wake up to urinate? Many women experience this as the uterus presses against the bladder when they are lying down. Even if the bladder is only partially full, added pressure from the uterus may signal the desire to urinate, causing you to awaken. Ingesting fluids within one hour of sleep increases the odds of being woken up by the bladder. Although not as often to blame, eating within two hours of sleep may also result in waking up since the body may be forced to digest food rather than relax while we are sleeping. While this might not sound like a big deal, it is like patting your head and rubbing your tummy at the same time for the digestive system—possible but awkward.

Tip #9: Avoid Coffee in the Afternoon

Remember the good old days when you could drink as much coffee as you liked, any time of the day? Well, sorry to break the news, but drinking coffee after 2:30 p.m. is one of the most frequent reasons why getting to sleep is so difficult for the middle-aged individual. Relax! It's not that the body is getting older, it's that it's getting louder, voicing its opinion of us when we neglect it. Coffee stimulates the upward movement of yang within the body—suitable for starting the day but not ending it. Yang energy starts to wane after 2:00 p.m., making it a time when many of us need a second wind of energy. If we perk yang up again, it usually has a difficult time coming back down when it's time to sleep. Try recharging your battery by drinking tea, taking a short cat nap, or simply focusing on taking deep breaths for about fifteen to twenty minutes after eating lunch.

Tip #10: Hug a Pillow!

Did you know that after heart surgery, some doctors give their patients a "heart pillow" and ask them to hug it at night? Light pressure from a pillow or hug is comforting to the heart and is likely why it feels so wonderful to hug someone with a big heart. Hugging a pillow at night relaxes the heart, making it easier to enter sleep. A smaller pillow may do the job for some, while others may enjoy the contact of hugging a life-size body pillow.

Tip #11: Try Acupuncture and Acupressure

A thorough review of forty-six randomized controlled studies involving 3,811 participants showed that acupuncture significantly improved sleep, with an even stronger effect than pharmaceutical medication on increasing sleep duration.[3] Along with assisting the flow of energy throughout the body, acupuncture needle insertion is also a way to calm and root the energies of the body. Patients who receive acupuncture for insomnia often feel relaxed and deeply rested following treatment, finding it easier to sink into a deep sleep at night.

I often utilize the points shown below to address insomnia, effectively providing relief for my patients throughout the years. These points correlate with different organs of the body, which play significant roles in the sleeping process. The HT8 point is located along an energy channel that flows from the heart, which is in charge of processing day-to-day emotion. Insomnia is often affected by the inability to process emotions efficiently, making the heart throb at night, attempting to relieve itself of the daily pressure. The LIV2 point resides along the liver channel and is responsible for releasing excessive heat from the liver, which is often responsible for hot flashes and restless sleep. These points are most effective if they are pressed several times daily, even in the absence of hot flashes.

HT8 (EIGHTH POINT ON THE HEART MERIDIAN): "SMALL STOREHOUSE"

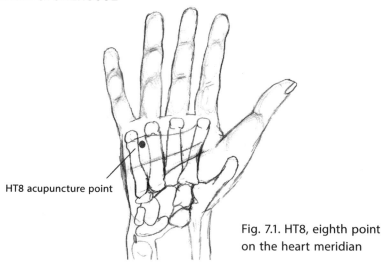

HT8 acupuncture point

Fig. 7.1. HT8, eighth point on the heart meridian

This point is located between the tendons of the pinky and ring fingers along the uppermost horizontal crease of the palm (see fig. 7.1 above). When a tight fist is made, the point is where the tip of the pinky touches the palm of the hand. HT8 calms the heart and facilitates emotional processing. Applying significant pressure to each point until it feels tender often yields better results than a light touch. Avoid using sharp metal objects that could penetrate your skin or applying excessive pressure.

* Use the index finger to apply direct pressure to HT8 while counting to ten and breathing slowly.
* Gently release and then switch to the other hand.
* Repeat this process up to five times.

☯ LIV2 (SECOND POINT ON THE LIVER MERIDIAN): "MOVING BETWEEN"

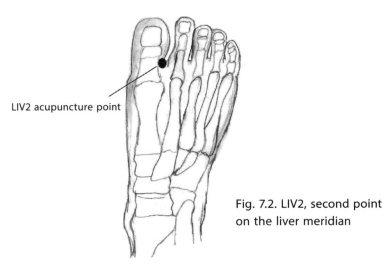

Fig. 7.2. LIV2, second point on the liver meridian

This acupressure point is the second point from the tip of the foot along the liver meridian and is located in between the first and second toes (see fig. 7.2 above). There is often a short crease that continues from the inner side of the big toe toward the upper part of your foot. LIV2 is located where this crease terminates. LIV2 releases heat from the liver, which cools those sleep-depriving hot flashes. Applying significant pressure to each point until it feels tender often yields better results than a light touch. Avoid using sharp metal objects that could penetrate your skin or applying excessive pressure.

✳ Use the index finger to apply direct pressure to LIV2 while counting to ten and breathing slowly.

✳ Gently release and then switch to the other foot.

✳ Repeat this process up to five times.

Tip #12: Find a Comfortable Mattress

Although this tip may seem like the most obvious one so far, it is also the most frequently disregarded. Buying a new mattress can easily become a daunting process. We are too often led to believe that comfort, rather than support, is a mattress priority, but months after buying the coziest mattress in the store, our back/shoulder/neck may begin to hurt again. At this point most of us would deny that our new

$3,000+ mattress could possibly be the problem and would swear by how comfortable we feel on it. Our new mattress may not be the issue, but if it is too soft and lacking support, then despite its coziness at the end of the day, come morning, we are as stiff as a board. A comfortable but unsupportive mattress is like comfort-food bingeing: it may give us temporary reprieve, but in the long run, it contributes to further discomfort. Before you go mattress shopping, make sure to do plenty of research, find out which are too firm or too soft, which are excellent for back pain, and which are made from enduring fill materials. Keep in mind that mattress shopping is rarely a successful love-at-first-sight scenario.

INSOMNIA AND THE YIN YANG BODY TYPES

How we get to sleep and stay asleep doesn't depend only on the events of the day and how we respond to them. A study done in 2015 discovered a genetic distinction between larks, or morning birds, and night owls.[4] The body's circadian clock runs on different schedules according to an individual's chronotype, or genetically defined internal rhythm. The early-bird chronotype naturally experiences a spike in cortisol, or stress hormone, early in the morning and a crash in the evening, so that they have less difficulty getting to sleep at night. Cortisone levels tend to kick in later for night owls, causing them to feel energized in the late evening but making it difficult for them to get up in the morning.

In Eastern medicine, creative energy is associated with the liver and gallbladder, which receive a wave of energy from 11:00 p.m. to 3:00 a.m. If we are awake during this time, creative thoughts often fill our consciousness, but if we are asleep, the liver stimulates dreaming and unconscious creativity.

Sleep quality is also influenced by different factors for each of the four yin yang body types. As we discussed in chapter 1, yin correlates with night and yang with morning. The yang types, born with excessive yang energy, are larks, and the yin types are often the night owls. Of course, there are exceptions to this, since many yin types are early birds and many yang types are late risers. Yet, generally speaking, even if yin types motivate themselves to wake up early, if they break this habit, then sleeping in easily becomes the new norm. The yang types may also feel sluggish in the morning, but this is only because they are extremely exhausted from lack of sleep the previous night, or because they have poor overall health.

YANG TYPE A

The menopausal Yang Type A is often even more easily angered than she was before the change began. She may find herself yelling at cars in a traffic jam, arguing with her family, or lashing out at the bank clerk for miscalculating her balance. Controlling her anger and hyperactive digestive system during menopause requires updated tactics, since attacking her anger head-on, or temporarily brushing it aside, only result in more anger. Her disregarded kidneys can no longer put up with uncontrolled anger, as health in this phase of life depends on her ability to discover calmness, quietness, and the ability to yield even when bursts of rage may seem appropriate.

Anger easily interferes with the Yang Type A's sleep because it pushes her yang energy further upward, bombarding the heart. Sleep requires that she let go of her desire for revenge, change, and/or rebellion. She naturally desires to solve her problems on the spot and move onward without just "sleeping on them" until a resolution is found. Like a wildfire, she rages through challenge and adversity. Yet sleep depends on do ryang (tolerance)—hidden within the gently subdued kidneys. Without accepting and yielding to her situation, she'll fight it night and day.

A hyperdeveloped digestive system also contributes to insomnia for the Yang Type A because of its tendency to overheat when she is stressed, under the weather, or angry. The digestive energy of a balanced Yang Type A smoothly flows downward to support the kidneys, her weakest organ, rooting and calming the mind along the way. It doesn't take much for her digestive system to overact, however, reversing the flow of energy. Upward-moving energy from the stomach, situated directly below the heart, easily induces anxiety, stress, and insomnia. A voracious, unsatisfied appetite is the first sign of digestive energy reversal.

Mantra for Better Sleep

If you have difficulty getting to sleep, try repeating, out loud or silently, the following sentence while slowly inhaling and exhaling, until you drift off into sleep: "My stronger spleen easily stirs up anger, but anger cannot help me sleep, so it's time to let it go."

Meditation for Better Sleep

Before going to bed, try sitting in a comfortable position somewhere other than your bed, dimming the lights, and putting on some relaxing music. Close your eyes and take deep breaths. When you breathe in, imagine that you are sending air all the way down to the lower abdomen, where calmness resides. While breathing out, imagine that you are releasing anger, stress, anxiety, and so on with each and every breath. I once had a Yang Type A patient who found it relaxing to listen to heavy metal music while getting acupuncture, reporting that it aligned her energies and made her think more clearly after her sessions. Many people, especially if they are not a yang type, may find it hard to imagine that anything but soft and slow music could be calming, but relaxation is different for each body type and individual. The point is that no matter what music you listen to, if it encourages balance and harmony, then it serves a valuable purpose.

Soothing Teas

In Eastern medicine, mint teas are said to calm the spirit and cool the stomach and liver energies. Drink two to three cups a day between meals to curb spells of anger and sadness, relax the mind, and/or reduce constant hunger.

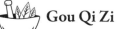 **Gou Qi Zi**
(Common: Goji Berry/Chinese Wolfberry; Latin: *Lycium chinense*)
It seems as if almost every herb mentioned so far in this book has had its own time in the spotlight of best natural remedies in the media, and Gou Qi Zi, or goji berry (aka wolfberry), is no exception. Claims for its ability to cure one disease or another can be found all over the internet. Some even refer to it as a "super fruit" that cures all ills. There is no doubt that goji plays a significant role in the Eastern medical

clinic. However, it is impossible to say that this or that herb is superior to others, since they all contribute in their own way toward balancing and harmonizing the body's energy depending on our constitution and the situation we are faced with. Goji is nonetheless very helpful for the Yang Type A because it nourishes and strengthens the kidneys, her weakest organ. In Sasang medicine, the kidneys help root the energy of the body, thus preventing rebellion of the Yang Type A's energy upward. Upward rebellion of energy may lead to insomnia, poor vision, headaches, and chronic sinus issues. Herbs that support the kidneys also assist in strengthening the bones. Goji can therefore also be used for the Yang Type A's bone-related issues.

Common Uses
Goji alleviates insomnia, visual disorders (blurry vision, weak vision), fatigue, anxiety, and osteoporosis/osteopenia.

Sources
Goji, also called Himalayan goji, packaged and in bulk, is currently available from just about any natural food store. You can also purchase it online from manufacturers such as Nuts.com and Navitas Naturals. Goji juice is available on the Healing Noni and Dynamic Health websites.

Preparation and Dosage
Raw wolfberry is another fine example of the culinary use of East Asian herbs. It can be sprinkled on salads or mixed with nuts, granola, or yogurt. In China, it is often sprinkled into soup made with chrysanthemum and dried jujube fruit to elicit a slightly sweetened flavor. Herbs that are also enjoyed as foods are safe for ingestion in higher dosages.

Caution
Since it is a fruit and contains sugar, diabetics should monitor sugar levels carefully when ingesting goji. Studies have suggested that goji may reduce the effects of warfarin and other blood thinners, so if you are taking a blood thinner, please consult a professional first.

The Yang Type A should not ingest goji if she is experiencing heat-related symptoms such as fever, sensitivity to heat, or pounding (vs. dull) headaches, because this herb is slightly warm-natured.

Mai Ya
(Common: Roasted Barley; Latin: *Hordeum vulgaris*)

Tea made of Mai Ya, or roasted barley, is a popular beverage in Japan and Korea, where it can even be purchased from vending machines! In the wintertime, roasted barley tea is consumed warm. In the summer, it is boiled, refrigerated, and then drunk cold. Barley itself has a very cold energetic nature. Roasted barley tea effectively cools excessive heat radiating from the yang types' hyperactive digestive system, which is often made worse by stress. In Sasang medicine, roasted barley soothes heartburn and abdominal distension while promoting blood circulation. Through balancing and redirecting digestive energy, roasted barley inhibits the reversal of stomach energy, preventing and addressing anxiety and insomnia.

Common Uses
Mai Ya clears excessive heat from the stomach to address heartburn, abdominal distension, and acid regurgitation. It inhibits the reversal of stomach energy to calm anxiety and promote sleep.

Sources
Bob's Red Mill produces barley flour that can be used as a baking ingredient or thickener for soups and sauces. While this form of barley is not as cooling as chilled barley tea, it is still somewhat effective and worth a try. Otherwise, roasted barley tea can be purchased on the internet. The Japanese brands House and Marubishi sell barley tea on Amazon, as does the Korean company Dongsuh. The Japanese name for roasted barley tea is *mugi-cha* and the Korean name is *bori-cha*.

Preparation and Dosage
Roasted barley tea usually comes in small cheesecloth bags. The bags are boiled in water but the tea itself is served chilled, thus enhancing barley's cooling characteristics. In both Korea and Japan, roasted barley tea is often further diluted with water and consumed throughout the day. I suggest drinking a glass of this tea while consuming a handful of goji berries two or three times a day, so that both herbs can enhance one another's energy rooting and digestion-balancing properties.

Caution

The cold nature of roasted barley tea may lead to diarrhea among the yin types. If you develop diarrhea after drinking barley tea, it is possible that you may actually be a yin type. In this case, it is important to discontinue it and retake the body type test. In some cases it is very challenging to figure out which body type you are, even after taking the test. It can also be challenging for the Sasang practitioner at times! Please refer to the test tips in chapter 2 for further guidance.

YANG TYPE B

As a part of her stronger lung (upper body) system, the Yang Type B's mind is constantly on the go. This trait often gives her enhanced insight and ingenuity. Yet a brilliant mind isn't necessarily equated with a sane one; in fact, the sanity of many ingenious Yang Type Bs of the past, including Vincent van Gogh, Lenin, and Leonardo da Vinci, has been questioned. Unlike the yin types, however, the Yang Type B's mind isn't focused on the events of the day but instead on the future. Dwelling on the events of the day often inhibits the yin type's ability to sink into sleep, whereas the desire to leap forward into tomorrow is what makes it difficult for the Yang Type B. Sleep depends on the downward flow of energy from the lung system to the liver and kidneys. With so much energy jumping around in her upper body, utter exhaustion from overactivity is sometimes the only way the Yang Type B gets to sleep. It is crucial for her to avoid going to this extreme by controlling her tendency to go overboard.

The notion that she is running out of time often weighs heavily on the menopausal Yang Type B's mind. She frequently compromises sleep in order to stay active, only to find herself crashing every few days. This cycle would eventually wear out the other types, making them appear and feel zombie-like, but after periodically crashing, the Yang Type B bounces right up again, looking and feeling brand new. Convincing her to slow down is easier said than done, but indeed worth trying, since little does she realize that this way of life is rapidly chipping away at her vulnerable and discreet lower body energies.

Heng gom—the ability to self-reflect—hides within her weaker liver, and without finding it the Yang Type B constantly focuses outward, saddened by the tainted world in which she lives, ignoring the basic needs of her own mind and body. The unbalanced Yang Type B becomes obsessed with distinguishing between right and wrong, correct and incorrect—a quality born from the ju check within her stronger lungs. Sleep depends on creating a smooth flow of energy from her lungs to the liver through reflecting on her own right and wrong actions, refraining from excessive sorrow, eating liver-supporting foods, and incorporating the tips below.

Mantra for Better Sleep

The insomnia-ridden Yang Type B has her gaze on the future, and what hasn't been accomplished today cannot wait for tomorrow. If you have difficulty getting to sleep, try repeating, out loud or silently, the following sentence while slowly inhaling and exhaling, until you drift off into sleep: "Tomorrow can wait. It's time to shut off my active mind."

Meditation for Better Sleep

Before going to bed, try sitting in a comfortable position somewhere other than your bed, dimming the lights, and putting on some relaxing music. Close your eyes and take deep breaths. When you breathe in, think about your future hopes, desires, and plans one at a time. While breathing out, release all expectations about your hopes/desires/plans one by one while saying something like "I do not have to accomplish this now," "I'll deal with this tomorrow," and/or "Here you go Universe/Heaven/God. It's in your hands for now." You may have to inhale and exhale several times for each hope/desire/plan, but try limiting yourself to three breaths for each one.

Soothing Teas

Mint teas, mentioned in the Yang Type A section, calm the spirit and cool the stomach and liver energies of the Yang Type B too! Drink two to three cups a day between meals to curb spells of anger and sadness and relax the mind.

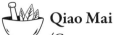 **Qiao Mai**
(Common: Buckwheat; Latin: *Fagopyrum* spp.)

Buckwheat is a cold-natured herb that helps calm the excessive yang energy of the Yang Type B. In the summer, buckwheat tea is often used to hydrate and cool the body. Buckwheat's cool nature soothes and relaxes the mind to assist with sleep. It also helps with other excessive yang conditions such as headaches, acne, and high blood pressure.

Common Uses
Buckwheat relieves insomnia, high blood pressure, headaches, acne, unsettled emotions (anger, frustration, stress), fever, and sensitivity to heat.

Sources
Buckwheat comes in several different forms. Buckwheat noodles, called soba in Japanese, are a popular summertime delicacy in Japan and Korea, where they are boiled and chilled and then eaten with a soy-based sauce. Buckwheat noodles are available from Annie Chun's or Eden Foods. Buckwheat flour for baking can be purchased from Bob's Red Mill and is often used as a gluten-free substitute for wheat flour. A very popular drink in Asia, buckwheat tea can be purchased from TeaSpring.

Preparation and Dosage
Buckwheat noodles: A recipe for preparing buckwheat noodles can be found on the Annie Chun's website. Buckwheat tea: Boil two teaspoons of dried buckwheat with two cups of water. Let simmer over low heat for five minutes. Buckwheat teabags can be boiled or steeped in warm water to make tea. Drink two to three cups of buckwheat tea daily. Try making a porridge with whole buckwheat grain by itself or with wheat and barley as kasha. Buckwheat flour can be used to make bread, cookies, and yummy pancakes!

Caution
Since buckwheat is used as food, it is generally considered a safe herb. However, its cooling effect may cause diarrhea or indigestion for the yin types, whose cool and/or cold-natured digestive systems benefit from warm, or hot-natured herbs.

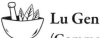 **Lu Gen**
(Common: Common Reed; Latin: *Phragmites communis*)

As we saw in our discussion of hot flashes in chapter 4, Lu Gen, or common reed, is often used to tame the excessive lung energy of the Yang Type B by transporting cool energy to the upper body and draining excess yang heat from the chest and lungs. Hence common reed addresses upper body heat-related issues such as hot flashes and insomnia.

Common Uses

Common reed relieves anxiety, worry, indigestion (stomach acid, heartburn, and/or vomiting), shortness of breath, and dry heaves.

Sources

A tincture of Lu Gen can be purchased from the Hawaii Pharm website.

Preparation and Dosage

Please follow the manufacturer's dosage guidelines. A Lu Gen tincture can be ingested after consuming buckwheat-derived foods or directly after a cup of buckwheat tea.

Brittany, the Yang Type B Superwoman

Brittany's friends were jealous of her overflowing energy. At the ripe age of sixty-one, Brittany woke up at 5:00 a.m. and worked as a director of her new organization nonstop until 7:00 p.m., six days a week, rarely taking the time to eat. On Brittany's time off from work, she would travel the world to hike the mountains of Machu Picchu, trek Mount Everest, climb Mount St. Helens, and much, much more. Brittany thought that sleep was a waste of time, and the only reason she slept three hours a night was because everyone else in her home was asleep. Occasionally Brittany noticed that her legs would suddenly give out, and she would fall to the ground without warning. In a flash, she would get up again and continue her task at hand, as if nothing had happened. After one of these episodes, Brittany began to feel uneasy, as she felt tired but not fatigued, uncomfortable but not in pain, and saddened but not depressed.

Yang Type Bs are known for looking and feeling robust and energized.

Yet if pushed too far, their legs will simply give out from under them, resulting in sudden tripping or collapsing. This condition, called *hei yok* in Korean, is often accompanied by a strange and uncomfortable sensation throughout the body. Western medicine doesn't have a diagnosis for this syndrome, as X-rays, MRIs, and the like cannot show why the Yang Type B may experience it. From the perspective of Sasang medicine, Brittany is running on empty, as her episodes of falling indicate lower body energy collapse, despite and being deceived by exuberant upper body energy. If Brittany does not address this soon by making an effort to get more sleep and tame her yang energy, she will eventually sink into depression and feel utterly exhausted . . . all the time.

YIN TYPE A

The inherently weaker lung system of the Yin Type A plays a major role when it comes to insomnia. The lungs help feed ample amounts of blood and energy to the heart when we are healthy. Weaker lungs may have trouble transferring enough energy to the heart. According to Eastern medicine, our heart is where our emotions are processed. So sleep for the Yin Type A is dependent upon an ample supply of blood and energy flowing toward her heart, which in turn helps her relax and feel emotionally balanced. When the lungs are in relatively good shape, they have little difficulty getting us to sleep at night. After dealing with chronic stress, physical/emotional trauma, or illness, the lungs may gradually weaken, initiating the vicious cycle of insomnia. For the same reasons, weaker lungs may also contribute to the onset of palpitations, feeling anxious, and being easily startled at night.

The stronger liver of the Yin Type A acts as a sponge, absorbing emotions and events of the past and having difficulty letting them go. Menopause is a time of reflection, weighing in on the events of the past to determine the role they play in our future. While this is a healthy and natural process, the Yin Type A tends to dwell on the past, storing emotions in her hyperabsorbent liver. Within her weaker lungs is the key to unlock the wisdom of ju check—the ability to determine right from wrong. With ample energy flowing from her liver to the lungs, she is able to resolve the question, "Is it 'right' for me to still feel this way?"

She may ask herself this question over and over again without resolution if the flow to the lungs is inhibited.

Lung energy is associated with the future, and liver energy with the past. The Yin Type A's menopause-related insomnia is a result of difficulty processing daily experiences and holding on to the past. Smooth energy flow from the liver to the lungs depends on the ability to release self-defeating thoughts like "If only I had done this . . ." or "Why did this happen to me?" In order for the Yin Type A to get in touch with her joyous nature, something has to give. If the past is plaguing her, then instead of wasting time trying to transform it into joy, she's better off just letting it go and giving sleep's gentle touch a chance to guide her away. At the heart of Asian philosophy is the concept of stepping back before advancing forward. For the Yin Type A this means ridding herself of toxic thoughts before attempting to find joy. If she does not cleanse her mind and body, joy will take on a twisted form that nags away deep into the evening. A smooth flow of energy from the liver to the lungs can also be promoted by daily cardiovascular exercise, consuming the lung-supporting foods listed in my book *Your Yin Yang Body Type*, and ingesting body-type-specific herbs for insomnia.

Mantra for Better Sleep

If you have difficulty getting to sleep, try repeating, out loud or silently, the following sentence while slowly inhaling and exhaling, until you drift off into sleep: "My stronger liver tends to hold on to emotions and thoughts, but now I am ready to release them."

Exercise for Better Sleep

Exercise-induced sweating is beneficial for all the yin yang body types but especially the Yin Type A because it encourages the release of toxins (via the skin pores) from her hyperabsorbent liver. While releasing toxins, it also facilitates the discharge of toxic, stressful thoughts. A little bit of sweat each day goes a long way for the Yin Type A, enhancing her ability to relax and enter a deep sleep. Exercising early in the morning is more effective than right before bed, since morning is associated with yang and movement, and evening with yin and calmness.

Soothing Teas

The following teas are especially helpful for the Yin Type A insomniac, since they calm her stronger liver—the source of dreaming and deep REM sleep.

Chamomile tea supports the Yin Type A's digestive system, encouraging the downward movement of energy. The stomach is responsible not only for digesting food but also for digesting experience. Excessive emotional stress will reverse the natural flow of stomach energy, causing it to rebel upward and bombard the heart energy. The ability to enter a deep sleep is dependent upon the descent of yin energy from the heart and lungs to the lower body.

Native to Europe and thriving in America, valerian root has been used for centuries to address insomnia, anxiety, and other emotional imbalances. Although this herb is not a member of the Sasang medicine pharmacy, my own research reveals that this herb is well tolerated and often effective for the Yin Type A suffering from these issues. Consult your physician if you are taking antidepressant medication since valerian root also has a mild sedative effect on the central nervous system.

 Suan Zao Ren
(Common: Sour Jujube Seed; Latin: *Ziziphus spinosa*)

Suan Zao Ren, or sour jujube seed, is commonly used in Eastern medicine to calm and soothe the heart and mind. These little red seeds nourish and support the function of the heart and lungs and are one of the most effective herbs to treat the Yin Type A's insomnia. For this reason, they are used in a variety of herbal formulas. Modern research has shown that sour jujube seeds contain ample amounts of flavonoids, alkaloids, and saponins, the combination of which likely contributes to their strong calming effects. A study in 2014 discovered that sour jujube is capable of enhancing REM sleep. This study also demonstrated that these effects were likely due to serotonin-mediating properties.[5] While pharmaceutical drugs that affect serotonin, like Zoloft and Paxil, also assist with sleep, they often have numerous unwanted side effects, whereas sour jujube is known to be relatively safe.[6]

Common Uses
Sour jujube alleviates insomnia, anemia, anxiety, nervousness, stress, night sweating, thirst, and palpitations.

Sources
Sour jujube is readily available in China and Korea, but it is difficult to obtain raw in the United States. It is, however, included within a popular and easily obtained formula that helps with sleep, Suan Zao Ren Tang (sour jujube decoction), which can be purchased from the Chinese Herbs Direct and Vita Living websites.

Preparation and Dosage
Please refer to the manufacturer for dosage instructions.

Caution
Consult a professional if you are taking other medications for sleep before trying sour jujube. If combined with other sleep medications it may cause excessive drowsiness.

Herbal Friend: Bai Zi Ren
(Common: Arborvitae Seed; Latin: *Platycladus orientalis*)

Bai Zi Ren, or arborvitae seed, is routinely prescribed with sour jujube in Sasang medicine for insomnia, anxiety, and stress. They both support heart and lung energy, addressing such issues as heart palpitations, shortness of breath, and chronic lung/heart-related illnesses. Arborvitae seed has the added benefit of addressing night sweats and promoting a smooth bowel movement. A combination of sour jujube and arborvitae seed can be found in the formula An Shen Ding Zhi Wan (Calm the Spirit and Support the Willpower Pill). Although this is not a Sasang-based herbal formula and contains a few herbs for other body types, it is primarily (more than 80 percent) made with Yin Type A herbs and is both safe and effective. It can be purchased on the Bio Essence Herbal Essentials website (bioessence.com; type "An Shen Ding Zhi Wan" in the search bar).

Laura, the Nocturnal Yin Type A

Laura is a renowned artist who thrives in the late evening; all her senses are at their peak and creativity streams smoothly and steadily after 11:00 p.m. But poor Laura can hardly function during the day. Her husband has to practically peel her out of bed every morning so that she can be at least somewhat functional by midday. Laura looks forward to the evenings, even to the point of checking her watch throughout the day in anticipation of the 11:00 p.m. hour, when she suddenly feels like a different person. I asked Laura if she ever went to bed early, and she recalled a phase when she had to get up for work by 6:00 a.m. and didn't feel fatigued during the day, but there was little to no creative energy flowing within her. If it came to choosing between daytime energy and creativity, Laura would choose creativity.

YIN TYPE B

The stronger kidneys of the Yin Type B give her a sturdy foundation of comfort and calmness, but when her kidneys are not balanced, she is prone to nervousness, fear, and insomnia. Her sluggish digestive system can easily make matters worse, as it takes her stomach longer to break down food, often hacking away at it until late in the evening. Indigestion may cause bodily energy to rebel upward and bombard the heart, which can also result in anxiety and/or insomnia. The adult Yin Type B, all too aware of this phenomenon, limits her food intake, often to the point of fearing food altogether. Going to bed on an empty stomach is just as detrimental as a full stomach, as the stomach energies swish this way and that in search of food. Determining when and what to introduce into her sensitive mind and body poses a continuous challenge for the Yin Type B that doesn't get any easier during menopause. The onset of menopause itself is like introducing a new food to the Yin Type B's cautious stomach. Aware of this, the balanced menopausal Yin Type B makes comfort her priority, not just a desire, and enhances her ability to tolerate, accept, and assimilate new foods, friends, and life transitions—qualities born from the do ryang residing deep within the kidney system.

While dignity and valiance come from the spleen and contribute to the Yang Type A's naturally poised appearance, *gung shim*—worry, distress, and anxiousness—also lurk within the spleen, awaiting the opportunity to wreak havoc. Without receiving ample flow from her stronger kidneys, the Yin Type B's spleen unleashes gung shim, and fear of even the smallest of life's challenges begins to surface. Through mastering do ryang she is capable of taming gung shim—a process that starts with calming and quieting her mind while still making an attempt to venture out and interact with others. Warmth is an excellent and effective way to promote calmness for the Yin Type B. Facing life's challenges is a lot easier with warm friends, a warm home, and one of the greatest gifts of all, a heating pad to warm her cold lower abdomen.

Timing Your Dinner

The sensitive digestive system of the Yin Type B makes it necessary for her to plan carefully when and what to eat for dinner. If she eats her last meal of the day after 7:00 p.m. or before 5:00 p.m., then getting to sleep may be difficult.

Mantra for Better Sleep

If you have difficulty getting to sleep, try repeating, out loud or silently, the following sentence while slowly inhaling and exhaling, until you drift off into sleep: "Thanks to my strong kidneys, I can be exceptionally secure and comfortable. It's time to let go of my insecurities."

Warming Up Your Abdomen

Excessive cold in her lower abdomen easily singes the embers of the Yin Type B's cozy but fragile fire, making heat a central part of staying healthy. Try placing a heating pad over your abdomen before sleeping at night to warm your center, and you'll be amazed at how comfortable and relaxing it feels. You may try buying an electric pad with a timer so that you can drift off to sleep while basking in delicious warmth. Otherwise, lying in bed with your heating pad on for twenty to thirty minutes before sleep will suffice.

Meditation for Better Sleep

While lying on your back with a heating pad, or another source of gentle heat, on your lower abdomen, take slow deep breaths, and imagine the heat radiating through your body like a bright light, warming and illuminating the cold darkness.

Soothing Teas

The following teas are especially helpful for the Yin Type B insomniac since they support and nourish her stronger kidneys—the source of comfort, calmness, and a good night's sleep.

Cinnamon tea is one of the healthiest drinks for the Yin Type B, for it warms her weaker digestive system and promotes the flow of energy to and through her stronger kidneys, enhancing calmness. The Yin Type B sleeps her best when the core of her body feels warm and her stomach is not preoccupied with digesting a heavy dinner.

Licorice tea is another one for the Yin Type B that warms the stomach and soothes the flow of energy throughout her body. Its calming and nourishing properties make it an appropriate choice for assisting with sleep, anxiety, and stress.

 ## Da Zao
(Common: Chinese Jujube; Latin: *Ziziphus jujuba*)

Da Zao, or Chinese jujube, a sweet-tasting fruit often used in Asian dishes, is said to nourish the heart and blood. In Eastern medicine, herbs that support the heart also help with insomnia, as the heart plays a major role in processing/releasing daily emotions and facilitating sleep. The true merit of Chinese jujube, though, comes from its ability to support the weaker digestive system of the Yin Type B. By balancing her digestive system, Chinese jujube can assist with her heart function. In Eastern medicine, it is often decocted with other herbs to balance and harmonize their properties. Recent studies suggest that Chinese jujube increases the flow of oxygen to the heart.[7]

Common Uses

Chinese jujube alleviates insomnia, indigestion, anemia, visual impairments (blurry and weak vision, floaters), anxiety, stress, and a lack of energy.

Sources

There are many ways to acquire Chinese jujube. For the gardener, purchasing a Chinese jujube tree might be the method of choice. Willis Orchard Company and Ty Ty Nursery offer mail-order Chinese jujube trees, also known as Li jujubes, which grow rapidly in almost all climate zones throughout the northern United States. Chinese jujube is also available in bulk or extract form from manufacturers such as ActiveHerb and Chinese Herbs Direct.

Preparation and Dosage

Raw Chinese jujube: Slice three dried fruits into thin sections and boil with two cups of water. Let simmer for thirty minutes over low heat. If the water level sinks rapidly, add another half a cup and then monitor. If the water level continues to sink, reduce or turn off the heat. Drink one cup up to four times a day for insomnia. Avoid drinking directly before bedtime so you aren't awakened for a trip to the bathroom.

Caution

Chinese jujube can cause fullness and distension of the abdomen in other body types. If you experience these symptoms consistently when ingesting Chinese jujube, then stop immediately. It is sometimes very difficult to determine your body type. Try taking the yin yang body type test again or log onto the Sasang medicine website for more tips on how to determine your body type.

Herbal Friend: Shan Zha
(Common: Hawthorn Fruit; Latin: *Crataegus pinnatifida*)

Shan Zha, or hawthorn fruit, doesn't only share the same color and shape of a human heart, it also nourishes and strengthens it! The Yin Type B's heart is by no means a constitutionally weaker organ, but it is nonetheless prone to injury if she struggles with anxiety, fear, and lack of comfort. Hawthorn helps return uprooted comfort to her kidneys, restoring vitality, warmth, and inner strength. Hawthorn and Chinese jujube enhance one another's ability to nourish and support the heart, calm the emotions, and nourish the Yin Type B's blood and essence. A nonalcoholic liquid extract of hawthorn can be purchased on the Piping Rock Health Products website. It can also be found in capsule form on the Nature's Way and Puritan's Pride websites. Please follow the manufacturer's recommendation for dosage. Ingest both Chinese jujube and hawthorn in one sitting for best results.

8

Minding the Waterline

Urinary Health

Frances was relieved to know that menopause had finally passed, putting an end to years of hot flashes, night sweats, mood swings, and insomnia. She convinced herself that these had been the worst of times and that things could only get better. Yet she was not prepared for what happened one evening when a friend joked about a goofy coworker. As soon as Frances started laughing, she noticed a sudden urge to urinate. Frances had read about urinary incontinence but thought that it would never happen to her. Seeing it as just a fluke, she tried forgetting about that episode only to realize that when she sneezed the following day, a tiny bit of urine again trickled out. Frances chalked this up to menopause and decided not to mention it to anyone, thinking that it would probably go away on its own.

When to See Your Doctor

- Blood in your urine may indicate a kidney infection or other kidney-related issue.
- Acute bladder infections should be addressed immediately to avoid the possibility of spreading to the kidneys.
- Urine output significantly greater than fluid intake may indicate the onset of diabetes.

What Frances didn't know was that there are ways to treat urinary incontinence and that if left alone, it may progress into more frequent and difficult episodes. While she and her friends talked for hours about other menopausal symptoms, nobody seemed to mention anything about urinary incontinence. This gave Frances the false notion that others around her were free of this issue, despite the fact that it occurs in three out of ten postmenopausal women.

WESTERN AND EASTERN PERSPECTIVES ON URINARY HEALTH

In Western medicine urinary incontinence is often explained to be a result of hormone loss. Estrogen is responsible for nourishing the uterine wall, which includes the cervix—where urine exits from the bladder. As estrogen decreases, so does the integrity of the bladder wall. Although this is likely the most common cause of urinary incontinence after menopause, there are other explanations, such as prolapse of the uterus due to the relaxation of the pelvic wall, UTIs, post-surgical issues, or nervous system disorders. If you are not sure what the source is, I recommend that you seek the advice of a medical professional.

Stress incontinence is the most common form of urinary incontinence, most often occurring in younger and middle-aged women who urinate or feel like urinating when coughing, sneezing, exercising, laughing, lifting heavy things, and other movements that put pressure on the bladder. Urge incontinence occurs without pressure on the bladder from the above issues and is marked by the urge to urinate when sleeping or hearing the sound of running water. This type of incontinence is more common after menopause and in those who have diabetes, stroke, dementia, Parkinson's disease, or multiple sclerosis. Other, less common types of incontinence include the occurrence of a bladder infection or other illness/handicap that interferes with the process of urination.

In Eastern medicine, stress and urge incontinence are often the result of yang deficiency. Yang energy typically moves upward, so when yang is deficient, energy within the body tends to sink downward, occasionally taking the bladder and other organs with it. In Sasang medicine, the source of deficient yang differs according to the body type, depending on each one's stronger and weaker organs, and is often due to an imbalance of organ-related emotion. Stronger organs produce excessive or intense emotions, while weaker organs may inhibit our ability to express or get in touch with certain emotions. The bladder gives us the ability to release excessive emotion and hold on to others that, as humans, we may need to experience and feel before letting them go. Health is the ability to hold on and let go depending on what each situation in life calls for.

THE YIN AND YANG OF URINARY HEALTH

In Sasang medicine, urinary issues are separated into two categories: excess and deficiency. Excess urinary issues are due to energy stagnation and accumulation, whereas deficiency-related issues are caused by weakness and lack of nourishment. Bladder pressure and heat will increase when energy stagnates within the bladder. Hence incontinence caused by a UTI is less likely a deficiency issue but rather heat stagnation within the bladder.

Since yang energy flows upward and yin energy flows downward, the former helps keep urine within the bladder, while the latter facilitates the flow of urine outward from the body. The continuous desire to hold on to certain things, people, and/or situations will eventually cause stagnation of heat within the bladder. When heat stagnates, inflammation of the bladder will follow, resulting in the inability to evacuate urine completely. This may also be accompanied by painful or burning urination with possible traces of blood. Bladder inflammation, too, is often due to stagnation of emotion, especially anger, sorrow, and lack of comfort. I'll discuss this further as it applies to each of the four body types.

Inflammation and infection of the urinary bladder are often the result of holding on to excess emotion, and weakness is commonly the aftermath of this process, when the body simply can't endure this excess any longer. Urination is one way that we get rid of unwanted thoughts and emotions. I once had a hiking buddy who made it a habit to urinate as soon as we reached the summit and the stunning scenery unfolded before our eyes. He told me that nothing ever felt so good! The lower half of our body rarely gets the attention it needs. We tend to hold it in at work or when out and about simply because we are so focused on the task at hand that the bladder signal goes unheeded. Sounds, smells, sights, tastes, and emotions enter our body through our head and exit via the lower abdomen. It's easier to focus on the external environment and what enters the body than it is to reflect inward and on what we need to release.

Sasang medicine associates the urinary bladder with the kidney system—the Yin Type B's strongest organ system—and calmness. By nature, the Yin Type B is the calmest of the four body types, and her bladder is the healthiest when calm. The kidneys represent inner calmness; the urinary bladder, outward calmness. It is easier for the Yin Type B to feel calm at home or in a quiet place but challenging for her to experience it outside or around other people, since she is extremely sensitive to her environment. A Yin Type B might say, "If only I could just be left alone" or "If others didn't interfere, my life would be quiet and peaceful." A lack of comfort in one's surroundings will eventually cause the bladder to lose its tone and integrity, leading to frequent urination or UTIs.

Anger, associated with the spleen and upward flow, prevents the Yang Type A's bladder from receiving energy, making it one of her weakest organs. Hence the Yang Type A is prone to urinary disorders and/or lack of bladder tone. Curbing her anger and finding the time to relax are essential factors in balancing and reinforcing energy flow to her bladder. Before we discuss this further, let's review several tips for supporting the urinary bladder no matter which yin yang body you are.

Tip #1: Practice Bladder Exercises

During the menopausal transition, the lining of the urethra begins to thin and the pelvic floor muscles may also start to weaken, often leading to urinary issues. Kegel exercises are 80 percent effective against urinary incontinence in postmenopausal women. There are several ways to perform these exercises, but the first step is to identify your perineal muscles—the muscles used when doing Kegel exercises. This is done by stopping your urine flow midstream. You may need to repeat this several times throughout the course of a day or week until they become familiar. Once you get acquainted with your perineal muscles, it's time to try Kegel exercises. For the beginner, start by lying down on your back with your knees bent and feet on the floor. Squeeze your pelvic and vaginal muscles inward and upward as you lift your lower back off the floor. Hold this position for three seconds and repeat four times. As you advance with Kegels, try holding this position longer or increasing the repetitions.*

The use of vaginal weights is another way to condition the muscles involved with urination and strengthen the pelvic floor, cervix, and vaginal wall, which are responsible for keeping the door to urine flow closed until it is time to urinate. There are several vaginal weight products out there, and I've found from my own research that one type is not necessarily better than the other. Some products are made from medical-grade silicone, while others are made from jade. Both products are effective, but jade itself has healing properties that may offer further benefit. In Chinese medicine it is said that, rubbed over the kidneys, jade helps alleviate kidney stones and bladder issues. Not to mention, it is natural! Silicone is more flexible and not as heavy as jade, making it an easier and potentially more comfortable way to start using vaginal weights. Nowadays there's an app for everything and vaginal exercises are no exception, with products like kGoal and Elvie that are inserted into the vagina and allow you to monitor your Kegel exercises via a cell phone.

Tip #2: Reduce Coffee Intake

I'm sure this is the last tip some of you would like to hear, since coffee is one of the most popular ways to start the day. Unfortunately, the combination of caffeine and diuretic properties within the coffee bean does not sit well with the bladder, since the former sends yang energy upward, away from the bladder, and the latter pushes yin downward, creating the urge to urinate. Hence coffee often makes urinary incontinence and UTIs even worse! I recommend reducing your coffee intake to less than a cup a day or switching to decaf. Eliminating coffee altogether would be the best option, since even decaffeinated coffee can

---

*Search for "Kegel exercises" on Youtube for several other variations. One good video is "How to Do Kegel Exercises That Strengthen Your Pelvic Floor.

interfere with your bladder. The same goes for other drinks with higher caffeine levels, such as black tea, Coca-Cola, Pepsi, and so forth.

Tip #3: Try Acupuncture and Acupressure

Acupressure and acupuncture are often helpful for urinary issues. A pilot study involving eighty-five women with bladder control issues showed that after four weekly treatments with acupuncture, they achieved significant improvement.[1]

Acupressure, or placing pressure on acupuncture points, is another way to support the bladder without the use of needles. There are over 360 points on the human body, each with a unique ability to stimulate the flow of bodily energy or qi. Bladder control issues are often a result of sinking yin energy or stagnant yang energy. The REN6 acupressure point revives the flow of yin within the body, while the DU2 point restores the natural flow of yang. Both points can be stimulated for yin and yang issues related to the bladder. The UB66 acupuncture point is often used for inflammation due to yang heat stagnation in the bladder.

When practicing acupressure, apply enough pressure so that you are feeling a dull ache but not to the point of producing sharp pain or significant discomfort. Applying significant pressure to each point until it feels tender often yields better results than a light touch. Those who are on the sensitive side may feel a gentle tingling sensation, indicating the stimulation of qi.

☯ REN6 (SIXTH POINT ON THE CONCEPTION VESSEL MERIDIAN): "SEA OF QI"

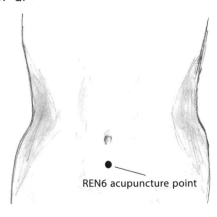

REN6 acupuncture point

Fig. 8.1. REN6, sixth point on the conception vessel meridian

This point is located one-and-a-half thumb widths directly below the midline of the umbilicus (see fig. 8.1 on the previous page).

* Use the thumb or pointer finger to apply direct pressure to REN6 for approximately twenty seconds.
* Gently release.
* Repeat three to five times.

DU2 (SECOND POINT ON THE GOVERNING VESSEL MERIDIAN): "LUMBAR TRANSPORTING POINT"

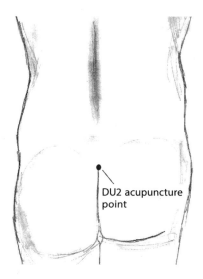

DU2 acupuncture point

Fig. 8.2. DU2, second point on the governing vessel meridian

This point is located in the center of the hiatus, at the base of the sacrum directly above the tailbone (see fig. 8.2 above).

* Use the thumb or pointer finger to apply direct pressure to DU2 for approximately twenty seconds.
* Gently release.
* Repeat three to five times.

UB66 (SIXTY-SIXTH POINT ON THE URINARY BLADDER MERIDIAN): "VALLEY PASSAGE"

This point is located on the lateral side of the foot along the crease of the fifth toe at the junction of red and white skin (see fig. 8.3 on the next page).

* Use the thumb or pointer finger to apply direct pressure to UB66 for approximately twenty seconds.

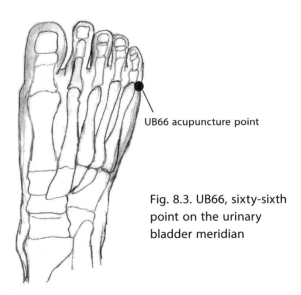

UB66 acupuncture point

Fig. 8.3. UB66, sixty-sixth point on the urinary bladder meridian

✳ Gently release and then switch to the other foot.

✳ Repeat this process three to five times.

Tip #4: Heed Nature's Call

If you feel the urge to urinate and have access to a bathroom, bush, tree, or bucket, then obey your body's message. Holding it in sets you up for UTIs and bladder wall irritation. If the urge to urinate comes way too often and/or urine output exceeds the amount of fluid intake, then you may be suffering from a UTI, bladder prolapse, or other condition worth discussing with your doctor.

URINARY HEALTH AND THE YIN YANG BODY TYPES

As mentioned above, each of the four body types has its own reason for bladder-related issues based on specific yin and yang characteristics. Born with a weaker urinary system and a lack of lower body energy, the yang types are prone to incontinence and dysuria, making it difficult for them to drink substantial amounts of water without frequently rushing to the bathroom. Insufficient kidney and bladder energy may also lead to inadequate urine flow, making it difficult for the yang types to completely void the bladder. The yin types, with a stronger urinary system and lower body energy, have a tendency to ignore the voice of their bladder and get away with it until it yells, "Urinate now or else!" Holding in urine for prolonged periods of time makes the yin types more susceptible to UTIs than the yang types. Despite such tendencies, both yin and yang types may experience the same urinary issues, such as UTIs and incontinence, making it crucial to determine the body-type-related root cause. Bladder treatment for the yang types in Sasang medicine is primarily aimed at strengthening the bladder; for the yin types, it's promoting the movement of energy to avoid bladder stagnation. Yet there are also situations that require bladder strengthening for the yin types and energy movement for the yang types, so read carefully before beginning your Sasang herbal regime!

YANG TYPE A

In Lee Je-ma's treatise on Sasang medicine, he states that the Yang Type A "has a well-developed, wide chest and broad shoulders but a loss of urinary bladder-area muscle tone."[2] The Yin Type B, on the other hand, has stronger urinary bladder muscle tone and a narrow chest and shoulders. This difference is a valuable tool for distinguishing between a Yang Type A and Yin Type B. When pressed lightly, the Yang Type A's lower abdomen (approximately one to two inches below the navel) easily sinks inward, but the Yin Type B's feels more resistant and full even if the bladder is empty.

The Yang Type A's stronger yang energy often bypasses the lower body organs, making a U-turn in the upper body before it reaches the kidneys. The Yang Type A's predominant emotion of anger and lack of yin comfort are the culprits, pumping yang energy upward and away from her weaker yin organs. The bladder has difficulty holding urine when yang doesn't mingle with yin. Ideally, these two energies should blend into one another, resolving their differences, but the reduction of yin energy during menopause often exacerbates the accumulation of yang in the upper body, giving rise to irritability and anger. Table 8.1 on page 230 and the sections that follow provide two Yang Type A bladder-issue scenarios and their resolution.

TABLE 8.1. THE YANG TYPE A'S BLADDER ISSUES

	Scenario A	Scenario B
Symptoms	Bladder infection, UTI, bladder inflammation	Bladder prolapse, frequent urination and/or incontinence without infection
Emotional Component	Anger and rage causing yang to accumulate in the spleen and kidney areas	Long-term anger and rage causing yang to accumulate in the upper body and vacate the lower body
Mechanism	Yang stagnates	Yin sinks
Organs Involved	Stronger spleen	Weaker kidneys
Other Potential Symptoms	Fever, reddish complexion, sensitivity to heat, excessive appetite	Fatigue, pale complexion, common-cold symptoms, weakness of the lower body

Yang Type A Bladder Issue: Scenario A

The Yang Type A's anger causes energy to rise upward, leading to stagnation and accumulation of yang energy in the upper body. Without enough circulating energy in the lower body, intestinal and bladder functions may be affected, resulting in constipation and disrupted urination. This is often, but not always, accompanied by a burning sensation with urination coming from the Yang Type A's excessive heat transferring from her stronger spleen to the weaker kidney system, which includes the urinary bladder and sacral area. Heat accumulation in the bladder may result in kidney, urinary tract, and/or bladder infections.

Resolution

Although it comes naturally for the Yang Type A, anger doesn't always result in illness. If the Yang Type A learns to release her anger rather than hold on to it, then bowel and urine will flow smoothly. Only when she has trouble letting go of anger does she experience heat-related issues. Letting go of anger doesn't mean vomiting it up and out but instead letting it sink into a comfort zone before you lash out. This takes considerable self-reflection—a challenge for every body type. Actually it's healthy excretion from the bladder and intestines that primarily determines the health of the yang types. Try drinking at least eight glasses of water a day and taking the time out of your busy schedule to urinate. And if someone rubs you the wrong way, take a deep breath in and then release.

Excessive anger leads to stagnation, and stagnation leads to bacterial accumulation and inflammation. The Yang Type A's UTI is commonly a result of her holding on to anger if a situation she is faced with lingers on without resolution. When she knows that a solution isn't immediately available, energy boils up within her, causing inflammation and accumulation. Lurking within her weaker bladder is *gwa shim*—the tendency to overreact, lash out at others, and be overcritical. By making an effort to tolerate and yield to others and accept her situation, she sends ample energy to the bladder, balancing gwa shim and avoiding bladder infections. Taking anger away from a Yang Type A is like plucking all of the quills from a porcupine. Not only would this be extremely painful, but it would inflict serious injury on both the porcupine and the plucker. When she takes a step back and reflects on it before lashing out, her anger has a much better chance of expressing itself appropriately. Channeling anger in the right direction can pump up more energy and promote humor, righteousness, clarity, ambition, and ultimately humility—the Yang Type A's virtue.

The following are herbs and foods that support the Yang Type A's weaker bladder and curb anger.

 ## Zhi Zi
(Common: Gardenia; Latin: *Gardenia jasminoides*)

In Eastern medicine, Zhi Zi, or gardenia, is used to clear heat from every nook and cranny of the body. It is especially effective in clearing heat from the urinary and digestive systems. Yang Type As have a tendency to accumulate heat in the stomach, which can easily spread to the bladder. Bacterial infection, inflammation, and accumulation of pressure are also correlated with excessive heat in the body. Hence gardenia is effective in reducing the Yang Type A's high blood pressure, among other heat-related issues. It has also been shown to increase the metabolic rate of obese middle-aged women taking hormone replacement.[3]

Common Uses

Gardenia alleviates urinary tract and bladder infections, high blood pressure, indigestion, anxiety, stress, nervousness, insomnia, inflammation of the muscles and joints, fever, and hot flashes.

Sources

Gardenia extract can be found on the Stakich website. Avid gardeners may purchase seeds from Tropical Oasis on Amazon. This plant is definitely worth the effort to cultivate for its beauty and fragrance. The fruits (flower bulbs) are collected in the fall and are sun-dried for tea.

Preparation and Dosage

Follow the dosage guidelines listed by each manufacturer. If the raw herb is used, prepare a tea by boiling up to six bulbs in two cups of water. Let the tea simmer for fifteen minutes. Drink half a mug of warm tea up to three times a day.

Caution

While gardenia fruit is very effective in reducing blood pressure, it is known to interfere with the effects of antihypertensive medication. Be sure to consult with a professional before taking this herb if you have been prescribed antihypertensive medication. Discontinue gardenia in cases of loose stools or loss of appetite. This herb is very cooling and should not be ingested by yin types, with their cooler energy.

Herbal Friend: Jin Yin Hua
(Common: Japanese Honeysuckle; Latin: *Lonicera japonica*)

Jin Yin Hua, or Japanese honeysuckle, has been used for thousands of years as a Chinese remedy for bacterial infection, as it contains chlorogenic acid, which is known to have powerful antibiotic and antioxidant effects. Pharmaceutical antibiotics have a tendency to disturb the natural balance of bacterial flora in the body. However, the antibiotic effects of honeysuckle in its natural form are much gentler on the system because they help restore the natural balance of the body. Honeysuckle is a helpful remedy for bladder infections of the

Yang Type A, and its antibiotic properties are greatly enhanced when combined with gardenia. Boil nine grams of dried honeysuckle with six bulbs of gardenia in two cups of water. Let the tea simmer for fifteen minutes. Drink half a mug of warm tea up to three times a day.

Not only are the flowers of Japanese honeysuckle beautiful, but they also emit a pleasant fragrance. Gardeners can purchase this medicinal plant online on the Nature Hills Nursery website, or you may also be able to buy this popular shrub at your local nursery. Japanese honeysuckle can also be purchased as a dried herb on the TeaSpring website.

Caution

Japanese honeysuckle has a very cold nature and is a strong natural antibiotic. It is therefore not recommended for use without heat-related symptoms. It is also not recommended for the yin types, who often succumb to cold-related issues.

Yang Type A Bladder Issue: Scenario B

Anger moves the energy upward within the body and depression sinks it downward. Taken to the extreme, the Yang Type A's untethered anger may morph into intense sadness and depression after burning itself out. In Sasang medicine, this is known as a yang explosion leading to a yin collapse, which may instigate stress incontinence or bladder prolapse. In Scenario A, the Yang Type A's anger is still in full force, but in this scenario it has run out of fuel.

Resolution

With excessive energy in the upper body and deficiency in the lower, the menopausal Yang Type A is prone to bladder and/or uterine weakness and prolapse—a situation where the uterus or urinary bladder sinks downward, causing a frequent urge to urinate without completely evacuating. This is the result of holding on to her predominant emotion of anger for several months, years, or decades, giving rise to the Yang Type A's outward expression of sorrow. At this point she's no longer able to hold on to anger, or urine for that matter, and is prone to utter exhaustion, sadness, and depression. If the menopausal

Yang Type A has yet to get in touch with and balance her anger, she'll be prone to feeling this way. It's never too late to address her anger, but when it gets to this point she'll first have to rekindle her energy through relaxation (meditation, yoga, Tai Chi, and so on) and the use of Sasang foods and herbs. The use of Kegel exercises is known to help prevent and possibly address bladder weakness and early stage prolapse (see general tips above). In Sasang medicine urinary frequency and prolapse are related to the sinking of yin in the lower body. The herbs listed below promote the flow of yin to the lower body and restore the health of Yang Type A's bladder.

Hai Cao
(Common: Seaweed, Kelp, Bladderwrack, Kombu, Wakame, Nori)
Seaweed is commonly used in Eastern medicine to nourish and strengthen the kidneys, making it one of the best foods for the Yang Type A. It contains high concentrations of iodine, which has traditionally been used in both Eastern and Western medicine to treat urinary tract disorders—hence the name *bladder*-wrack given to one type of seaweed. Iodine has also been shown to prevent certain types of breast and stomach cancer. Studies suggest that seaweed inhibits the growth of endometrial and breast cancers since these diseases are rare among Japanese women, who consume it in high amounts.[4]

Common Uses
Seaweed addresses bladder weakness (prolapse, lack of muscle tone, urinary incontinence, decreased urine flow without infection) and lower body weakness.

Sources
Seaweed can be purchased in capsule form from Swanson Health Products and from Life Extension. Sushi nori, or sheets of dried seaweed, sold in snack-sized packages or as larger sheets, can be used to make rice balls and homemade sushi or can simply be consumed as a snack food. If you live near the ocean and have access, fresh seaweed is always the best option.

Preparation and Dosage

If you are taking seaweed as a supplement, please refer to the manu-facturer's suggestions and the caution section below. Otherwise, enjoy a daily seaweed snack or mix seaweed with rice as kimbap, sushi, or another Korean or Japanese dish.

Caution

Avoid seaweed if you have an overactive thyroid condition such as hyperthyroidism or cardiac problems and/or during pregnancy and breastfeeding. It is not recommended for children under five years old. The recommended daily intake of iodine is 90 micrograms for children from five to eight years, 130 micrograms for children up to thirteen years, and 150 micrograms for adults.

Herbal Friend: Hei Mei
(Common Name: Blackberries; Latin: *Rubus fruticosus*)

Because they help nourish and strengthen the kidneys, blackberries are one of the best foods for Yang Type As. They are often used in combination with herbs in Eastern medicine to address kidney and urinary disorders. Blackberries can be consumed regularly to pre-vent UTIs, assist with urinary incontinence, and support sore or weak lower back and legs. Seaweed and blackberries work together to strengthen the kidneys and bladder, preventing and supporting the healing of urinary issues. Double up on bladder support by eating a handful of blackberries after a seaweed-complemented meal.

YANG TYPE B

The Yang Type B's center of energy is in the uppermost part of her body. This area, controlled by the lungs, provides her with ample upper body strength but weaker and sometimes nonexistent lower body strength. Hence the muscles that contract the urinary bladder are often lacking integrity, causing both urine retention and a consistent urge to urinate. Lee Je-ma stated that regular urination frequency is a sign of health for Yang Type Bs since it indicates that their excessive upper body energy is capable of descending without collapsing.

The Yang Type B's predominant emotion of sorrow sends energy upward from the lungs to nourish the brain. When sorrow is balanced, this energy flows smoothly upward and is then sent downward to nourish the rest of the body. Yet uncontrolled sorrow causes lung energy to rebel upward, overwhelming the upper body and disregarding the lower. Unbalanced sorrow is the biggest culprit behind urinary disorders of the Yang Type B. Unlike the yin types, her sorrow is not associated with loss but rather with the inability to achieve and turn into reality what her powerful mind has in store. Disappointment and lack of accomplishment weigh extremely heavily on the mind of a menopausal Yang Type B.

The ascent of yang energy from the lungs stimulates the Yang Type B brain and enhances her ability to think logically. The other body types are often awed by her quick-witted insight and sharp mind. Intuition and the ability to perceive independent of reasoning, however, come from yin type territory, the lower body, and the cultivation of jei gan—the deep-seated feeling of connection and balance with one's environment—in the lumbar spine. Instead, the Yang Type B has her gaze on the heavens above, rarely finding the time to connect with anything and anyone below. Table 8.2 and the sections that follow provide two Yang Type B bladder-issue scenarios and their resolution.

TABLE 8.2. THE YANG TYPE B'S BLADDER ISSUES

	Scenario A	Scenario B
Symptoms	Bladder infection, UTI, bladder inflammation	Bladder prolapse, incomplete urine stream and/or incontinence without infection
Emotional Component	Sorrow, despair	Anger, rage
Mechanism	Yang stagnates	Yin sinks
Organs Involved	Stronger lungs	Weaker liver
Other Potential Symptoms	Loss of balance and lack of coordination in the lower body	Vomiting after meals, acid reflux, dry heaves, inability to digest meat

Yang Type B Bladder Issue: Scenario A

The Yang Type B's jung emotion of anger may lead to stagnation of the lung's energy and blood, causing yang heat energy to accumulate in the chest rather than descend, resulting in constipation and lack of smooth urination. A burning sensation may also accompany urination due to excessive heat transferring from the lungs to the lower body.

Resolution

Sorrow comes naturally for the Yang Type B, but it does not always result in illness. If the Yang Type B learns to work with her sorrow rather than hold on to it, then bowel and urine will flow smoothly. Unbalanced sorrow causes the Yang Type B to feel as if others are untrustworthy. Holding on to sorrow causes her to hold on to urine, while channeling it in the right direction encourages the smooth flow of urine. The balanced Yang Type B may still grieve often, but she uses this emotion to love and understand the suffering of others. Her love is capable of being extremely powerful as long as she lowers her gaze and shines the light of her heaven-engrossed energy toward humanity.

The following are foods and herbs that help balance grief and support the Yang Type B's bladder.

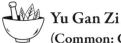 **Yu Gan Zi**
(Common: Gooseberry; Latin: *Phyllanthus emblica*)

Yu Gan Zi (meaning "sweet fruit remaining"), or gooseberry, has been used for thousands of years in Chinese medicine and even longer in Ayurvedic medicine to address diarrhea, jaundice, inflammation, and stomach weakness and for moistening the throat to alleviate a dry cough. In Sasang medicine, it is used to cool and encourage the downward flow of the Yang Type B's excessive upper body yang heat. It is also known to have natural antibiotic, antioxidant, and hypolipidemic (fat-tissue-reducing) properties. Gooseberry is very high in vitamin C, which increases the acidity levels of urine, creating an unfavorable environment for bacteria growth. A recent study also suggests that high levels of antioxidants and the ability to decrease monoamine oxidase levels in the brain make gooseberry a viable remedy for depression.[5]

Common Uses
Gooseberry relieves bladder infections, dysuria (difficult or painful urine flow), burning urination, diarrhea, jaundice, inflammation, stomach weakness, dry throat, and depression.

Sources
Admittedly, gooseberry is not the easiest fruit to get hold of unless you'd like to have this beautiful fruit growing in your yard. Check availability at your local nursery. If you're not ready to start an herb garden, then give dried gooseberry a try. You can find an organic source at Nuts.com. Gooseberry extract, under its synonym *amla,* can also be purchased from Swanson Health Products.

Preparation and Dosage
Snack on a handful of fresh or dried gooseberries daily to prevent UTIs, or use in capsule form if an infection has already manifested. For capsules, please follow the manufacturer's suggested dosage.

Caution
This is a cold-natured herb that cools the excessive yang heat of the Yang Type B but freezes the already cold organs of the yin types. The Yin Type A may get away with consuming gooseberry once in a while, but the Yin Type B, more sensitive to cold, should avoid it altogether.

Yang Type B Bladder Issue: Scenario B
The Yang Type B's deep sorrow may morph into intense anger—her jung emotion—causing yang energy to rebel upward from the lungs, vacating the lower body and bladder. As a result, it loses its ability to store urine and/or maintain bladder wall tone. Expressing her anger at this point is just as detrimental as holding it in. The anger-ridden Yang Type B is fed up with others and the direction her world is going in. She is no longer interested in doing what is right but instead implements her own self-seeking agenda. As time goes on her anger and upward-bearing energy intensifies, eventually leading to urinary incontinence and possible bladder prolapse.

Resolution

There is so much in our world today that could easily bring us down and cause anger. The Yang Type B is particularly sensitive to these issues, especially since she feels it is her responsibility to make everything better! She easily fails to see things from others' point of view and instead forces her opinion on them. This tendency comes from *tal shim*—the impure aspect of the urinary bladder that surfaces when it is ignored. Also residing within the bladder is bang ryak. *Bang* means "direction" or "path," and *ryak* "to regulate" or "control." Therefore, bang ryak is defined as the ability to control one's mind and to follow one's life's path. The Yang Type B desires to walk before she can crawl, swallow before she chews, and finish before she even gets started. By taking a deep breath and returning to the drawing board, being patient with others and especially herself, she will naturally send more energy to the bladder and improve her overall health. Below are two fruits that could also help calm her anger and help rebellious yang energy descend.

 ## Mu Gua
(Common: Chinese Quince; Latin: *Chaenomeles lagenaria*)

Mu Gua, or quince, is a fruit with a taste somewhere between that of a pear and an apple if mixed with honey or sugar. Without sweetener, it is astringent and bitter, and it is seldom consumed fresh. In Sasang medicine, the dried fruit (including the peel) is often used to treat the Yang Type B's indigestion, lower body weakness, and lower back and knee joint pain. Quince's strong ability to strengthen the lower body makes it a commonly used herb for urinary incontinence and bladder weakness. Quince is also a good source of vitamin A, fiber, and iron.

Common Uses

Quince alleviates indigestion, bladder weakness (urinary incontinence, bladder prolapse), joint pain of the lower body, weakness of the legs and hip area, and swelling of the legs, knees, and/or ankles.

Sources

Quince fruit tea mixed with honey is often sold in Korean markets. If you do not live near one, try ordering it from the PosharpStore website.

Gardeners can purchase quince trees from Willis Orchard Company. A delicious quince jelly fruit spread is available at Nuts.com, while you can find quince fruit liquid extract from Hawaii Pharm.

Preparation and Dosage

Quince can be consumed often as a tea or as jam. For quince fruit tea, follow the preparation instructions on the label. Quince fruit extract should be ingested according to the manufacturer's suggestions.

Did You Know?

The Croatians traditionally planted a quince tree when a child was born to symbolize fertility, love, and life. It was also a ritual offering during weddings in ancient Greece. Hence it was called the "fruit of love, marriage, and fertility."

 ## Shi Zi
(Common: Persimmons; Latin: *Diospyros kaki*)

According to Eastern medicine, the primary function of Shi Zi, or persimmons, is to direct the energy of the body downward—a process that is particularly challenging for the Yang Type B. The movement of energy downward can assist with the flow of urine and can also encourage the descent of food within the upper and middle digestive tracts, making it a common remedy for hiccups and acid regurgitation too.

Common Uses

Persimmons aid urine flow and blood cell growth and alleviate hiccups and acid regurgitation.

Sources

Juicing with fresh persimmon and quince to start the day is an ideal way to keep the Yang Type B's bladder energy flowing. Yet finding these fruits, especially in season, could be a challenge. So if you have difficulty locating fresh persimmons, your best bet is to purchase persimmon leaf tea from sources such as Hankook Tea; the company calls it "persimmon leaf tisane."

Caution

Persimmons may cause bladder irritation among individuals with interstitial cystitis. Moreover, despite their ability to promote the downward flow of urine and food in the stomach, persimmons contain tannins, whose strong astringent properties affect the intestines, possibly instigating an episode of constipation. For this reason and because they solidify the stools, persimmons are occasionally eaten to alleviate diarrhea. Ripe and soft persimmons are sweeter and not as astringent, making them less likely to cause constipation.

YIN TYPE A

The Yin Type A's stronger liver system correlates with joy, making all members of this type radiate toward joyfulness. Yet not all Yin Type As are joyful, and if the constant need for joy isn't met, their health will be compromised. As I mentioned above, the urinary bladder correlates with comfort. The Yin Type A achieves comfort through joy by sending energy from her stronger liver to the kidneys and bladder. When joy is sought but not achieved, she will go straight for comfort, often becoming indolent and harboring the desire to escape from her circumstances. Table 8.3 and the sections that follow provide two Yin Type A bladder-issue scenarios and their resolution.

TABLE 8.3. THE YIN TYPE A'S BLADDER ISSUES

	Scenario A	Scenario B
Symptoms	Bladder infection, UTI, bladder inflammation	Bladder prolapse, frequent urination and/or incontinence without infection
Emotional Component	Frustration, anger, disappointment, stagnation from lack of joy	Escaping from one's circumstances and challenges in search of comfort
Mechanism	Yang stagnates	Yin sinks
Organs Involved	Stronger liver	Weaker lungs
Other Potential Symptoms	Fever, reddish complexion, sensitivity to heat	Fatigue, pale complexion, common cold symptoms

Yin Type A Bladder Issue: Scenario A

The Yin Type A's unachievable joy may lead to stagnation of the liver's energy and blood, causing the accumulation of heat, inflammation, and blockage in the middle and lower abdomen. Constipation and difficulty with urination are common symptoms of this scenario. There may also be a burning sensation when urinating due to excessive heat transferring from the liver to the kidneys and then the bladder. UTIs, dysuria, and bladder infections are often a result of the Yin Type A's stagnant liver energy.

Resolution

The Yin Type A never loses joy, since it is an integral part of who she is, but she may lose track of it and feel as if it is impossible to manifest. This type, more than any other, needs to ignite joy in her everyday life in order to stay healthy and happy and be herself. The first step toward rediscovering joy is to realize that you embody it, even in the worst of times. When you are in the midst of despair, it is easy to forget that you were once full of joy and that it is possible to reclaim it. Joy is always waiting to be activated within the Yin Type A's stronger liver, but during and after menopause, the switch that activated her joy might not work as well. What made her joyful in the past may not be as important to her now. Redefining what makes her joyful might take longer than anticipated, and, desperate for joy, she may rush into situations that initially offer her solace but in the end steal it away. When all is said and done, true joy can only be found within the confines of her own mind and body. Heng gom, or self-reflection, also residing within her liver, provides her with the ability to find joy within.

The following are foods and herbs that promote the smooth flow of liver energy and help bring back joy.

Ju Hua
(Common: Chrysanthemum; Latin: *Chrysanthemum morifolium*)
After entering the body, Ju Hua, or chrysanthemum, quickly travels to the liver and promotes its function. This herb has strong natural antibiotic properties, and when taken regularly, it can reduce the frequency of bladder infections. It also relieves and encourages healing of the kidneys and addresses nonacute bladder infections.

Common Uses
Chrysanthemum protects against bladder infections, addresses eye disorders, and alleviates sinus infections, colds, flu, and a sore throat.

Sources
Chrysanthemum tea can be purchased from manufacturers such as Mighty Leaf and TeaSpring.

Preparation and Dosage
Steep three to five flowers in one cup of hot water. Let the tea sit for four minutes until the water turns light yellow. Drink warm. To enhance its effect, the leaves may also be chewed after finishing the tea. Up to four cups a day may be consumed.

Caution
Studies have shown that chrysanthemum is a relatively safe herb. However, if you are taking this herb within the recommended dose range and experience indigestion or allergy-related symptoms (such as sinus inflammation, rash, or runny nose), you may be allergic to chrysanthemum or simply not a Yin Type A.

Herbal Friend: Pu Gong Ying
(Common: Dandelion Root; Latin: *Taraxacum officinale*)

Dandelion root and leaf tea can be taken with chrysanthemum tea for added effect against a UTI. Drink equal portions of both herbs, reducing and adding water according to your taste. Organic dandelion root tea can be purchased from the Traditional Medicinals website.

 ## Apple Cider Vinegar

With its abundant yang energy, high acidity, and potassium and enzyme content, apple cider vinegar can help prevent and address UTIs, creating an unfavorable environment for bacteria to grow within the bladder. In Sasang medicine, vinegar is often mixed with other herbs to promote blood flow and cleanse the liver. The Yin Type A is often faced with circulatory issues because her stronger liver frequently absorbs more than it needs, taking blood and energy away from the other organs. Turmeric is often used with vinegar to enhance its circulatory and anti-inflammatory effects. Vinegar also helps prevent and reduce high blood pressure. There are more than twenty different types of vinegar, each derived from different sources. Vinegars produced from cider have a higher acetic acid content, said to have cholesterol- and blood-sugar-reducing effects.

Common Uses
Apple cider vinegar alleviates infection (kidney, bladder, sinus), high blood pressure, circulatory issues (cold extremities, numbness of the extremities, weight gain), and indigestion.

Sources
Naturally fermented apple cider vinegar is available at most supermarkets.

Preparation and Dosage
Add two tablespoons of apple cider vinegar to one cup of water. Stir well and drink it up. Take twice daily for optimum efficiency. A teaspoon of honey, maple syrup, or molasses can be added to moderate the sour flavor.

Caution
Apple cider vinegar is very acidic, aromatic, and potent. This is how it helps get energy flowing better throughout the body. However, this property may cause burning of the tongue and throat in some individuals. Make sure to dilute vinegar with a substantial amount of water when starting an apple cider vinegar regimen. The ratio mentioned under "Preparation and Dosage" should be adjusted appropriately to avoid a burning sensation. After it is ingested, apple cider vinegar turns alkaline, making it compatible with alkaline dietary regimes.

Yin Type A Bladder Issue: Scenario B
The Yin Type A's overwhelming desire to escape from life's responsibilities may cause her to drop (pun intended) everything, including

urine, and in some cases the bladder too. In Sasang medicine, this is referred to as "yin sinking," which may instigate stress incontinence or bladder prolapse. Bladder prolapse and urinary incontinence may be the result of putting her own joy aside for the sake of helping others find it. Decades of labor-intensive work or an exercise routine that required continuous and/or heavy lifting may have also played a significant role. Before seeking comfort, finding joy is essential for the Yin Type A. Likewise, without ample flow from her liver, the kidneys cannot function normally. Without joy, yin energy simply drops downward, leading to urinary incontinence, prolapse, and/or heaviness/weakness of the lower extremities.

Since Scenario B is a sign of deficiency, the Yin Type A's weaker lung system is usually involved even if she doesn't have any respiratory issues. About half of those who suffer from urinary incontinence and/or bladder prolapse will experience frequent colds, wheezing, chronic allergies, chronic coughing, and so forth. Hence the herbs below address her weaker lungs and encourage them to pull her yang energy upward again, returning the bladder to its original position and restoring its ability to hold urine.

Resolution

Even though we all could use a vacation to recharge our batteries from time to time, the overstressed Yin Type A may take this opportunity to the extreme. Rather than face the heat, this individual constantly wishes to escape from her circumstances. Despite the challenges she faces, the Yin Type A who stays engaged will certainly reap the benefits in the end. Yet staying engaged doesn't mean bearing a situation that is causing her pain and anguish. For the Yin Type A, menopause is a time for reclaiming and redefining her joy. At this juncture in life, she can finally let go of situations that have caused her grief over the years, but caution should be heeded against refusing ones that challenge her to grow. Recognizing whether or not a challenging situation is a source of growth or grief takes considerable thought and wisdom. Shik kyun, residing in the upper body, is the ability to distinguish between right and wrong, positive and negative, and advantage and disadvantage. Even though it comes naturally for the Yang Type B with a strong upper body, the Yin Type A has to take time and effort to master it, which happens when she consistently makes her own health and wellness a priority in life.

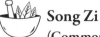 ## Song Zi
(Common: Pine Nuts; Latin: *Pinus* spp.)

Pine nuts promote kidney function and nourish and promote the integrity of the bladder muscles. In Sasang medicine, they are useful for sending energy from the Yin Type A's liver to her kidneys, enhancing comfort through joy. The bone-strengthening properties of pine nuts make them a suitable remedy for joint pain related to osteopenia or osteoporosis, and they are especially beneficial for joint issues in the lower body, including the lower back, knees, ankles, and toe joints. Each pine nut has up to 35 percent of its weight in protein, making them a great source of gluten- and cholesterol-free cellular energy.

Common Uses

Pine nuts alleviate urinary incontinence, uterine prolapse, osteopenia/osteoporosis, aging teeth, lower body joint pain (e.g., ankles, knees, hips), dry skin, and menstrual issues.

Sources

European pine nuts, also called stone nuts, are slender and longer than the Asian variety. Despite a difference in shape, the two varieties are equally beneficial for the bones. Pine nuts can be purchased in bulk from Nuts.com. Organic pine nuts can be found at Woodstock Foods and Trader Joe's.

Preparation and Dosage

Pine nuts make a good snack and are also a valuable ingredient in numerous delicious recipes. In Korea, pine nuts are often sprinkled into teas to add a pleasant nutty taste. Try it with your favorite tea! Consume ten pine nuts a day to support your bones and bladder function.

Herbal Friend: Yin Xing Yi
(Common: Ginkgo; Latin: *Ginkgo biloba*)

In Eastern medicine, ginkgo is said to make the lower body more stable, enhancing bladder integrity and preventing incontinence by assisting lung energy movement (see the explanation on page 245). The earliest recorded use of ginkgo in China goes back as far as 2600 BCE, and since then it has been highly prized for its ability to alleviate asthma-related symptoms. Modern research supports the use of ginkgo to boost memory by enhancing the circulation of blood to the brain. In support of these findings, Sasang medicine holds that the lungs control the flow of energy to the brain. This is another example of how Eastern and Western medicine have reached the same conclusion by completely different means! Ginkgo leaves and nuts contain ginkgoloid, a substance known to promote blood circulation. A study in 2006 suggested that ginkgo has a biphasic effect on estrogen (estradiol) levels within the body, meaning that it promotes the reception of estrogen while reducing its cancer-producing effects.[6]

Ginkgo nuts are commonly used for urinary incontinence, uterine prolapse, asthma, allergies, restoring lung function, and eliminating phlegm. Ginkgo is readily available online in pill form from companies such as Vitacost and Puritan's Pride. Whole ginkgo nuts are more difficult to get hold of but can occasionally be found at Asian food markets or herb supply stores. You should follow the manufacturer's dosage suggestions carefully when using ginkgo supplements. Ginkgo nuts have a sweet and slightly acrid flavor when fried until golden brown. For incontinence and/or bladder prolapse, you may also try consuming five fried ginkgo nuts a day. Make sure to remove the ginkgo nut shell before preparing. For best results try consuming five ginkgo nuts with ten pine nuts a day.

Caution

Raw ginkgo nuts are poisonous and should not be consumed. Even cooked ginkgo nuts in excessive amounts have been known to cause headaches, nausea, gastrointestinal upset, diarrhea, dizziness, and allergic skin reactions. Take no more than five whole ginkgo nuts a day and make sure to fry them until they turn yellowish brown.

When taking ginkgo in capsule form, follow the manufacturer's recommended dosage closely. Ginkgo intake is contraindicated during pregnancy. Its circulation-enhancing properties make ginkgo inadvisable if you're taking blood thinners or following an aspirin regimen. For more details about the side effects of ginkgo, do a search of ginkgo side effects on the National Institutes of Health website.

YIN TYPE B

With her stronger kidney and bladder, it may be difficult to imagine the Yin Type B having urinary issues, yet strength is not always a sign of health. If the Yin Type B does not embrace her predominant emotion of calmness, then the stronger kidneys feel anxious and unsettled, as if to say, "We're supposed to be calm; what happened?" Do ryang, or the ability to embrace others and be open-minded, is the key that unlocks the Yin Type B's comfort. The incontinent Yin Type B may prefer to isolate herself from others and feel anxious and defensive when in public. This condition, called *wei dun* or "outward escape," involves the escape of kidney energy through the bladder, resulting in irritability and frequent urination. Each body type has an energy escape route, and for the Yin Type B, it's the bladder. Table 8.4 (page 249) and the sections that follow provide two Yin Type B bladder-issue scenarios and their resolution.

Yin Type B Bladder Issue: Scenario A
The Yin Type B's lack of comfort may lead to stagnation of her stronger kidney energy, causing kidney and/or bladder infection, inflammation, and congestion of energy in the lower abdomen. Constipation and difficulty with urination are also common symptoms of kidney energy stagnation. There may also be a burning sensation when urinating as abundant yin cold from the kidneys takes over, and yang heat escapes to the bladder. Scenario A of the Yin Type B is often characterized by a sensation of heat in the upper body and burning urination even though the lower body remains as cold as ice. If the area directly below the umbilicus feels cold to the touch even when fever and burning urination are present, it's a telltale sign that you're dealing with a genuine Yin Type B. The absence of comfort and warmth within her cold kidneys is to blame for these symptoms.

TABLE 8.4. THE YIN TYPE B'S BLADDER ISSUES

	Scenario A	Scenario B
Symptoms	Bladder infection, UTI, bladder inflammation	Bladder prolapse, frequent urination and/ or incontinence without infection
Emotional Component	Unsatisfied need for comfort causing anxiety, stress, and fear	Giving up on the ability to feel comfortable, falling into despair or loss of touch with reality
Mechanism	Yang stagnates within the bladder	Yin sinks to the lower part of the body and chases yang out
Organs Involved	Stronger kidneys	Weaker spleen
Other Potential Symptoms	Fever, reddish complexion, sensitivity to heat	Fatigue, pale complexion, common cold symptoms

Resolution

The Yin Type B never loses comfort, since it is an integral part of who she is, but she often loses track of it and feels as if it is impossible to achieve, giving rise to anxiety and a lack of self-esteem, or gung shim—qualities unleashed from her weaker spleen when it is disregarded. This type, more than any other, needs to reestablish comfort in her everyday life in order to stay healthy. Comfort for the menopausal Yin Type B usually consists of more time devoted to self-care and tranquility. Yet Lee Je-ma cautions this type against staying home too long, isolating herself, and disengaging, because doing so will only further entrap the yang within her kidneys, making it even more difficult to socialize. The kidneys' yang is never completely secure when surrounded by abundant yin cold. Only when it is reinforced by warm emotions, exercises, foods, and, occasionally, herbs can her yang energy flow freely to and from its cold kidney home.

Coupled with the desire for quiet and solitude comes a strong drive for accomplishment and success. Hence an inner battle is waged between these two forces, occasionally driving the Yin Type B bonkers. Her lofty idea of success is blended with fictional notions of an ideal world built within the confines of her own mind. By this phase in her life, she has spent too much time either in a cocoon or engaged but without recharging her kidneys. As she continues along the Sasang path, the Yin Type B's definition of comfort will naturally expand. She'll slowly transform her comfort from conditional to conforming; the former requires a certain set of circumstances like staying home and away from work and being alone, while the latter means adjusting to each situation, finding calmness in chaos, and taking comfort with her wherever she goes.

The foods and herbs below send warmth to the kidneys and support the function of the Yin Type B's urinary bladder, helping to bring back calmness.

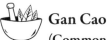 **Gan Cao**

(Common: Licorice Root; Latin: *Glycyrrhiza uralensis*)
The Korean equivalent for the expression "jack-of-all-trades" is "licorice root in the medicine cabinet," since this herb was traditionally used for so many health-related issues! It also has a unique way of balancing the properties of other herbs in a formula that no other herb could rival. One of licorice root's greatest merits is its ability to gently but effectively treat bacterial and fungal infection. Hence it is commonly used to treat kidney, bladder, and other infections of the Yin Type B. As an added benefit, it also assists with her weaker digestive system. Researchers have discovered that licorice root has estrogen-like effects, reduces body fat,[7] has a significant effect on serotonin reuptake—potentially benefiting women with postmenopausal depression[8]—and enhances the healing of blood vessels in cardiovascular disease.[9]

Common Uses
Licorice root alleviates infections (kidney, bladder, sinus) and common colds (sore throat, fever) and acts as an antifungal (candida).

Sources
Organic licorice tea can be purchased from suppliers like Traditional Medicinals and Alvita. Organic tinctures are available from Nature's Answer and Herb Pharm.

Preparation and Dosage

Drink a cup of tea—one cup of boiling water steeped with one licorice tea bag—twice a day. Please follow the manufacturer's suggestions for tincture dosage.

Caution

In higher doses, glycyrrhizin, the most well-known component of licorice root, may cause a condition referred to as "pseudoaldosteronism," which can lead to headaches, fatigue, water retention, and even high blood pressure. In the fifteen years of my practice and prescription of thousands of formulas, I have never witnessed any side effects from licorice, and I actually consider it to be quite safe for the Yin Type B. This caution illustrates the importance of ingesting herbs according to your body type. If you experience any of these symptoms, stop using licorice root immediately and consult a specialist.

Herbal Friend: Rou Gui
(Common: Cinnamon; Latin: *Cinnamomum cassia*)

Do you remember Rou Gui, commonly known as cinnamon, from the discussion of osteoporosis in chapter 5? Well, it can also be used with licorice root in Sasang medicine for the Yin Type B's urinary bladder infections. These two herbs complement one another's ability to cultivate and prevent stagnation of yang energy within the body. Hence Lee Je-ma credits cinnamon with "filling the inner (kidney) and outer qi (urinary bladder) of the lower body." Cinnamon has also built a reputation as an effective antimicrobial agent. A 2017 study showed that an active component of cinnamon, trans-cinnamaldehyde, helps prevent and reduce the occurrence of UTIs.[10]

Cinnamon bark can be purchased from most supermarkets throughout the United States. Suppliers such as Nature's Answer, Solaray, and Gaia offer a capsulated extract form of cinnamon. Raw cinnamon bark tea is prepared by boiling three two- to three-inch slices of bark in two cups of water. Let the tea simmer over low heat for fifteen minutes. More or less cinnamon can be added depending on your taste preference. If you're using capsules, refer to the manufacturer's dosage guidelines. To enjoy cinnamon and licorice root together, try Egyptian

Licorice tea by Yogi or Licorice and Cinnamon from Pukka Herbs. Both manufacturers add other ingredients like cardamom and fennel that are also compatible with the Yin Type B.

Yin Type B Bladder Issue: Scenario B

The Yin Type B's overwhelming desire for peace, quiet, and calmness may eventually lead to isolation from the outside word, mistrust, and fear of being around others. Within the body, this situation is reflected by a lack of communication between the Yin Type B's comfortable and secluded kidneys and her weaker, socially oriented spleen. At first she'll find refuge being alone and away from the chaos around her, but eventually she'll lose a sense of reality and connection with the outer world. With nowhere else to go, her kidney energy retreats further and escapes downward through the bladder. In Sasang medicine, this is referred to as "yin sinking," which may instigate stress incontinence or bladder prolapse.

Resolution

The Yin Type B often has a difficult time realizing that calmness is not limited to isolation or being in the comfort of her own home. It can be found at work, in a store, and even on a busy city street where car horns are the primary mode of communication. If the Yin Type B embraces rather than fears these situations, she can unlock a level of comfort that no other body type could experience no matter how hard she tries. I've met numerous Yin Type B patients who enjoy frequent spiritual/religious retreats, especially during and after the menopausal transition. For the Yin Type B who spends a lot of time outside of her comfort zone, an occasional retreat can offer rejuvenation and solace, making it easier to commingle. Yet she can easily get addicted to the relaxation she feels while retreating and dread returning to society. The balanced Yin Type B will quickly recognize this tendency before going too far, and although she may treasure her time alone, she still makes it her priority to stay engaged.

Wi eui, or dignity, resides within the Yin Type B's weaker spleen, waiting to be fed by her stronger kidneys. Consequently, dignity and self-worth don't come easily for her, especially if she's faced with criticism or ridicule. The Yang Type A's stronger wi eui provides strength and empowerment in this situation as it feeds her anger and desire for change. Like a snail, the Yin Type B simply retreats back into the comfort of her shell. Her self-criticism can also be an impetus to challenge and improve herself. The change of life is a perfect time to reflect on her unique qualities and what makes her special. I've met many amazing Yin Type Bs who have achieved so much in life without believing in themselves, and Yang Type As who are extremely overconfident and overproud. The Yin Type B's humility can be extremely powerful if she learns how to master it, and self-defeating if she doesn't. Despite rejection or ridicule, the balanced Yin Type B pushes her chest out, stands strong, and isn't afraid of failure. In doing so, she'll send ample yang energy upward from the kidneys to the spleen. The herbs below are also capable of assisting this process.

Cong Bai
(Common: Green Onion/Scallion Root; Latin: *Allium fistulosum*)
Just when you thought the compost pile was the most appropriate place for this part of a green onion, think again! Cong Bai, or green onion root, is a commonly used herb in Sasang medicine, consumed in tea form to promote yang movement in the lower body of the Yin Type B, stimulating the movement of urine and reducing water retention. By ascending yang, this herb addresses urinary frequency, incontinence, and urinary bladder prolapse. Green onion root is also an effective remedy for early-stage common colds since the stimulation of yang gives the Yin Type B's immune system a boost. As an added benefit, the findings of a study performed in 2014 by the Medical University of South Carolina suggested that frequent onion consumption may have bone-strengthening effects in perimenopausal women.[11]

Common Uses
Green onion cultivates and strengthens kidney and bladder yang energy, clears phlegm from the throat and sinuses, and boosts immunity for early-stage colds.

Sources
Good news for green onion lovers: if you place the cut roots of green onion in a cup of water, they'll grow again! If you'd like to grow them

yourself, purchase non-GMO organic scallions seeds from Everwilde Farms.

Preparation and Dosage

Cut the white portion and small hair-like roots from six green onion stalks and retain them. Lightly rinse them in water and then place them in a pot with two cups of water and bring to a boil. Let simmer for five minutes and drink half a cup four times a day until the condition improves.

Herbal Friend: Yi Zhi Ren
(Common: Black Cardamom Seed; Latin: *Alpinia oxyphylla*)

Yi Zhi Ren (meaning "seed that enhances wisdom"), or black cardamom, was given its name thanks to its ability to strengthen and fortify the kidneys—a source of wisdom and knowledge. Its powerful ability to support and raise the Yin Type B's weaker yang energy makes it a frequently used herb in formulas that address bladder issues caused by yin sinking. In Sasang medicine, Yi Zhi Ren is said to warm the kidneys and solidify the *jing*—the essential body fluids produced within the kidneys. Try consuming twenty drops of Yi Zhi Ren tincture (available on the Hawaii Pharm website) three times a day mixed with, or directly before/after, green onion root tea.

9

Untangling the Fishing Net

Uterine Fibroids

"What do you mean I have fibroids?" Shauna, age forty-five, asked her doctor. When she had made the appointment, she had attributed her bloating sensation with indigestion, but now her doctor was telling her that she has a whopping fibroid, seven inches in diameter! No significant pain was involved, just a subtle feeling of bloating, but when she pressed on her abdomen, she could feel a faint sensation of something roundish and harder than its surroundings. It was around this time that Shauna started wearing looser clothing to self-consciously hide her abdomen. Soon afterward, she began to notice spotting of darker blood in between cycles but again thought it was just a sign of impending menopause. It was only when the bleeding and bloating worsened that she went to visit her doctor, who didn't share her disbelief. "Yes, you and about 40 percent of all other women entering perimenopause have fibroids," her doctor continued, "but I wouldn't be too worried. Since fibroids are estrogen-fed, most of the time they shrink naturally after menopause, and most importantly, they are benign, not cancerous tumors. I wouldn't be concerned about your fibroids unless they are causing you pain or distress." Shauna's doctor discussed with her several options, such as waiting until menopause to see what happens, cryotherapy, uterine ablation, or fibroidectomy. Shauna was relieved that he didn't mention the need for a hysterectomy, but she still felt uneasy about the other options. Instead she was able to reduce the size of her fibroid from seven to two inches by modifying her lifestyle through exercise and diet years before she reached menopause.

When to See a Professional about Your Fibroids

Uterine fibroids are generally not life threatening but could cause significant health issues if not addressed appropriately. If you experience extreme pain, heavy bleeding, frequent UTIs, anemia, and/or non-menopause-related infertility, then I suggest consulting a health professional.

By age fifty, fibroids, also called myomas or fibromyomas, occur in approximately 80 percent of African American women and 40 percent of Caucasian women, while obesity increases the odds of occurrence. There are four types of fibroids: The first, most common type is called intramural, protruding from the inner wall of the uterus. The second most common, and often the largest type, is subserosal, which grows from the outside wall of the uterus. The third is submucosal, which grows within the lining of the uterus wall. The last, least common type is called cervical because it grows at the cervical opening to the uterus. Every year, almost four out of ten women below the age of sixty undergo hysterectomies, and close to 200,000 hysterectomies are performed in the United States for the sake of removing fibroids.

Most of the time fibroids are symptom-free, but occasionally they involve one or more of the following:[1]

- Heavy bleeding (which can be heavy enough to cause anemia) or painful periods
- Feeling of fullness in the pelvic area
- Enlargement of the lower abdomen
- Frequent urination
- Pain during sex
- Lower back pain

Why do so many women get fibroids during perimenopause? To answer this question, we need to discuss how hormone levels within the body fluctuate rapidly during this transition, with estrogen peaking right before menopause. Among its various functions, estrogen is responsible for retaining moisture within the uterus and thickening the uterine wall in preparation for pregnancy. This process occurs naturally during the monthly cycle. With elevated levels of estrogen and reduced levels of progesterone during perimenopause, the uterine lining sometimes thickens out of control, causing blood and moisture to stagnate within and/or around the uterus. In the first chapter, we discussed how estrogen is associated with yin, which correlates with moisture, cold, reduced circulation, and contraction. Hence sudden increases in estrogen and yin may contribute to circulatory issues during perimenopause.

The average woman has approximately five hundred monthly cycles in her lifetime, which technically makes her capable of having hundreds of babies! Yet a 2015 census suggests that the average mother gives birth to 1.87 children. So that's only one or two eggs out of five hundred that get fertilized! Yet despite these odds, the body consistently prepares itself every month for approximately forty years for the possibility of conception. With so much attention and energy devoted to preparing the uterus, things do not always go smoothly.

The perimenopausal transition is a time for impregnation of a different nature involving a shift from nurturing the life of another to embracing our own needs and desires. For many women, this is a period of uncertainty as they intuitively feel the need to shed old skin but are not so sure what the new coating will look like. They may choose to hold on, letting the lives of their husband or child(ren) occupy their every thought, or pour themselves into work despite inner signals suggesting that they need more time for themselves. Internally, their uterus may also cling to old blood as if it were a fetus, causing the formation of a fibroid. Perimenopause is an opportunity to rid ourselves of toxic or unnecessary thoughts and shed the lining of our past.

WESTERN AND EASTERN PERSPECTIVES ON UTERINE FIBROIDS

The source of uterine fibroids is still a topic of debate in Western medicine. Reasons such as family history, excess adipose tissue, abdominal trauma, or hormonal imbalance have been the top contenders. Although these factors may contribute to the formation and growth of uterine fibroids, they aren't always the culprit. Treatment is equally ambiguous and options are limited, usually leaving surgical removal of fibroids as a last resort. Since most women would rather opt out of surgery, doctors often suggest that their patients wait until menopause begins and estrogen levels rapidly decrease, which often reduces the size of fibroids. This option may work for some but not for others who have higher levels of estrogen and/or other complications due to extensive fibroid growth. Other treatments, usually reserved for more acute cases, include the use of progesterone via birth control pill or hormonal IUD to counteract the effects of estrogen; gonadotropin-releasing hormone to artificially induce the onset of menopause; uterine ablation, which involves the removal of the uterine lining to prevent excessive bleeding; or embolization, a method used to seal off blood supply to the fibroid. While one or more of these procedures may be the only option(s) for some women with acute fibroids, they aren't infallible. Fibroids have a tendency to regenerate even after they are minimized or removed.

In Eastern medicine uterine fibroids are a result of energy and blood stagnation in the lower abdomen from physical and emotional imbalance, and if left on their own, they could lead to other energy blockages down the line. The uterus is located along an intricate network of energetic pathways that flow throughout the body. Eastern medical practitioners take into account these pathways, tracing their flow via the patient's pulse or other traditional diagnostic methods. The reason for blood stagnation in the lower abdomen differs according to the individual, and while easily detected in some women, in others it is not so apparent. Layer upon layer of physical/emotional imbalance may point to other areas of the body that are indirectly related to the uterus. Treatment is implemented whether or not menopause is approaching and often involves the integration of specific foods, herbs, acupuncture, and exercises that enhance blood circulation through the lower abdomen and address other potential energy imbalances.

THE YIN AND YANG OF UTERINE FIBROIDS

In Sasang medicine, the uterus is associated with the kidney system, which is responsible for circulating energy and blood through the lower abdomen. As we've discussed earlier, the kidneys are the source of yin and cold, and with an abundance of thick yin fluid and congealing cold, circulation through the kidney system presents a challenge for anyone, healthy or not. Uterine fibroids are a result of long-term yin and blood stagnation in the lower abdomen that eventually accumulates and solidifies. The emotional and physical center of a woman's body, the uterus, and the flow of yin and blood through it, is particularly dependent on comfort—the emotion of the kidney system. The ability to feel comfortable with others and with one's self is a major part of staying healthy. In the hustle and bustle of modern-day life, it is so easy to forget the seemingly not-so-urgent things and disregard the more intimate aspects of our lives and bodies. A woman's uterus is like an inner child that, even though it may not be harvesting a fetus, needs to be nourished, cared for, and heeded on a daily basis through self-reflection, self-love, self-appreciation, and self-care.

Before we go into body-type-specific methods for addressing fibroids, let's take a look at a few general tips that help promote the flow of yin and blood in the lower abdomen and send love and energy to the uterus regardless of your body type.

Tip #1: Exercise Them Away!

Well, actually, exercise itself does not reduce the size of fibroids, but it stimulates several processes that can. Hormonally speaking, exercise increases testosterone levels but decreases estrogen levels in women. In Eastern medical terms, this is described as increasing yang and decreasing excess yin within the body. Since fibroids are considered to be a result of excessive yin accumulation and entrapment within or around the uterus, an increase in yang energy causes a decrease in yin accumulation.

Cardiovascular exercises in particular are effective at increasing metabolism and burning calories. Studies show that excessive weight gain contributes to the onset of fibroids and hence the need for exercise. Cardiovascular exercises such as walking, using a treadmill or elliptical, swimming, or bicycling are the fastest ways to work up a sweat, which is the best indication that we are burning off calories and balancing estrogen levels. Make sure to pace yourself when exercising because high-impact movements may aggravate fibroid-related pain. If you do not experience pain when exercising, then don't worry about worsening a fibroid situation.

Tip #2: Massage Your Abdomen with Essential Oils

Enhancing the movement of abdominal energy is essential for addressing your fibroids. Try lightly tapping your lower abdomen before you get out of bed each morning, while inhaling and exhaling deeply. Then circle the palm of your hand around your abdomen in a clockwise direction, with the uppermost point being your belly button and the lowermost point your pubic bone. For added effect, you may also want to apply essential oils, such as tea tree oil, castor oil, and/or lavender at the same time.

Tip #3: Guided Imagery

Studies have shown that guided imagery assists the healing of wounds and the lowering of stress levels.[2] In Eastern medicine we often include it as a method to enhance the flow of energy to different parts of the body. Imagine a bright light emitting outward in all directions from the uterus around your fibroid (if you are not sure of its location, then an approximation will do). This exercise can also be done by placing your hands on your lower abdomen while performing this exercise.

Tip #4: Try Acupuncture and Acupressure

Acupressure promotes the flow of energy throughout the body. Each acupressure point on the body acts as a valve, enhancing flow where it is needed and slowing it down when it is out of control. Used for thousands of years to balance emotion and energy, acupuncture and acupressure utilize the same points on the body.

🌓 *LIV3 (THIRD POINT ON THE LIVER MERIDIAN): "GREAT SURGE"*

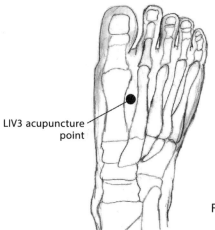

LIV3 acupuncture point

Fig. 9.1. LIV3, third point on the liver meridian

The LIV3 point is located on the liver energy meridian between the first and second toes (see fig. 9.1 above). Lightly run your finger along the web between these toes. At approximately one inch down you'll come to a V-shaped junction between them. LIV3 is directly below this junction in an area that feels soft when pressed.

❋ Use your index finger to apply direct pressure to LIV3 for approximately twenty seconds. Apply enough pressure that you feel a dull ache but not so much that you produce a sharp pain or significant discomfort. Those who are on the sensitive side may feel a gentle tingling sensation, indicating the stimulation of qi.

❋ Gently release, and then switch to the other foot.

❋ Repeat three to five times.

UTERINE FIBROIDS AND THE YIN YANG BODY TYPES

As with other health issues, each body type has its own unique fibroid source, which originates from an imbalance of flow from stronger to weaker organs. This flow is restored and maintained with the use of body-type-specific foods, herbs, exercises, and, most importantly, emotional balancing. Since estrogen, which feeds fibroids, is a yin hormone, fibroids are more commonly present in the yin types. The yang types, however, are not completely off the hook. Whereas abundant yin in the lower body may contribute to the accumulation and blockage of flow, weaker yin may also result in lower body blood and energy stagnation due to a lack of downward flow from the upper body. Hence flow for the yin types needs to be directed upward from the lower body, while flow for the yang types should be directed downward from the upper body.

YANG TYPE A

The Yang Type A's predominant emotion of anger flows strongly upward from the spleen, feeding the chest and head. Hence it is a fundamental challenge for the Yang Type A to relax and feel comfortable while sending energy downward to her weaker kidneys. The ability to embrace and tolerate others, or do ryang, is a quality also associated with the kidneys. The Yang Type A's tendency to ridicule and judge others gets in the way of manifesting do ryang, inhibiting the flow of fresh, warm energy to the lower body. This may lead to the accumulation of stagnant blood and other fluids in the lower body. The Yang Type A's fibroids are a result of long-term unsettled anger and a lack of flow to her sexual organs.

As the Yang Type A transitions through menopause, she may find it even more difficult to overlook others' shortcomings, criticizing their every move. Rather than embracing others, the Yang Type A may start losing her temper and distance herself from them, throwing intimacy out the window (see the the discussion of libido in chapter 11). Yet unlike the Yin Type B, she doesn't discover much comfort in distancing, so she finds herself back to square one. The menopausal transition is an opportunity for her to shift into a more tolerant attitude, accepting others despite their faults. This doesn't mean she has to stay married to an abusive husband or hang out with "friends" who make her feel uncomfortable. Instead, she can cultivate an inner sense of acceptance, one that allows her to chill out and feel more comfort with her own life and circumstances. This comes not from *finding* the time to slow her life down, but from the decision to *make* the time for it, without exception.

The following herbs help the Yang Type A embrace others and send energy downward to the uterus.

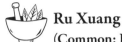 ## Ru Xuang
(Common: Frankincense; Latin: *Boswellia* spp.)

While many herbs in Eastern medicine are unique to the region, frankincense is certainly an exception. This herb, along with myrrh, was mentioned in the Song of Solomon section of the Hebrew Bible. The word *frankincense* means "pure fragrance," and it has been used as an incense in religious ceremonies for centuries. It is frequently prescribed in Eastern medicine, along with its friend myrrh, for issues related to blood stasis. As a cold-natured herb, it is ideal for the heat-induced stagnation of the Yang Type A and can address menstrual difficulties, nonhealing sores, trauma, and fibroids. There are over three hundred known active components of frankincense, among them boswellic acid, prized for its strong anti-inflammatory properties.

Common Uses

Frankincense relieves dysmenorrhea (the lack of menstrual flow often accompanied with darker red, brown, or purplish clots), fibroids, blood stasis, pain, and traumatic injury.

Sources

Frankincense is readily available as an essential oil from suppliers such as doTERRA, Swanson Health Products, and Puritan's Pride. Please keep in mind that several other manufacturers mix frankincense with turmeric. Although turmeric is also effective in promoting blood circulation and reducing accumulation, as a warming herb, it isn't compatible with the Yang Type A.

Preparation and Dosage

Please follow the manufacturer's suggestions.

Herbal Friend: Mo Yao
(Common: Myrrh; Latin: *Commiphora myrrha*)

Frankincense and myrrh are inseparable friends in both Eastern and traditional Western herbal medicines, since they enhance and assist one another in promoting blood flow, reducing inflammation and accumulation, and healing wounds. Surprisingly, I have yet to find a supplement on the market that combines these two ingredients into a simple formula. Myrrh can be purchased in capsule form from Nature's Way as "myrrh gum" and as a tincture from Eclectic Institute. Follow the manufacturer's suggested dosage and take with frankincense.

YANG TYPE B

The Yang Type B's energy is similar to the Yang Type A's in that it spends most of its time in the upper body, especially the neck and head. The Yang Type B, however, is slightly worse off because her weakest organ, the liver, is responsible for sending energy to her uterus. This is precisely why the Yang Type B often suffers from infertility. A weak uterus is also a side effect of having so much upper body energy and an unsurmountable desire for forward and upward movement.

Menopause may give the Yang Type B an overwhelming sense that time is running out as she chooses to speed things up even more. Yang Type Bs have a weaker liver, the organ associated with heng gom—the ability to reflect on one's actions. Hence the unreflective Yang Type B often hastily takes matters into her own hands, doing as she pleases without considering others. As she moves through the change, this approach no longer seems to work as well as it did in the past. The defiant Yang Type B will keep going without heeding the messages from her friends and within her own body. The ability to self-reflect can effectively change the course of her ship in full throttle.

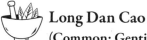 **Long Dan Cao**
(Common: Gentian Root; Latin: *Gentiana* spp.)

Long Dan Cao (meaning "dragon's gallbladder"), or gentian root, has a strong effect on the energy of the liver and gallbladder. Dragons represent strength and vigor in Asian philosophy and the term *dragon* is applied to several herbs, all of which have a strong effect on the body. Gentian root is often used in Eastern medicine to clear stagnant heat within the liver. Sasang medicine, in particular, uses it to treat swelling in the lower body, manifesting as cysts, fibroids, or pelvic inflammatory disease. In both Sasang and Chinese medicine, it is also used to treat red and painful eyes—often a result of excess heat within the lungs and liver. Gentian root contains glycosides, gentiopicrin, and amarogentin, all of which are extremely bitter even when diluted fifty thousand times. Studies show that these substances help protect the liver, making them particularly suitable for the Yang Type B's weaker liver function.[3]

Common Uses
Long Dan Cao addresses eye disorders and reduces toxicity, swelling, and inflammation due to accumulation of heat in the abdomen.

Sources
Gentian root is offered in capsule form by Solaray and as an extract from Nature's Answer.

Preparation and Dosage
Please follow the manufacturer's suggestions.

Caution
This is an extremely cold-natured herb that is very efficient at cooling the Yang Type B's excessive heat but can easily *freeze up* and inhibit the function of the Yin Type B's inherently cold digestive system. Reduce or discontinue use of this herb and retake the yin yang body type test if you are experiencing indigestion, diarrhea, lack of appetite, or a common cold.

Marla, the Fireball Yang Type B

What took Marla, age forty-five, a single day would take the average person a month to accomplish. Not only was she the mayor of her small town, but she was also a part-time psychic and full-time employee. On the weekends she spent most of her time preparing for work, devising new and efficient ways to promote sales. On a hot summer morning in July, things suddenly changed. Marla felt utterly exhausted and had to cancel work for the first time in her life. As the days passed, her energy continued to flatline, and she noticed a significant amount of mid-cycle dark bleeding. Marla was stunned when her gynecologist discovered a twelve-centimeter uterine fibroid, since she hadn't had any previous discomfort. Other than fertility issues, she couldn't recall a single health issue since childhood, although she did admit to consistently feeling out of touch with her lower body—as if it wasn't connected to the rest of her. A week after her fibroid diagnosis, Marla's fatigue became so intense that her legs felt like heavy weights. Shortly thereafter she decided to try Eastern medicine rather than wait, as her doctor suggested, until menopause for the possibility that her issues would naturally go away. I identified her as a Yang Type B with an extremely weakened liver and prescribed a formula containing Long Dan Cao (gentian root) and Mu Gua (quince fruit) to fortify her lower body and descend excessive upper body yang energy. After one month of taking these herbs and slowly reducing her workload, Marla noticed a significant increase of energy. Her three-month follow-up appointment with the gynecologist also went very well, revealing that her fibroid had shrunk to half its original size!

YIN TYPE A

While insufficient flow to the liver may contribute to fibroids of the Yang Type B, excess liver absorption presents the same issue for the Yin Type A. In both Eastern and Western medicine, the liver is responsible for absorbing and filtering digestive by-products from the blood. The

Yin Type A's stronger liver often absorbs more than it can excrete, holding on to by-products and toxins from the blood. Her weaker lungs are responsible for differentiating between profit and loss, friend and foe, and right and wrong through a process called ju chek. The Yin Type A may find it difficult to filter out unnecessary relationships or get herself out of unprofitable situations. Her uterus may also find it hard to let go of old blood, which then accumulates over time, leading to scanty periods, blood clots, PMS, ovarian cysts, and/or fibroids. Menopause is a time to let go of regret, pain, and sadness and start anew for the sake of enhancing her ability to decipher and distinguish.

Letting go of the past might imply turning away from friends who have a tendency to soak up her energy and no longer serve her needs. The Yin Type A's predominant emotion of joy easily manifests around like-minded people—a trait born from dang yo, or group orientation. She also prefers familiar situations over ones that require substantial adaptation and modification. She may decide to hold on to these situations just for the sake of holding on. Little does she know that if she can shed her old skin, new and improved dang yo awaits her. She can enhance this process through purifying her diet, simplifying her life, and learning how to say no to toxic situations and negative influences.

The following are herbs that help filter the liver and treat the Yin Type A's fibroids.

 ## Pu Huang
(Common: Cattail Pollen; Latin: *Typha angustifolia*)

Pu Huang, or cattail pollen, is commonly used in both Chinese and Sasang medicines to address a variety of blood-related disorders. Its ability to promote blood circulation and stop bleeding makes cattail pollen one of the most versatile herbs in the medicine cabinet. It is often used for dissolving accumulations within the body, such as fibroids, cysts, hematomas, and scar tissue caused by traumatic injury, while preventing excessive blood loss—a common issue with submucosal fibroids. With its ability to invigorate blood flow, cattail pollen cleanses the Yin Type A's easily congested liver and counteracts abdominal blood stagnation and accumulation. A recent study demonstrated that cattail pollen is effective in reducing both acute and chronic inflammation.[4] As an added benefit, it contains flavonoids and sterols that have cholesterol-lowering and antiatherosclerotic effects![5]

Common Uses
Cattail pollen alleviates blood stasis (fibroids, hematoma, amenorrhea, inhibited blood circulation) and bleeding disorders (fibroids, excessive bleeding associated with the monthly cycle, traumatic injury).

Sources
Due to its infrequent use in the West, Pu Huang isn't readily available, but a tincture can be found online on the Hawaii Pharm website, which offers both alcohol-based and non-alcoholic tinctures.

Preparation and Dosage
Please refer to the manufacturer's recommendations for effective and safe dosage.

 ## Jiang Huang
(Common: Turmeric; Latin: *Curcuma longa*)
In Sasang medicine, turmeric is used to counteract the strong absorbing nature of the Yin Type A's liver, making it an effective herb to promote circulation and reduce accumulation in the lower body. Curcumin, the most active component of turmeric, is known to suppress the growth of fibroids by acting together with the body's own peroxisome proliferator-activated receptor gamma to regulate the process of cell division and suppress inflammation.[6] From my experience turmeric is well tolerated among the Yin Type Bs, too, likely because it enhances the circulation of yang throughout the body—a quality that both yin types can enjoy.

Common Uses
Turmeric promotes blood circulation, alleviates pain, and reduces swelling.

Sources
Turmeric can be purchased from most supermarkets as a powder or condiment, of which two teaspoons a day will suffice. Turmeric extract

can be purchased in capsule form online from Life Extension, Puritan's Pride, and Nature's Way. CuraPro is a high-quality source of turmeric that can be purchased from the EuroMedica website.

Preparation and Dosage

Follow the manufacturer's dosage guidelines on the above product labels. For added benefit, take with cattail and black cohosh (see "Herbal Friend: Sheng Ma" below).

Herbal Friend: Sheng Ma
(Common: Black Cohosh; Latin: *Actaea racemosa*)

In Sasang medicine, Sheng Ma, or black cohosh, is primarily prescribed for its ability to clear heat and congestion from the liver. By promoting the flow of liver energy, it is also used to reduce the size of uterine fibroids. A study involving 122 participants with fibroids undergoing a twelve-week controlled dosage of black cohosh extract showed a 30.3 percent decrease in tumor size.[7] Black cohosh is commonly used for other liver-energy-related symptoms such as tinnitus, nausea, hot flashes, excessive stomach acid, acne, and fever. It is also used to treat sore throat and sinus congestion, making it suitable for use whether headaches are due to lung weakness and/or liver stagnation. Because of its common use for hot flashes and postmenopausal symptoms, black cohosh is readily available and is carried by Nature's Way and Planetary Herbals. This herb can be taken with turmeric and cattail to enhance its ability to inhibit fibroid tumor growth. Please follow the manufacturer's label for dosage guidelines.

Caution

Black cohosh is a cold-natured herb. If you cannot drink cold fluids without sneezing or getting a stomachache, diarrhea, or indigestion, then black cohosh may not be suitable for you. These symptoms will occur after ingestion of black cohosh if there is not enough heat in the body. Very high doses of black cohosh may cause a slower heart rate, lower abdominal cramps, dizziness, tremors, or joint pain.

YIN TYPE B

With stronger kidneys, correlating with peacefulness and calmness, Yin Type Bs would be satisfied living as a hermit and avoiding the complexities of public life. The ability to publically govern and administer affairs, however, comes from the Yin Type B's weaker spleen. While some of us may succeed at the hermit's life, most require at least minimal interaction with others. Our connection with others is reflected in the relationship between each of our organs. As the lowermost of the yin organs, the kidneys often prefer to get by on their own, hidden underneath the hustle and bustle of the other organs. Yet just as people need to connect and communicate with one another, so do the organs. The kidneys of the socially disassociated Yin Type B will eventually isolate themselves from the other organs, causing accumulation of cold energy in the lower abdomen, eventually forming cysts, fibroids, or related intestinal issues.

The menopausal Yin Type B may feel an overwhelming urge for peace and quiet, easily feeling anxious and irritable, looking for that perfectly quiet place. Without her own space and comfort, the Yin Type B will lose her mind and the lower body, the seat of comfort, will also suffer. Yet knowing whether or not she is truly deprived of these things is particularly difficult for the Yin Type B, requiring considerable self-reflection. The Yin Type B may feel deprived of quietness and aloneness even if she has spent ample uninterrupted time by herself. She who craves the hermit's life despite distancing herself from others may lose the sense of her need to coexist, eventually feeling remorse and loneliness. The balanced Yin Type B finds comfort and peace within herself, even when she is with others.

A warm abdomen is the secret to keeping the Yin Type B healthy since heat facilitates blood circulation, bowel movement, and the ascent of yang energy. A lack of comfort, anxiety, excessive intake of cold-natured foods, and exposure to cold temperatures can all contribute to abdominal cold and toxic accumulation. This can be avoided by regularly drinking ginger tea, eating hot-natured foods, and trying the herbs below, which promote comfort and flow in the Yin Type B's lower abdomen.

Dang Gui/Dong Quai
(Common: Chinese Angelica Root; Latin: *Angelica sinensis*)

With its many functions, Dang Gui, or Chinese angelica root, is one of the most commonly used herbs for Yin Type Bs. Its most significant claim to fame in Eastern medicine is the ability to promote blood flow, especially in the lower abdomen. This unique property makes it a great candidate for addressing various gynecological issues. Chinese angelica root also generates and circulates blood throughout other areas of the body to heal wounds, address vascular issues, and alleviate anemic disorders, headaches, and menstrual cramps. It also supports the function of the Yin Type B's weaker spleen, thus assisting with digestion.

Chinese angelica root looks like a dried squid and emits an aromatic, earthy smell. If left sitting on a shelf, it will eventually cause the whole room to smell like an Asian medical pharmacy! A small piece of it placed inside the mouth will leave behind a tangy taste and sensation for hours, giving a hint of its power. Try chewing on a little piece for a quick pick-me-up!

Common Uses
Chinese angelica root alleviates circulatory issues (like fibroids) menstrual cramps, cold extremities, numbness of the extremities, heart palpitations, anemia, vision disorders (blurry vision, floaters, eyestrain), indigestion, insomnia, and irregular menstruation (scanty, early, or late cycle), and it heals cuts and wounds.

Sources
An encapsulated form of Dang Gui root can be purchased from Nature's Way under the name "Dong Quai." A liquid extract can be purchased from Nature's Answer.

Preparation and Dosage
Follow the dosage guidelines specified by the manufacturer.

Caution
Excessive intake of Chinese angelica root can lead to gas and bloating even for Yin Type Bs. Start with smaller dosages and work your way

up to the recommended dose. Volatile oil extracts of Chinese angelica root have been known to cause skin sensitivity to the sun, leading to a greater risk of skin cancer. Because the liquid extract sold by Nature's Answer and the capsule form sold by Nature's Way are not volatile oils, they don't present this risk.

Do not ingest Chinese angelica root if you are currently taking blood thinners, such as warfarin, because as mentioned above, it promotes circulation and could interfere with prescription-drug effects, causing excessive bleeding. The Nature's Answer version may cause bruising because of its potential blood-thinning effects. There are several different species in the *Angelica* genus that are native to North America. Most of these plants have high levels of toxicity and should not be ingested.

Herbal Friend: Yan Hu Suo
(Common: Corydalis; Latin: *Corydalis yanhusuo*)

Yan Hu Suo, or corydalis, is one of the most effective herbs in Eastern medicine to promote blood movement and break up stasis and accumulation within the body. Along with Dang Gui (Chinese angelica root), Yan Hu Suo supports the Yin Type Bs' circulation and dissolves accumulation, warms their weaker spleen, and assists with digestion. Higher doses of Yang Hu Suo may cause dizziness, drowsiness, and abdominal distension. Doses over 60 grams have also caused difficulty breathing, low blood pressure, and muscle spasms, so make sure you don't go overboard! Fortunately, most readily available sources don't even come close to this dosage range. Hawaii Pharm offers a tincture of Yan Hu Suo on its website, and Biotech Nutritions offers it in capsule form. Follow the manufacturer's guidelines for the correct dosage and take together with Dang Gui for added effect.

Diana, the Reclusive Yin Type B

Diana, age fifty-four, spent most of her life running away from relationships. Despite her attractiveness, she managed to stay single, celibate, and satisfied. Diana found men desirable, but all it took was a few hours with them and she'd turn and walk the other way. While this frustrated others, it didn't seem to faze Diana, who felt just fine being alone and focusing on her own introverted pleasures. It wasn't until she turned fifty-two, with an erratic monthly cycle and a sense that menopause loomed ahead, that she experienced a deep feeling of loneliness. Moreover, Diana's appetite decreased further, a telltale sign for a Yin Type B that something isn't right. Filled with anxiety and uncertainly, she visited her doctor. One test led to another, until finally she was diagnosed with three medium-sized uterine fibroids. I explained to her that an unbalanced desire for comfort and solitude could backfire, leading to stagnation and accumulation of energy within the body. Uterine health depends on our ability to be intimate with others, not just ourselves. Without embracing others and letting them in, the lower abdomen remains cold and damp. Sensing this was Diana's case, I prescribed an herbal formula with Dang Gui (Chinese angelica root) and Yan Hu Suo (corydalis) to warm up and befriend her uterus, and I encouraged her to slowly, but consistently, warm up to others. After ingesting her herbs, Diana said that she felt a gentle warmth fill her lower abdomen. Eventually this feeling intensified and became apparent whenever she cuddled with her new boyfriend. A checkup with her gynecologist three months later showed that Diana was fibroid free.

10

Shouldering the Ropes

Frozen Shoulder

Cindy, age fifty-six, is an avid swimmer who has spent most of her life in a swimming pool, engaging in numerous swimming competitions and improving her performance as she grew older. As she approached menopause, Cindy started to notice occasional upper back and shoulder pain after swimming, though it never seemed to stick around. She would simply wake up the next day, jump into the water, and swim the pain away! It wasn't until a fateful Monday morning that Cindy woke up with excruciating pain in her left shoulder, so intense that she was afraid to move it. Needless to say, she did not swim that morning, hopeful that her pain and stiffness would quickly fade away. By that afternoon it was still there, so she decided to place her arm in a makeshift sling to keep it secure, thinking that the arm must be tired after so much swimming. That evening, her shoulder pain worsened, waking her up throughout the night. Believing that something was seriously wrong, she made an appointment to see her doctor, who immediately suggested that she take muscle relaxants and, if the pain did not subside, schedule an MRI. Cindy decided to go straight for the MRI, since she did not want to take medication, and to her surprise the MRI results didn't show any tears or tendon/ligament damage. Frustrated and confused, she continued to skip swimming, and any upper body exercise, for that matter, consistently protecting her shoulder with a sling.

Cindy came to our clinic a week later feeling as if her life had been taken from her and that this was the beginning of the end. After carefully examining her shoulder, I concluded that she had an acute case of frozen shoulder and suggested that she receive a combination of acupuncture and herbs to ensure a speedy recovery. I also mentioned that keeping her shoulder immobile was partly why it wasn't getting any better, since movement is the only way to awaken the tendons and improve her circulation. I prescribed body-type-specific acupuncture and herbs to nourish her tendons and increase circulation to her shoulder and arm. Even though Cindy's doctor predicted that it could take between one and three years to recover, with the above combination and shoulder exercises, she completely recovered in six weeks.

I encouraged Cindy to use her shoulder or lose it, not to fear added injury, and to slowly chip away at her remaining shoulder tension with exercise while being careful not to push it too far. Even though acupuncture and herbs are capable of getting the frozen shoulder healing process started, it is the steadily increased range of shoulder motion via stretching and exercise that ultimately leads to recovery.

WESTERN AND EASTERN PERSPECTIVES ON FROZEN SHOULDER

Most Western menopause sources would not include frozen shoulder among its symptoms, but Eastern medicine has a different perspective. Frozen shoulder is actually referred to as "fifty-year shoulder," or *wu shi jian,* in Chinese because it frequently occurs around the age of fifty, the average age of menopausal onset. My patients around menopausal age are often surprised to find that shoulder tightness suddenly manifests for otherwise unapparent reasons. As we saw in the first chapter, a loss of estrogen contributes to a reduction of moisture within the body. Larger muscles, like the hamstrings, store larger amounts of estrogen, while narrow muscles, tendons, and ligaments store smaller amounts and are prone to tightness and injury during and after menopause. There are two inherent factors that do not work in favor of the shoulder joint during menopause. The first involves the fact that it has a greater range of motion than practically any other joint in the body. Hence it has a lot of moving parts, making it prone to injury. Second, it is suspended from a group of tendons much like a marionette hangs from strings, constantly pulling downward from the shoulder joint. Persistent tension, along with a lack of nourishment from estrogen, contributes to tighter "frozen" tendons. Menopause is not the only perpetrator of frozen shoulder, since shoulder trauma, immobility, diabetes, cardiovascular disorders, thyroid disorders, and/or Parkinson's disease can also contribute.

In the West, frozen shoulder is also referred to as "adhesive capsulitis," a name describing inflammation and adhesion of the ligaments that enclose and connect the humerus (tip of the shoulder bone) to the scapula. Despite its ability to detect, diagnose, and monitor frozen shoulder, mainstream medicine does not have a cure. Doctors routinely suggest anti-inflammatory drugs, cortisone injections, or, as a last resort, arthroscopic surgery to break up adhesions within the joint capsule. Even though these approaches occasionally provide long-awaited relief, they often produce side effects, such as stomach irritation, immunosuppression, and/or scar tissue buildup. Drug effects tend to diminish over time, causing dependence and addiction. While mainstream medicine often chooses to suppress and weaken various biological functions to kill pain, Eastern medicine aims to enhance the body's natural ability to heal itself. The former approach doesn't take into consideration what lurks behind the observable, while the latter ventures beyond the physical, delving into energetic and emotional pain-related components.

According to Eastern medicine, different areas of the body are either prone to or protected from injury depending on the extent of energy and blood flow. There are a total of twelve major channels of energy, or meridians, that flow from each bodily organ outward toward the muscles, tendons, and skin. Where there is ample energy and blood flow along a meridian, healing will occur faster than where this flow is impeded.

THE YIN AND YANG OF FROZEN SHOULDER

In Sasang medicine, each of the yin yang body types hosts meridians that flow more smoothly or are more prone to obstruction depending on their stronger and weaker organ systems. Yin Type As, for example, are most prone to frozen shoulder because the energy meridian associated with their weaker lungs travels through the shoulder (see fig. 10.1 below). The yang types, with a stronger upper body, experience frozen shoulder less frequently but instead succumb to lower body weakness and/or discomfort during menopause because of their weaker organ channels. Yet even the yang types can be plagued with frozen shoulder syndrome, since the stronger organ systems may hoard too much energy, excessively absorbing and blocking energetic flow from the shoulder to the rest of the body.

Before getting into the details of each body type, let review a number of tips that might be helpful regardless of your body type.

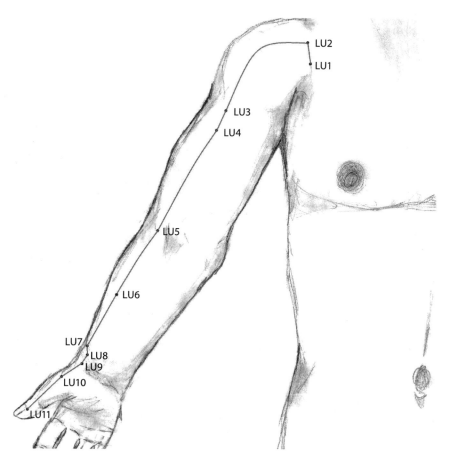

Fig. 10.1. The pathway of the lung meridian

Tip #1: Use It or Lose It

Since it is shaped like a swivel, the shoulder joint is designed to rotate freely, and it requires frequent movement in order to avoid stiffness. If you experience pain and/or stiffness in your shoulder, then try using it more. The secret is to encourage rather than force it to move. If your shoulder simply cannot move further, don't force it! Instead, try again later, perhaps after taking a shower to warm up the tendons. A little soreness, however, goes a long way. There will inevitably be some discomfort involved as you thaw out those tight shoulder tendons.

If you recently suffered a shoulder injury, heard a snapping sound inside your shoulder joint following shoulder movement, and/or suddenly experienced tightness and stiffness of the shoulder joint leading to reduced range of motion, it is recommended that you seek professional care, since it may indicate a shoulder tendon or ligament tear, and if significant enough, this may require reattachment through surgery.

Tip #2: Stretch

Whether you have frozen shoulder syndrome or not, I recommend stretching your shoulders daily to avoid stiffness. There are a couple incredibly simple but effective stretches for your shoulder tendons to keep them elastic and flexible. Both of the following stretches should be performed on and off throughout the day.

☯ SHOULDER STRETCH USING A DOORKNOB

* First, make sure that the door is securely closed.
* Hold on to the doorknob with your palm facing upward and gently rotate your body away from the door. Make sure that you do not stretch too far beyond any possible discomfort.
* When you start to feel the shoulder stretch working, nudge the stretch slightly further. Your shoulder might start to feel slightly tender, so take three deep breaths and then release the stretch slowly.
* Repeat this stretch three times, and each time see if you can stretch it slightly more without causing pain, which is a step further beyond tenderness or discomfort.
* Repeat on the other side.

☯ *SHOULDER STRETCH USING THE WALL*

✳ For the second stretch, face a wall and lean your palms against it over your head, with your elbows slightly bent outward.

✳ Place your feet about shoulder width apart with one leg in front of the other, with the front leg one to two feet from the wall. It doesn't matter which leg is in front to begin.

✳ Now slowly sink the torso at a 45-degree angle to the wall, leaning toward the floor, while breathing outward. Try to keep your elbows almost fully extended throughout this exercise.

✳ Then gently push your body away from the wall toward your original position, breathing inward.

✳ Repeat these movements while slowly breathing in and out, three breaths with one leg in front and three with the other. If you have difficulty raising your arms above head level, then simply lower your arms to a more comfortable starting position.

Tip #3: Try Acupuncture and Acupressure

There are several acupressure points along the lung and large intestine meridians that release tension from the shoulder by stimulating the flow of energy. The diagrams below illustrate three points that I often use in my clinic for shoulder issues. I suggest applying pressure to all three points in the order presented below to address the entire shoulder. Focusing on one meridian or a single tendon may give only temporary relief from shoulder discomfort, since all of the rotator cuff tendons work together, intricately affecting one another. Applying significant pressure to each point until it feels tender often yields better results than a light touch. Avoid applying excessive pressure or using sharp objects, which could potentially penetrate your skin.

☯ *LU9 (NINTH POINT ON THE LUNG CHANNEL):*
"GREAT ABYSS"

This acupressure point is located at the crease of the wrist just below the thumb (see fig. 10.2 on the next page). To find it, run your finger from the outside (thumb side) of the wrist crease toward the inside until you feel a soft spot, approximately one-eighth of the distance from where you started. This is where

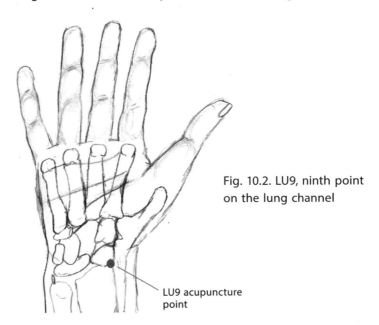

Fig. 10.2. LU9, ninth point on the lung channel

LU9 acupuncture point

the LU9 acupressure point is located. LU9 helps release tension from the anterior shoulder, relaxing the anterior deltoid and the long- and short-head biceps tendons.

* Use your index finger to apply direct pressure to LU9 while slowly counting to ten.
* Gently release, and then switch to the other hand.
* Repeat this process up to five times, rotating the shoulder three times after every round.

LI1 (FIRST POINT ON THE LARGE INTESTINE CHANNEL): "YANG STOREHOUSE"

Imagine two lines, one from the tip of your index fingernail, located on the side facing the thumb, extending straight downward, and another across the bottom of the nail perpendicular to the first line. LI1 is located at the point where these two lines intersect (see fig. 10.3 on the next page). LI1 helps release the medial portion of the shoulder, relaxing the medial deltoid and biceps tendons.

* Use your fingernail, a toothpick, or the tip of a pen to apply direct pressure to LI1 while slowly counting to ten.
* Gently release, and then switch to the other hand.
* Repeat this process up to five times, rotating the shoulder three times after every round.

☯ SJ1 (FIRST POINT ON THE SAN JIAO OR
TRIPLE BURNER CHANNEL): "PASSAGE HUB"

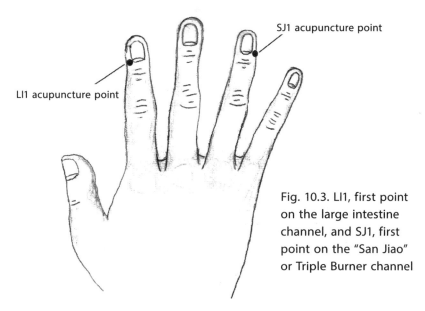

SJ1 acupuncture point

LI1 acupuncture point

Fig. 10.3. LI1, first point on the large intestine channel, and SJ1, first point on the "San Jiao" or Triple Burner channel

Imagine two lines, one from the top of your ring fingernail, on the side facing the pinky, extending straight downward, and another across the bottom of the nail perpendicular to the first line. SJ1 is located at the point where these two lines intersect (see fig. 10.3 above). SJ1 helps release the posterior portion of the shoulder, relaxing the posterior deltoid and triceps tendons. SJ stands for "San Jiao," a channel of energy that transverses the upper, middle, and lower parts of the body and is primarily responsible for water metabolism. The San Jiao channel flows through the shoulder and is often employed to treat energy stagnation and pain in this area.

* Use your fingernail, a toothpick, or the tip of a pen to apply direct pressure to SJ1 while slowly counting to ten.
* Gently release, and then switch to the other hand.
* Repeat this process up to five times, rotating the shoulder three times after every round.

FROZEN SHOULDER AND
THE YIN YANG BODY TYPES

Whether it is trauma, a lack of estrogen, and/or your body type that contributes to frozen shoulder, as long as there is ample energy flow through your shoulder joint, it is capable of healing. In my experience acupuncture and Sasang medicine, often performed together, are effective ways to encourage the flow of energy through this joint. Getting energy to flow through the shoulder is a different story for each type. The yin types, for example, benefit from warm- or hot-natured herbs to encourage yang energy to ascend toward the shoulder, while the yang types benefit from cool- or cold-natured herbs to descend their deficient yin energy away from it. To ascend yang energy, the yin types also benefit from balancing yin emotions such as joy and calmness to address and work through such unresolved yang emotions as anger and sadness. To descend yin energy, the yang types benefit from balancing anger and sorrow to address disregarded emotions such as joy and calmness.

You may recall that in chapter 3, "Weathering the Storms: Emotions and Menopause," I discussed how the shoulders correlate with the spleen system and with wi eui, or dignity/self-confidence. Born with a stronger upper body, the yang types access self-confidence and dignity more easily than the yin types. Yet just because someone may look confident doesn't mean that they truly believe in themselves. There are many outwardly successful people who, on the inside, are feeble and insecure. Uncultivated individuals make an intense effort to appear and feel strong around others but lack the ability to appreciate who they are when they're alone. Still others may appear feeble and insecure on the outside or when with others but internally are firm and strong when they are alone. It is easier for the yin types to be inwardly focused and firm compared to the yang types, who radiate strength and dignity. Yet since they are not dignified by nature, the yin types may lack confidence in themselves and inhibit energetic flow from their stronger lower body to the weaker shoulders.

Self-confidence and dignity are affected by our body type's innate strengths and weaknesses. Wi eui comes more easily for the yang types, while the yin types have to work harder to believe in themselves. Yet even if they do, the yin types may still come across as soft and gentle. The wi eui of the yang types, on the other hand, is like a sword that, when mastered, emits strength and valor even if it isn't wielded. Radiant dignity and valor have their place but are not always called for. A hairstylist who shaves all the hair off a client who asked for a trim, or a waitress who slams a machete through the dinner table when asked to cut a piece of steak, could obviously use a more yin-like approach. Yet for another hairstylist who judiciously trims away at a single piece of hair, or the waitress who leisurely slices through the meat with a dull knife, a more yang-like methodology would be more effective. A balance of yin and yang is what brings out wi eui and enhances flow through the shoulder no matter what type we are.

Each body type relates to and manifests wi eui in their own way by taking advantage of their innate strengths. Dignity for the yang types may entail force and valor, whereas the yin types may find it through calmness and gentleness. Sure, the yang types may be gentle and calm, but if this is done superficially, then wi eui will be left untapped. The yin type who tries to be forceful and authoritarian will also have difficulty bringing about wi eui and instead be perceived as snobbish or arrogant. We each have unique emotional strengths that, if utilized, can balance out our weaknesses. Hence despite having a weaker upper body and shoulders, the yin types are fully capable of manifesting wi eui and strengthening this section of their body, just as the yang types could potentially impair it if a balance isn't struck.

YANG TYPE A

Born with developed shoulders associated with her stronger spleen system, the Yang Type A rarely experiences chronic shoulder-related issues. Yet as a yang type, she is relatively more prone to estrogen-level plunges during menopause compared to the yin types, making frozen shoulder a potential scenario. As mentioned above, estrogen is a yin hormone, produced within the kidney system that nourishes the tendons of the body. A lack of yin energy and weakness of the kidney system contributes to the Yang Type A's potential tendon tightness and discomfort during menopause. In order to master her innate wi eui, the Yang Type A must temper her self-confidence and dignity, which otherwise may overpower others, making her seem authoritarian and bossy. Balanced wi eui is the result of yielding and empowering others without feeling humiliated and angered by them. The unbalanced Yang Type A wields the sword of wi eui against anyone and anything in sight, seeing herself as superior to others, emboldened by her mission to rebuke or punish wrongdoers. Yielding is the last thing on her mind, since she feels that others are ignoring and looking down on her.

The Yang Type A's shoulder energy flows smoothly when she is able to respect others and treat them without disdain. It comes from the ability to feel respected and honored, and reciprocating this toward others. After decades of being the matriarch of the family, the menopausal Yang Type A may start to question whether or not her husband, mentors, and/or friends are worthy of respect. Fluctuating yin and yang within the body may also cause her to take offense more easily and get angrier over otherwise mundane or easily surpassed issues. The Yang Type A does not have to change her circumstances per se; she can just rediscover, recognize, and regulate her wi eui.

Qiang Huo
(Common: Notopterygium Root; Latin: *Notopterygium incisum*)

Qiang Huo (translated as "strong life,"), or notopterygium root, is an herb with incredible dignity, vibrancy, and strength. The fragrance from even a tiny piece of this herb can be detected from more than ten feet away. This peculiar fragrance is often sensed as soon as one enters an Eastern medical pharmacy. Naturally, this herb also has a powerful effect on the body, as it plows through stagnation of blood and energy in the upper body and is often used for neck, shoulder, elbow, and wrist pain. Notopterygium root's potent aroma is also capable of chasing stubborn pathogens away from the upper body, assisting with common colds, sinusitis, and persistent sore throat issues. Lastly, it is efficient at curbing the Yang Type A's anger by releasing stagnant emotion and heat trapped inside her stronger spleen. It helps reignite her wi eui, sending ample energy to and through the shoulders.

Common Uses
Notopterygium root alleviates joint pain and arthritis in the upper body (neck, shoulders, elbows, wrists), common colds, sore throat, sinus congestion, and inflammation.

Sources
Despite its common use in the East, this herb is hard to come by in the West, but luckily Hawaii Pharm offers a tincture on its website.

Preparation and Dosage
Please follow the manufacturer's suggestions.

Caution
Excessive intake of notopterygium root may lead to nausea and vomiting.

Herbal Friend: Du Huo
(Common: Pubescent Angelica Root; Latin: *Angelica pubescens*)

Qiang Huo almost always appears with its favorite acquaintance, Du Huo, or pubescent angelica root, in Sasang herbal formulas. They even share the same last name—*huo,* meaning "life"—and enliven the flow of energy and blood, but Du Huo has a slightly stronger effect on the lower body, supporting the kidney function. Together they sprint through the body, blasting away at anything in their way, assisting with joint pain in both the upper and lower body. Hawaii Pharm offers a tincture form of Du Huo on its website. Ingest both Qiang Huo and Du Huo in one sitting as recommended by the manufacturer.

YANG TYPE B

While the Yang Type B has more strength in her shoulders and neck than the yin types, her shoulders are not as developed as those of the Yang Type A, who has the strongest shoulders of all the body types. In general, this means that the Yang Type B heals relatively quickly from shoulder injury. With abundant upper body strength and plenty of yang energy, however, she tends to abuse her shoulders, and no matter how strong they were to begin with, repeated injury will eventually give way to inflammation, arthritis, and/or tendon issues. As the most developed area of the Yang Type B's posterior body, the muscles and tendons of her neck and cervical spine often contract, pulling her shoulder muscles and tendons upward, potentially giving rise to frozen shoulder syndrome.

The Yang Type B often engages in wi eui, or self-confidence, a process associated with the shoulders that requires a healthy dose of sorrow and anger to achieve. If her sorrowful temperament is balanced, then she'll have just enough anger to stay dignified and stand up for herself. Yet if she lets sadness take control, then it will morph into anger and burst outward while engaging in wi eui, as she believes that only she is capable or worthy. Imbalanced sorrow, in this case, stagnates the energy of the cervical spine, impeding its flow downward to the shoulder and potentially resulting in frozen shoulder syndrome.

Menopause unleashes a sense of urgency for the Yang Type B, making her feel as if time is running out. This could also cause an imbalance of her sorrow, as she laments about time constraints and unaccomplished tasks. The balanced Yang Type B may decide to take on new tasks and responsibilities, giving her a renewed sense of duty and purpose. Yet the hasty Yang Type B will often overlook the needs of those who are closest to her, which, combined with a sense of urgency, may eventually lead to isolation, obstruction, and finally a loss of self-confidence and flow to her shoulders.

Song Jie
(Common: Chinese Red Pine/Masson Pine; Latin: *Pinus massoniana*)
Pine nodes—the tiny joints of the pine tree where the branch meets the prickly leaves—have numerous advantageous properties. They help prevent and soothe allergies and colds, alleviate joint pain due to swelling, and assist in the flow of lung energy through the upper extremities. While other body types may benefit to some degree from this herb, it is especially suitable for the Yang Type B person whose stronger lungs hoard energy from the other organs—a condition that may lead to stagnation of energy and blood in the upper body. The Yang Type B's temperament of sadness is often behind this situation, and since pine is capable of stimu-

lating the flow of lung energy, it is also a mood booster.

Most pine supplements utilize the entire bark of the pine tree, which contains the nodes. The bark and nodes of the Masson pine tree contain a flavonoid that can be found in Pycnogenol, a trademarked formula that has both anti-inflammatory and antioxidant properties. It is also believed to help support immune activity and strengthen the blood vessel walls. Since pine nodes by themselves are hard to come by, its bark can be used instead.

Common Uses

Masson pine alleviates joint pain (e.g., shoulders, knees, etc.), allergies, common colds, water retention, and muscle and/or tendon pain.

Sources

Masson pine bark extract is available on the Planetary Herbals and Puritan's Pride websites. Pine bark extract from other sources is often mixed with ingredients that are not suitable for the Yang Type B.

Preparation and Dosage

Please refer to the manufacturer's label for dosage.

The Yang Type B Who Carried the World on Her Shoulders

Life was always a struggle for Lynn, who never seemed to have enough time to eat or sleep, let alone sit back and enjoy a single moment. She had many friends, but those closest to her always felt uneasy since being the leader of the pack was always her modus operandi and she seemed to have no time for intimacy. Yet Lynn was always ready to offer a helping hand and would often go out of her way to do so. She was always the go-to when heavy items needed to be lifted, or bottles needed to be opened. As a child, she routinely stood up for those who were bullied and ridiculed, never afraid to take a swing at the naughty big boys. Nobody would have ever imagined that, as soon as Lynn hit fifty, she would suddenly lose all motion in her dominant arm. Immobility turned her into a raging bull prior to a bullfight as it kicks at the fencepost before getting released into the arena. Friends started distancing themselves from Lynn, as her anger would lash out when least expected. Lynn's shoulder was telling her that it was about time she decided how to relax and slow her life down a bit, if only she heeded its call.

YIN TYPE A

Frozen shoulder syndrome frequently affects the Yin Type A, since her shoulders are the least developed area of her posterior body. X-rays and MRI images often fail to show anything significantly wrong with her shoulder, leaving more questions than answers about its stiffness and pain. Unfortunately, images can only portray a small part of the picture, since they cannot reveal how she is doing emotionally and how her energies are flowing from organ to organ. Balancing wi eui is particularly difficult for the Yin Type A, who typically lacks dignity and self-confidence and occasionally requires a healthy dose of yang emotion such as anger to take action. She would rather seek the yin type emotions of joy and comfort than face her fears or deal with "unpleasant" emotions. Heng gom (self-reflection), associated with her stronger liver, also plays a role as she can be overly self-critical, belittling herself in the company of others.

The unbalanced Yin Type A's shoulders become a repository for stored emotions associated with sadness or anger. The menopausal phase of life often brings these emotions to the surface, as her shoulder(s) cries for help. Hence it is an opportune time to improve her self-image by addressing them. The healing process unfolds when the Yin Type A acknowledges and accepts that her shoulder pain will resolve in time, as she patiently and consistently stretches, exercises, and addresses her shoulder's underlying energetic and emotional needs. The herbs below support the function of the lungs, send energy to the shoulders, and perk up the Yin Type A's mood.

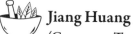 **Jiang Huang**
(Common: Turmeric; Latin: *Curcuma longa*)

The use of turmeric in Indian (Ayurvedic) medicine dates back to approximately 1900 BCE. As a sacred plant in the Hindu religion, it is often used in ceremonies. Turmeric's beautiful flowers and powerful medicinal function contribute to its significant role in Indian and Chinese history. Curcumin, the most active component of turmeric, has an equal or greater effect than ibuprofen in relieving joint pain.[1] From my own experience turmeric is well tolerated among the Yin Type Bs, too, likely because it enhances the circulation of yang throughout the body—a quality that both yin types can enjoy.

Common Uses
Turmeric addresses upper-body joint pain (e.g., shoulder, neck, elbows, and/or hands), inhibits the growth of fibroids, alleviates menstrual pain from stagnation, and relieves traumatic injury that causes bruising.

Sources
Turmeric can be purchased from most supermarkets as a powder or condiment. Turmeric extract can be purchased in capsule form online from Life Extension, Puritan's Pride, and Nature's Way. CuraPro is a high-quality source of turmeric that can be purchased from EuroMedica.

Preparation and Dosage
Turmeric can be used as a condiment in soups, stews, and salads and is a component of curry powder, used in curries and other Indian dishes.

Herbal Friend: Apple Cider Vinegar

Along with turmeric, apple cider vinegar is also an effective blood and energy flow stimulant. Together they clear inflammation and stagnation of blood and energy within the joints. Historically, 30 to 50 grams of fresh turmeric was steeped inside a 24-ounce bottle of apple cider vinegar for several weeks before the vinegar was ingested in 8-ounce doses. If fresh turmeric root isn't available at a health food store near you, then I recommend taking it in capsule form and following it down with up to two tablespoons of vinegar mixed with one cup of water, twice daily.

Grief and a Yin Type A's Shoulder

Jeannie, a sixty-three-year-old Yin Type A, was about to enter her typical acupuncture-induced relaxation state when she suddenly felt an immense amount of sadness well up inside her, which she said felt like it was pouring outward from her frozen shoulder. Tears kept streaming from her eyes as she thought about a situation in the past that she had very little previous recollection of. "It's pouring out of my shoulder!" she cried. "What's going on?" I explained to her that Yin Type As have a hard time dealing with grief since their hyperdeveloped liver, correlating with joy, has an aversion to it. They often stow away their grief within the soft tissues of their body, and since the lungs are their vulnerable organ, it gets packed away in the lung channel. Grief is an emotion often connected to the Yin Type A's frozen shoulder syndrome.

Jeannie is tough, always standing strong for the sake of her family, never showing them her vulnerable side. Yet here she was, with tears flowing, as she wept and wept even more. After about thirty minutes, she cried her last tear, saying that her body felt tremendously lighter. When I asked her to move her shoulder, we were both surprised by how freely she moved it without pain. As in Jeannie's situation, acupuncture and Sasang herbal therapy are often capable of facilitating the release of physical and psychological stagnation and pain. In my early years of practice, I used to avoid certain acupuncture points that I was told could release emotions but eventually discovered that they are released when it's time to let go. This can be an arduous process, especially if we do not have a support network of close friends, a therapist, and/or family members.

YIN TYPE B

With a weaker upper body, the Yin Type B is next in line, directly behind the Yin Type A, when it comes to shoulder issues. Her shoulders are often narrowly structured, placing stress on the surrounding tendons and muscles of the neck and upper back. Backpack and pocketbook straps, designed for broader shoulders, routinely slide downward, forcing her to lift her shoulders higher, placing added stress on the shoulder tendons and surrounding ligaments and muscles. Yang energy flow to the upper body is further impeded during menopause, making the shoulders and neck area more vulnerable to tightness and injury. This is a phase when the Yin Type B's already deficient yang energy may further weaken, leaving her extremities feeling cold and stiff. Warming the body up with ample cardiovascular exercise, hot-natured foods and herbs, and direct application of heat are assured ways to crank up her yang energy.

The uncultivated Yin Type B is far from being dignified—a trait that barely trickles out from her weaker shoulders. Instead, she slumps her shoulders and stares at the ground as if to say, "I am not capable enough and would rather just be left alone." Dignity for the Yang Type A gets more attention than for the Yin Type B, amplified by an angry-natured, hyperdeveloped spleen. Without the spleen's support, the Yin Type B's dignity is hidden beneath layer upon layer of self-consciousness. The cultivated Yin Type B builds her self-confidence by feeling secure and calm amidst adversity, establishing a portable safe haven for herself when with others.

Whenever the Yin type B is faced with a challenge, she has a tendency to feel as if she is going at it alone. The menopausal transition is no exception, often making her feel lonely and disregarded—a result of her own self-effacing choice to distance herself from others. Dignity cannot be achieved in isolation, making it crucial to discuss her feelings with and get closer to others. It is a time to loosen her grip on herself and open up about her feelings and emotions. She may never be as extroverted as a yang type, but rising above her timid nature can bring about a profound sense of pride and dignity.

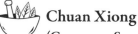 **Chuan Xiong**

(Common: Szechuan Lovage Root; Latin: *Ligusticum striatum*)
Chuan Xiong, or Szechuan lovage root, is commonly used in the Eastern medical clinic to treat headaches and pain in the upper body thanks to its blood-invigorating and energy-stimulating capability. In Sasang medicine, Szechuan lovage root is said to raise the Yin Type B's weaker yang energy upward to the head and shoulders. As a warm-natured herb, it is also capable of addressing and preventing the cold-induced

pain usually felt after catching a cold and/or during the colder months. The Yin Type B's frozen shoulder responds well to this herb's warm, yang-ascending, and blood-invigorating properties. Ferulic acid, a component of lovage root, has anti-inflammatory, antioxidant, and lipid-reducing potential.[2] Two lactones found in lovage root—senkyunolide and Z-ligustilide—have been known to effectively treat various cerebrovascular diseases and migraines.[3]

Common Uses
Chuan Xiong invigorates yang energy and blood flow to reduce upper body pain, alleviates headaches, and boosts immunity.

Sources
Both alcohol-based and nonalcoholic tinctures of lovage root can be purchased from the Etsy and Hawaii Pharm websites.

Preparation and Dosage
Please follow manufacturer's dosage recommendations on the label.

Herbal Friend: Yan Hu Suo
(Common: Corydalis; Latin: *Corydalis yanhusuo*)

As we saw in the discussion of fibroids in chapter 9, Yan Hu Suo, or corydalis, is commonly used in Eastern medicine to treat pain of all types, thanks to its strong blood-invigorating properties. Together, Yan Hu Suo and Chuan Xiong symbiotically enhance circulation in the upper body and reduce pain. Higher doses of Yang Hu Suo may cause dizziness, drowsiness, and abdominal distension. Doses over 60 grams have also caused breathing difficulty, low blood pressure, and muscle spasms, so make sure you don't go overboard! Fortunately, most readily available sources don't even come close to this dose range. Hawaii Pharm offers a tincture of Yan Hu Suo on its website, and Biotech Nutritions offers it in capsule form. Please follow the manufacturer's suggested dosages for both Chuan Xiong and Yan Hu Suo, and remember to ingest them both in one serving.

11

Rocking the Boat

Libido

"I just don't have much interest in sex anymore," Melissa said. It started soon after she skipped her last cycle, which she thought was a reason to celebrate as she remembered the days when a cycle would get in the way, causing mood swings and pain in her lower abdomen. Melissa used to plan her entire life around her cycle and now all of that had come to an end. She and her husband were snuggling in front of the TV when he made his usual clumsy advances toward her. She would usually get the message, and off they'd go giggling to their cozy bed. But now things were different: although she knew what he was up to, Melissa felt no desire in response, so instead, she just brushed his hand aside. She would never have come to see me if her husband hadn't begged her to try something, anything, to get things going again. "My love for him hasn't changed at all! Actually I am still sexually attracted to him after thirty years of marriage," she said, sobbing. "Intercourse for the sake of satisfying your husband is not intercourse," I said. "There are many happily married couples who no longer have sex. The issue is whether or not *you* would like to resume having intercourse. Menopause is an opportunity for you to reclaim what is precious and shed what is not."

Like many other women her age, Melissa's desire for sex had waned. We could easily blame this on a decline in estrogen, a word that gets its name from the Greek word *estrus,* meaning "sexual passion." Fortunately however, hormone reduction doesn't paint the whole picture when it comes to postmenopausal libido. A survey conducted by the National Council on Aging revealed that 70 percent of sexually active women age sixty and over were even more satisfied with their current sex lives compared to when they were younger.[1] In her book *Women, Sex, and Desire,* Elizabeth Davis describes how many older women continue to have sex as often as they did before menopause, and that it frequently gets even better for them. She admits that changes inside and outside of the uterus could easily make women shift their attitudes around sex, seeking gentler ways to reach orgasm, without causing pain or irritation. The secret to a satisfactory sex life after menopause, according to these women, is adjusting to the change and not giving up on their sex organs.

For many women, the menopausal transition and the changes that occur in this phase of life affect sexual desire. At times, heightened testosterone levels may induce a heightened desire for sex. Plunging estrogen levels, on the other hand, often result in the opposite scenario. The discomfort associated with vaginal dryness or hot flashes may also contribute to a lack of desire to engage in sexual activity. These changes may occur gradually or fluctuate daily, seemingly without rhyme or reason.

WESTERN AND EASTERN PERSPECTIVES ON LIBIDO

According to the North American Menopause Society, sexual health is divided into three components: drive, beliefs, and motivation. Drive is the physiological aspect of sexual health that includes involuntary arousal of sex organs and sexual attraction. Belief is the psychological component, which involves one's own ideas about sex in general. And motivation is the incentive to engage in sexual activity.[2] Even though all three of these components play a significant role in libido, one can fill in for the other. Drive, for example, is usually stronger with the yin types, since their lower body in general is fed more energy. Even if their belief system steers them elsewhere, a healthy drive will eventually spur them on. Yang individuals with a weaker drive can still enjoy sex if they are motivated or believe it is an important part of their life. We will talk more about this in the section below.

Although Western medicine acknowledges that libido can be influenced by both psychological and physiological factors, an established treatment approach has yet to be implemented. With an emphasis on physiological components, researchers have examined hormone function, specifically testosterone, in the enhancement of sexual desire in men and have only begun to explore its role in women. Studies involving testosterone supplementation to enhance libido in women have either been inconclusive or showed moderate results. Moreover, significant side effects from long-term administration have been noted.[3]

In Sasang medicine, sexual health issues are divided into two major categories: excess and deficiency. Excess issues involve the stagnation of energy in our stronger organs, requiring outward energy flow from the genitals. Deficiency issues are due to a lack of energy, calling for more energy flow to the reproductive organs. The yin types are more often faced with the former condition, and the yang types with the latter. Take the Yin Type B, for example, who is so sensitive that the slightest issue surrounding sex can tick her off, slamming the door shut. So if you lack sex drive, don't automatically think it is a weakness! The inability to balance one's predominant emotion may be responsible, causing the stronger organs to absorb bodily energy for themselves, eventually stealing energy away from the genitals.

Although all body types may be affected by stress-related sexual health issues, each has its own tendencies that can contribute. The yang types succumb to sexual health issues more easily than the yin types because yang energy correlates with the upper body, where the majority of it flows. The yin types have a stronger lower body, making it easier for energy to flow to the genitals, igniting arousal. The yang types tend to equate sleep rather than sexual intercourse with relaxation and stress release, whereas the yin types often think less about sleep and more about intercourse as a means of relaxation. There are many exceptions to this rule, since there are yang types who equate sex with relaxation and yin types who would rather just sleep after a long day at work. The challenge is to know where you stand in the sexual health spectrum. Is your upper body hoarding all of the energy flow, or are you simply tired and wanting sleep? Knowing your body type and its unique requirements can help improve not only your sex life but also your health in general.

Other Factors That May Contribute to a Lack of Libido

- Certain medications, such as antibiotics and antihypertensive drugs
- Excessive caffeine intake, which may eventually cause the energy in your lower body to weaken
- Other dietary factors, such as food allergies or body-type-incompatible foods

---

The following tips may be helpful in jump-starting your sex drive.

Tip #1: Find the Optimal Time

Yang corresponds with the morning and yin with the evening. Yang energy flows upward and yin downward. Yang represents activity and yin calmness and quiet. Do you see a pattern here? Most people have sex in the evening, during yin time, when their body is ready to slow down. When we are younger, yang energy may be abundant at all times of the day, but as we age, the ebb and flow of energy throughout the day becomes more apparent. We need plenty of yang energy to engage in sex, so if you are feeling sluggish in the evening, then reserve Sunday morning for a little fun between the sheets.

Tip #2: Be in the Moment: Bringing Energy Down to the Genitals

The center of bodily energy, according to Eastern philosophy, is the dan tian, which is located about one inch below the navel and is approximately three inches wide. The hustle and bustle of daily life causes our center of energy to slowly rise upward, to the point that when menopause arrives, it is somewhere in the chest or even higher, in the head. This is one reason why hot flashes are so common among menopausal women. Sex is another form of meditation, requiring our energy to be rooted in the dan tian.

While inhaling, imagine air flowing from your nose to the dan tian, and when exhaling, encourage it to flow outward from this area.

Repeat this step over and over again while freeing your mind from the stresses of the day.

Tip #3: Warm Up and Put All Expectations Aside

You do not have to be aroused or even reach an orgasm to have a satisfying sexual experience. Making the time to clear your mind while spending it with your partner is more than enough. Most of us do not give or take this time, and our relationships suffer. Give yourself thirty minutes a day to chill with your partner, refraining from playing with the iPod or watching TV; simply focus on each other. Make physical contact during this time with no expectation or goal in mind, just letting it flow.

One way to get away from feeling inadequate and defeated by sexual expectation is simply to stop expecting! If our mind is always focused on the finish line, then the process is wasted. Mention ahead of time to your partner that orgasm is not the goal and that spending intimate time with them is what you desire the most. Simply placing your hands on each other is enough to stimulate and balance the flow of yin and yang.

Tip #4: Get Rid of "Have To's"

Sex is not a validation of love, nor is it a requisite. A lack of libido itself is not a problem, nor a disease. If you are an otherwise healthy female, then chances are you can switch it on again. Yet before you blame yourself or your partner, keep in mind that many couples are still deeply in love with each other without having intercourse. The question is, "Could you still love your spouse without making love to them even once more throughout your life?" If the answer is a definite yes, and you are concerned about libido, then it's just a matter of time. Women tend to blame themselves for an unsuccessful sex life. Most of the patients who come to see me about libido are women who are concerned about satisfying their husbands. I hardly ever see their husbands, and when I do, there's a much higher success rate when both partners seek treatment.

Tip #5: Try Something New

One thing that keeps us feeling young is the desire to keep learning and trying new things. Ask your partner what turns them on. Is it a particular spot on the body? A new position? Is there a particular time of day or month when they feel like having sex? Reveal to your partner what turns you on and how you would like them to satisfy you. Reflect on this yourself, since there may be new parts of you that have yet to be discovered. Human touch is the most powerful healing energy there is! Search for the right spot by slowly rubbing your fingers along your body. You may want to try this with your partner, too. We all have places along our energy meridians that increase health and well-being. Surprising your partner by changing into something silky and sexy and/or bringing out a sex toy may also spark things into action. In Christiane Northrup's book *The Secret Pleasures of Menopause*, she explains how these methods don't have to be implemented with a partner. Getting in touch with one's own sexual energy is the first, if not the only, step necessary to satisfy one's sexual needs. Lastly, the use of lubricants, as you'll see in tip 7, is another way to spice things up in bed.

Tip #6: Talk Openly and Be Patient with Your Partner

There is nothing more romantic than simply being with your partner, setting everything else in life aside. A healthy relationship is one that is open, expressive, and verbal. If something is bothering you about your partner, don't hold it back for the sake of your relationship. On the same note, be open about yourself with your partner. Make the time to simply talk, agreeing not to argue or get on each other's nerves. Only when both of you communicate and share energies can the spark of libido be reignited.

Tip #7: Recognize If Pain Is the Perpetrator

A loss of libido is not necessarily a result of lacking motivation; it can also be a result of vaginal dryness, causing significant pain during intercourse. After several episodes of pain, the body may simply say enough is enough, reducing your sexual desire. Luckily, there are numerous gentle and safe lubricants available, such as Wild Yam Cream, Sylk, Astroglide, and Key-E, which have offered many women significant relief. Emerita is another source that specializes in natural products, such as Oh! Warming Lubricant and Response Arousal Cream to enhance sensations. The application of a prescription plant-based or bioidentical estrogen and/or progesterone cream may also provide comfort in more acute cases.

THE YIN AND YANG OF LIBIDO

Yin and yang play an important role in libido, and deficiency in one or the other can interfere with sex drive and/or performance. Yin, for example, correlates with the desire to submit oneself, be penetrated, or let it all loose during sex, whereas yang is the desire to initiate sex, penetrate, and take control. Neither of these aspects is exclusive to men or women; yin and yang are not absolute, and both contribute in their own way to libido. Intercourse itself is the courting of yin and yang, giving and taking, submitting and controlling.

When yin and yang are abundant, sexual desire comes naturally, but if they are stagnant or deficient, it can be challenging to get our juices pumping. Stagnant yin is frequently the result of trauma to a woman's feminine nature—when she submits or lets go prematurely, feeling defeated and taken advantage of by others or by events in her life. She may feel violated or raped not necessarily physically, but by circumstances beyond her control. Yang stagnation often happens when she gives every ounce of her effort to initiate, penetrate, or take control of something but does not succeed. Yin and yang stagnation take her away from the moment and instead fill her with regret, remorse, and distance from her partner.

Stagnation eventually morphs into deficiency—where regret and remorse become fatigue and exhaustion. Yin and yang naturally decrease slightly during the menopause transition, but as long as she is still living, these energies flow within her. Reduction of yin and yang does not equate directly with a lack of libido; instead, it forces her to reflect on her relationships and find a deeper, stronger sense of love. After raising children, working for decades, and waking up next to the same person day after day, it becomes a challenge for many to appreciate their partner and the process of making love. Deficient yin and yang nevertheless still need to be nourished and fortified, and satisfying sex with your partner may do the trick, as both of you fill in the gaps. If the flame of love is still flickering between partners, then hope for a healthy sex life is still there. When we are younger, sexual intercourse is primarily a means to release pent-up, stagnant, and agitated energy. Even though intercourse can serve this role as we advance in life, it also becomes a way to further unite and supplement our energies.

LIBIDO AND THE YIN YANG BODY TYPES

Sasang medicine holds that libido has two components: emotional and physical. The former component drives the latter, and hence our emotions are the key to unlocking sexual potential. Each body type has its own unique way of sending energy to the genital area by balancing emotions. The body-type-specific herbs listed in this section can also encourage flow to this area.

Each body type has its own reason for libido issues, depending on which organ is inherently stronger and which is weaker. As mentioned earlier, the yin liver and kidneys feed energy to the lower half of the body, and the yang spleen and lungs feed it to the upper half. Yin energy moves downward, nourishing and strengthening the reproductive organs. Born with stronger yang organs, the yang types are more prone to lower body issues such as sexual dysfunction than the yin types. But the yin types may have issues too, especially if their lower body energy stagnates and lacks yang. As an upward-moving energy, yang gives the sexual organs a boost and assists with arousal. Hence the yin types benefit from yang-stimulating herbs, and the yang types from those that are yin nourishing.

Whether you are yang or yin deficient, the symptoms of libido loss may be exactly the same, making it crucial for you to address them according to your body-type-related source. Strengthening yin or yang when there is already too much to go around can make things go from bad to worse. If you have any doubts about which body type you are, please retake the yin yang body type test or have a close acquaintance take it for you. If you are still not sure, then look to the "Continuing the Voyage" section (page 335) for further options.

YANG TYPE A

Sexual desire for the Yang Type A often departs as quickly as it arrives, and if she or her partner misses the cue, it could be too late to get the action going. Fluctuation in sexual interest is not the only situation when the Yang Type A switches gears quickly, since she is constitutionally on the cusp of yin and yang energies. The Korean name for the Yang Type A is So Yang, which refers to change, transformation, and fluctuation. If you have a Yang Type A partner or are one yourself, it is important not to feel offended by or ashamed of such rapid fluctuations.

Adapting to the changes of menopause is another skill that the Yang Type A easily acquires. Others admire how she rarely complains or dwells on her symptoms. Yet adjusting to menopause does not correlate with an increased interest in sex. A lack of libido is likely to disturb her partner more, since the Yang Type A's focus is always on what lies ahead, not in the moment. A focus on the future causes the energy within the Yang Type A's body to forge upward, toward the yang portions. As with all the body types, however, health is determined by the smooth flow of energy in both the upper and lower parts of the body. Excessive energy flow to the upper body will further weaken their kidneys, bladder, and uterus. Sexual activity, and the intimacy that it involves, can activate the lower body energy, strengthening these organs.

Solution

Slow down and listen to your body. Your sexual energy is deep within you, waiting to be accessed and engaged. Because it encourages the flow of energy down to the lower parts, abdominal breathing is a perfect practice for this. Menopausal symptoms are a reminder that you are living your life too fast and need to apply the brakes. Try eating and thinking more slowly, and taking the time to interact with your partner instead of solving everything in haste. Sex can offer you a chance to slow down and root your energy, sending it to your weaker kidneys. It is easy to write off sex as an unproductive activity compared to immediate imperatives, like washing the dishes or getting dinner ready. These activities, however, do not activate your lower energies like sex can.

Table 11.1 on the next page provides a quick view of Yang Type A's sexual advantages and disadvantages.

TABLE 11.1. AT A GLANCE: SEX AND THE YANG TYPE A

Advantages	Disadvantages
She can feel just fine living her whole life without sex.	Reproduction and spousal satisfaction are at risk.
She doesn't waste time getting things started.	The show is usually over before it gets started.
She can stay in love without the need for intimacy.	Convincing her partner of this isn't always easy.
She is capable of sexual arousal and enjoyment.	She rarely takes the time to feel it, and when she does, it's often gone before she recognizes it.

The following are herbs that send energy to the Yang Type A's sex organs and nourish the kidneys.

 Mu Dan Pi

(Common: Cortex of Tree Peony Root; Latin: *Paeonia suffruticosa*)
In Sasang medicine, Mu Dan Pi, or tree peony, is used to promote the flow of energy toward the lower half of the body, igniting sexual energy and nourishing the reproductive organs. Along with this function comes the ability to assist with digestion, which also relies on the smooth downward flow of energy. The cold nature of tree peony makes it suitable for the hot-natured Yang Type A, cooling her temper and unsettled emotions. Coldness nourishes and supports bodily yin, making it suitable for the yin-deficient Yang Type A. It is also used for the Yang Type A's menstrual cramping and lack of menstrual flow, which are both considered the result of blood stagnation in the lower body. The cold nature of tree peony is also effective in alleviating the Yang Type A's hot flashes.

Common Uses
Tree peony alleviates libido issues (weakness and/or lack of flow toward the sexual organs), indigestion, and hot flashes.

Source
Hawaii Pharm offers a tincture of Mu Dan Pi on its website.

Preparation and Dosage
Follow the manufacturer's suggestions.

Caution
Tree peony is a cold-natured herb, making it suitable for the Yang Type A but not for the yin types, who benefit from warmer-natured herbs. Cold-natured herbs may cause constipation, diarrhea, and/or indigestion for the yin types. Since this herb promotes the flow of blood and energy, it is not recommended in cases of excessive uterine bleeding.

Herbal Friend: Sheng Di Huang
(Common: Rehmannia or Chinese Foxglove;
Latin: *Rehmannia glutinosa*)

Sheng Di Huang, or rehmannia root, can be combined with Mu Dan Pi (tree peony) to strengthen the Yang Type A's lower body. Sheng Di Huang is also commonly used for nourishing the blood, supporting kidney function, and strengthening the lower back, knees, and ankles. It can be purchased as a tincture from Herb Pharm. The Sasang-based formula Dokhwal Jihwang Tang, which contains both Mu Dan Pi and Sheng Di Huang along with several other herbs, can help nourish and support the reproductive organs. This formula is available on sasangmedicine.com: click "Sasang Store" from the main menu and then the "Add to Cart" icon beneath "Herbal Pills." Type "Dokhwal Jihwang Tang" under "Ordering Instructions."

It's Not Over Till It's Over:
A Yang Type A's Story

Joanne was convinced that her sex life was over and expected to live out her postmenopausal years without having one more sexual encounter. Yet life never fails to throw surprises at us, and in Joanne's case it was a new boyfriend, who "just showed up" twenty years after she had divorced her husband. Joanne told me that after meeting him, she occasionally had "weird feelings" that came and went before she could recognize what they were. She said it felt like a "tickle" coming from her lower abdomen that would occasionally catch her attention when she was alone with him. When I mentioned that it could be her sexual energies talking, she giggled and responded, "I never knew that half of my body still existed!" I prescribed a Yang Type A formula (Dokhwal Jihwang Tang) that included Mu Dan Pi and suggested that she entertain these feelings by slowing her mind down and breathing deeply into them. We discussed how over the years her stronger spleen had taken over, hoarding the energy away from her kidneys and liver—where sexual energy arises. Joanne admitted that she simply dismissed any signs of intimacy with her boyfriend since there were always other things that needed to be done. After taking this formula for several weeks and making a sincere effort to slow her life down, the tickle she felt when with her boyfriend morphed into sexual desire and a reignited sex life.

YANG TYPE B

The Yang Type B's weaker liver is often behind sexual health issues, as it governs the flow of energy to her genitals and interferes with fertility and monthly-cycle regulation. It is also common for the Yang Type B to have very little or no motivation toward sexual activity since she has "more important" things to do. The Yang Type B faces the biggest challenge when it comes to sexual intimacy since she spends most, if not all, of her energy on public responsibility, or sa mu, depriving her of close relationships.

The menopausal Yang Type B is further pushed toward her outward goals and accomplishments. If she has not completed the bulk of her public work by this point, then anger and frustration will set in. The balanced Yang Type B will relax her goals, especially the ones that, in the end, hurt those who are close to her. The idea that time is running out no longer makes her sad and angry. She views life as a continuum, realizing that not everything has to get done right here, right now. For the Yang Type B, menopause is a time to discover her joy once and for all.

Solution
The Yang Type B has the profound ability to detect when others are being truthful to one another, a trait born from the sa mu within her

stronger lungs. Yet by the time menopause sets in, many untruthful people have come her way, which upsets her tremendously, sending yang energy bursting upward toward her head. In order to activate her sexual energies, the Yang Type B must renew her belief in humanity, appreciating those who are truthful and forgiving those who aren't. Dang yo, or group orientation, associated with her weaker liver, is particularly difficult for the Yang Type B, who tends to be overcritical and sensitive to the faults of others. She benefits from finding commonality with, rather than distancing herself from, others, but forcing herself to do so will only cause more grief and anger. Sexual energy awaits the Yang Type B who gets in touch with her soft side and finds joy in occasionally yielding to her partner.

Table 11.2 provides a quick view of Yang Type B's sexual advantages and disadvantages.

TABLE 11.2. AT A GLANCE: SEX AND THE YANG TYPE B

Advantages	Disadvantages
Sex rarely causes her confusion or stress.	This is only because sex is the last thing on her mind.
She doesn't have to worry about getting pregnant . . .	But this is because over 90 percent of Yang Type Bs are infertile.
Sex can stimulate her weaker liver energy, reduce sorrow, and enhance joy.	Convincing her of this is not easy, as it requires that she preserve her bedroom energy.

The following are herbs that send energy to the Yang Type B's sex organs and nourish the liver.

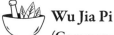 **Wu Jia Pi**
(Common: Devil's Club; Latin: *Oplopanax horridus*)
One of the most spectacular sights when hiking the mountains of the Pacific Northwest is the majestic devil's club. Its humongous leaves kneel down and pay tribute to a stem filled with bright white flowers bursting out from the center, indicating its profound medicinal power. Devil's club gets its name from the prickly appearance of its

thorny stem, which resembles a devil's club. For thousands of years, the local Native American population made use of devil's club for its healing properties. As a plant native to East Asia, it also plays a major role in Sasang medicine: it grounds the excessive yang of the Yang Type B, sending energy to her lower parts and strengthening her sexual organs. Like its cousin ginseng, it also has the ability to support and strengthen the immune system and has been traditionally used to combat pneumonia, tuberculosis, tumor growth, and diabetes.

Common Uses
Devil's club addresses deficient libido, immunodeficiency (common colds and allergies), headaches, paralysis or weakness of the lower extremities, soreness/numbness of the muscles, and cramps and spasms of the legs.

Sources
Devil's club is available from manufacturers such as Herb Pharm and HerbalRemedies.com.

Preparation and Dosage
Follow the manufacturer's suggested dosage guidelines.

Caution
The prickly spine of devil's club may cause topical allergies if touched. Devil's club also has the potential to lower blood sugar levels and should be used with caution while taking medications for diabetes.

Herbal Friend: Mu Gua
(Common: Chinese Quince;
Latin: *Chaenomeles lagenaria*)

Quince fruit is another frequently prescribed herb for the Yang Type B's weaker lower body. This herb, which is mainly prescribed for pain in the lower body, is not as effective as devil's club in strengthening the lower body. Yet they get along very well together, enhancing each other's effects. Quince fruit tea mixed with honey is often sold in Korean markets, but if you do not live near one, try ordering it from the PosharpStore website. You can also purchase quince trees from Willis

Orchard Company or a delicious quince fruit spread from Nuts.com. Look for quince fruit extract at Hawaii Pharm. For best effect, devil's club and quince fruit should be consumed together in one sitting.

YIN TYPE A

With over 70 percent of all Americans being Yin Type As, their ability to reproduce and perform in the bedroom cannot be underestimated. Yet not all Yin Type As are ready to jump into bed and get it on! Born with a stronger liver, they tend to absorb environmental toxins more than the other types. Toxic fumes, foods, and even emotions tend to stick around and inhibit the flow of energy to their genitals. The objective is to get their liver energy flowing again. Actually, the liver's most powerful function, filtering blood, is a result of wanting nothing other than to be pure and free of restriction. Yet this desire often gets it into trouble, since there is no such thing as absolute purity, and nobody can be completely free of bacteria, toxicity, responsibility, and negativity.

The menopausal liver has already had its fair share of dealing with toxicity, and it is common for the Yin Type A to have difficulty ridding herself of it all. Often the liver will be so focused on eliminating the accumulation of the old that it has no time to take in the new. No matter how many vitamins and/or minerals the Yin Type A ingests, if her liver is congested, she may still be deficient. The more she lets go, the more she is capable of absorbing. Knowing what to let go of and what to take in is a fundamental challenge for Yin Type As because this ability, called ju chek, is associated with their weaker lung system.

Solution

The liver relies on the emotion of joy to flow smoothly and function normally. Without joy, the liver loses its bearings and absorbs excessive by-products from food and life. Joy that comes from the lower body is sustained more easily than that which is derived from the upper body. Lower body joy stems from intimacy and immersion, whereas upper body joy is momentary and fleeting. The genitalia need to feel joy to be stimulated. Fleeting moments of joy and sorrow actually confuse sexual energy, engaging the sympathetic nervous system and making you feel on edge most of the time. Bringing joy back to your genitalia requires that you free yourself from old and unproductive thought patterns and habits. It means that you have to let your liver out for a walk and relieve itself from constant burden.

Table 11.3 provides a quick view of Yin Type A's sexual advantages and disadvantages.

TABLE 11.3. AT A GLANCE: SEX AND THE YIN TYPE A

Advantages	Disadvantages
Sex can be particularly joyful and fun for this type.	Her idea of joy and fun might be different from her partner's.
Relaxation can reignite the libido for most Yin Type As.	Responsibility and obligation can easily reduce her libido.
Orgasm is an excellent way to release her pent-up liver energy.	Her stronger liver often absorbs excessive stress, stealing energy from her genitals and blocking libido.
She's an animal in bed! (Her sexual energy is surprisingly robust once it gets going.)	It takes a while for her to warm up.

The following are herbs that release liver tension for the Yin Type A and promote the flow of sexual energy.

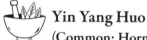 **Yin Yang Huo**
(Common: Horny Goat Weed; Latin: *Epimedium* spp.)
As its name implies, this innocent-looking weed was discovered when goats by the hundreds became more sexually active after consuming it. In Eastern medicine, this herb has been used for thousands of years to stimulate sexual energy in livestock and humans alike! Horny goat weed's warming and yang-tonifying properties are also useful for the yang-deficient individual with sterility issues, making it suitable only for the yin types. This property also helps strengthen the lower body and assists with arthritic pain of the waist, knees, and ankles. After ingestion, horny goat weed travels to the kidneys and liver to support their function. Acrid in flavor, it also supports the pathogen-dispersing

function of the lungs and immune system. In Sasang medicine, it is used to promote the flow of lower body energy upward to the lungs, stimulating sexual energy along the way. A recent study showed that this herb has testosterone-like properties, contributing to the Eastern idea that yang and testosterone correlate with one another.[4]

Common Uses
Horny goat weed addresses decreased libido, impotence, sterility, erectile dysfunction, and chronic lower body weakness and pain (e.g., waist, knee, ankle).

Sources
A capsule form of horny goat weed can be purchased from the Nature's Way website. It can also be purchased in liquid extract form from the Amazing Herbs website.

Preparation and Dosage
Follow the manufacturer's suggestions.

Herbal Friend: Tu Si Zi
(Common: Cuscuta; Latin: *Cuscuta chinensis*)

Tu Si Zi, or cuscuta, is another herb used to stimulate the yang energy of the liver and kidneys that is often prescribed for a lack of libido and other symptoms due to yang weakness, such as vaginal discharge, urinary incontinence, and diarrhea. Cuscuta and horny goat weed together enhance each other's ability to support yang energy and address libido. Swanson Health Products offers a capsule form of cuscuta on its website. Both herbs can be taken at the same time according to manufacturer's recommended dosages.

Between the Sheets of a Yin Type A

Melissa, a Yin Type A, started to cry when she told me that her sex life had "gone down the tubes." When I inquired what had made things get so sour, she simply replied, "Life." Melissa lamented about how she and her husband used to jokingly refer to Sundays as "sex days," but now those days were long gone. Now every time she tapped her husband's shoulder, he just snored away, and when he tapped hers, she replied, "Not now, I'm tired." I was relieved to know that both she and her husband still had a desire for sex, even though it was hard to get the show on the road. After I met her husband and asked him a few questions, it turned out that her husband was also a Yin Type A. I explained to her that the yin types sometimes have difficulty getting foreplay started because of deficient yang energy. I then prescribed both of them a decoction with horny goat weed and cuscuta to ascend yang and promote movement of sexual energy. After about two weeks of taking the herbs, Melissa told me that on Sunday she was about to tap her husband's shoulder only to find him awake and smiling at her. "Not only that," she told me, "it happened again on Monday!" Sometimes all it takes is a little spark to ignite the flame again.

YIN TYPE B

With stronger kidneys, responsible for willpower and consistency, the Yin Type B tends to retain a healthy sexual desire later on in life compared to the other body types, but her shy and timid yin nature could put a damper on things, keeping this energy hidden within her kidneys and expressed only when she is by herself. Lee Je-ma stated that the Yin Type B needs to get out of the house more, while the Yang Type A needs to spend more time there. "Getting out of the house" can be interpreted literally, but also figuratively. The expression of sexual energy for the Yin Type B is a challenge often plagued with feelings of "my partner is probably not interested" or "I shouldn't feel this way." Little do most Yin Type Bs know that simply feeling sexy around others can enhance their sex appeal.

The menopausal Yin Type B is often tired of dealing with people, wishing to live like a hermit, away from the hustle and bustle of society. For most of us, sex occupies a very intimate place in the heart, and the Yin Type B, living in her fantasy world, may find it satisfactory to hide there, under lock and key. On the occasions when the Yin Type B feels lonely or yearns for intimacy, she often lacks the courage to express it. Maybe she's been hurt too many times by doing so, or perhaps she has found it safer just to keep things inside. Menopause is a time when a woman's inner world gets turned inside out, when she no longer has the ability simply to keep her inner thoughts unexposed. The Yin Type B is faced with a choice: to retreat further or exit her comfort zone.

Solution

The self-conscious Yin Type B may fear the changes that menopause brings and sink deeper into isolation, choosing to find intimacy alone rather than with a partner. Yet menopause has a sneaky little way of reminding you that the tides are changing, and it's time to jump on board. It is time to challenge your limitations and emerge from the status quo. With immense hidden energy inside your kidneys, there is an ocean of intimate potential knocking at your door and waiting to come out. Trust your instinct and take action. True, the first few attempts may end in failure, as your partner (or you) may be too tired, too stressed, or too busy, but don't give up. Use your bang ryak, or innate strategic ability, to figure out a way. Lee Je-ma said that the Yin Type B cannot simply live her life by clinging to the comfort of home. Although comfort is a priority, it can also entrap her.

Table 11.4 provides a quick view of Yin Type B's sexual advantages and disadvantages.

TABLE 11.4. AT A GLANCE: SEX AND THE YIN TYPE B

Advantages	Disadvantages
Thanks to stronger kidney energy, she is easily stimulated.	This can lead to undue sexual frustration and stress when fantasy doesn't become a reality.
Sex is an excellent way to release excessive fear and worry from her stronger kidneys.	But sexual interaction itself can easily become a source of fear and worry for her.
Her stronger kidneys enhance the ability to be intimate and warm.	She is extremely sensitive to others' lack of intimacy and warmth.
Of the three factors influencing libido, most Yin Type Bs have a strong drive and motivation.	The third factor, belief, is frequently her greatest challenge.

The following are herbs that calm the kidneys of the Yin Type B and stimulate sexual yang energy.

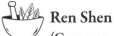 ## Ren Shen
(Common: Ginseng Root; Latin: *Panax ginseng*)

Ren Shen, or ginseng, is one of the most powerful herbs for the Yin Type B, as it strongly stimulates the spleen and gives her a jolt of energy. After a dose of ginseng, the Yin Type B may feel as if she can be more engaging and social—the spleen's domain. The added energy also assists with flow in her lower body and sexual organs, which tend to get blocked by her excessively introverted nature. With more energy flowing to and from the genitals and a boost in social energy, the Yin Type B has a better chance at improving her sex life. Ginseng, a root shaped like the human body, is one of the most prized herbs in Eastern medicine, embodying the concept of "like treats like." It is used to assist in recovery from chronic illness, support digestion, and encourage wound recovery.

Common Uses
Ginseng addresses fatigue, deficient libido, indigestion, chronic diarrhea, lack of confidence, dryness, and delayed wound healing.

Sources
There are numerous sources of ginseng on the internet, and it is often found in combination with other herbs to stimulate energy. I would recommend steering clear of these formulas if you are not sure whether or not the other ingredients are compatible with your body type. Korean ginseng from Nature's Way and Chinese ginseng from Herb Pharm are both reliable single-herb sources. A slightly more expensive route would be to purchase a Korean brand of ginseng extract pill that is used widely amongst Koreans from the LuckyVitamin website; search for "Korean ginseng extract pill."

Preparation and Dosage
Please follow the manufacturer's suggestions.

Caution
Even though ginseng may sound like an elixir for the Yin Type B, it comes with a catch. Yin Type Bs are very sensitive to everything, especially when

it comes to food and drink. Ginseng sends energy from the lower to the upper sections of the body, and for sensitive Yin Type Bs, it could easily bring on headaches. Start with a low dose and slowly work your way up to the standard dose if needed. Most Yin Type Bs can get away with lower doses, which saves them money and headaches. This property of ginseng makes it unsafe for the other body types, as it can possibly lead to high blood pressure and other upper body pressure-related disorders, such as headaches, visual disorders, anger, irritability, and so on.

Herbal Friend: Rou Gui
(Common: Cinnamon; Latin: *Cinnamomum cassia*)

Rou Gui, or cinnamon, and ginseng are great friends that travel hand in hand throughout the lower body, stimulating the flow of energy. Cinnamon is slightly warmer and less yang stimulating than ginseng, yet both herbs have their stimulating and warming effects. Used together, these effects are greatly enhanced. The Sasang-based formula Kwangye Doksam Palmul Tang contains both ginseng and cinnamon with several other herbs to strengthen yang and promote energy movement in the lower body. This formula is available on sasangmedicine.com: Click "Sasang Store" from the main menu and then the "Add to Cart" icon beneath "Herbal Pills." Type "Kwangye Doksam Palmul Tang" under "Ordering Instructions."

12

Sailing through the Mist

Brain Fog

Cindy was a master multitasker, impressing her coworkers and friends with her ability to remember just about anything despite always having so much to do. It wasn't until shortly after her fifty-third birthday, when she arrived at her car without the keys, that she felt an intense fear building up. "I never forget my keys! It's downhill from here on!" she thought. Life seemed to return to normal quickly until the next episode, when she left the house without feeding her fish, who greeted her after work with loud slurping sounds, opening and closing its mouth so wide that it could have swallowed her finger. "Alzheimer's!" she blurted out. "I'm following in my mother's foot-steps!" Things reached a crisis one morning when she fed her fish the car keys and took its food with her to the car while rushing out of the house. After days of unplanned fasting and strange foreign objects sinking to the bottom of its tank, Cindy's fish was not the only one in desperate need of a solution.

Cindy's visit to her doctor left her feeling old and helpless as he explained that her condition was likely due to a menopause-related estrogen deficiency, despite the fact that she was already undergoing hormone therapy. Unsatisfied with this explanation, she sought a sec-ond opinion from a doctor specializing in postmenopausal treatment.

He diagnosed her with brain fog, or mild cognitive impairment, but otherwise had nothing extraordinary to impart. One evening while staring remorsefully at her underfed and grossly emaciated fish, Cindy made up her mind to seek an alternative approach. When she arrived at my clinic, I saw before me a bright, energetic, but anxious woman, eager to complete all of the unfinished tasks piled up behind her.

What Exactly Is Brain Fog?

Brain fog, also known as "cloudiness of consciousness," "mental fog," and "cognitive dysfunction," is defined as forgetfulness and difficulty concentrating and thinking clearly. Here are some possible contributing factors as noted by Healthline:[1]

- Low energy
- Stress
- Lack of sleep
- Hormonal changes
- Diet
- Medications
- Accompanying medical conditions

After a thorough review of her history and current symptoms, an otherwise clear bill of health made it apparent that Western medicine couldn't come to her rescue. After I got to know Cindy and discovered her constitution, however, it seemed "natural" for her to feel this way. She spent practically every waking minute of her life juggling five to ten different tasks. As this is one of her Yang Type A strengths, Cindy had been able to multitask *this* far, but ultimately something had to give.

Memory loss and lack of focus are common occurrences during menopause, affecting six out of ten women. While, as we will soon see, there are numerous possible causes, brain fog is an issue faced by more and more women in the modern era. It may be that brain fog is, to a certain degree, the side effect of living in an increasingly fast-paced and industrialized society. Most of my patients with brain fog have several irons in their fires as they attempt to balance work and family or to simply quiet the screeching voices within their own minds. Brain fog can also be a result of being overwhelmed by internal responsibilities, like dealing with chronic pain or illness. In short, brain fog is frequently a side effect of feeling overwhelmed and inundated by one's circumstances.

Factors such as depression, hot flashes, and trouble sleeping may play a significant role in instigating brain fog. Stress is another prime suspect that inhibits the neurotransmitter dopamine (happy hormones) and enhances the production of cortisol levels within the body, suppressing the immune system and making us feel drowsy, unhappy, and unfocused. Attention deficit hyperactivity disorder, or ADHD, may also be a trigger, but primarily in women who have a history of this disorder, since adult onset is rare.

WESTERN AND EASTERN PERSPECTIVES ON BRAIN FOG

While Western medicine hasn't yet pinpointed the source of menopausal brain fog, studies do indicate that it occurs primarily in conjunction with reduced estrogen levels. Yet how estrogen deficiency affects memory loss and focus is still a subject of debate. We are now beginning to discover that estrogen influences more areas of the body than previously thought, such as facilitating the processing of verbal memory and the organization of thought. Estradiol (E1), the most active form of estrogen, plays an essential role in fine motor control, learning, memory, sensitivity to pain, and motor coordination.

After menopause, estradiol reduces to approximately 10 percent of its premenopausal amount, forcing the body to rely on estrone (E2)—another form of estrogen stored and produced in fat tissue after menopause. Before we blame estrogen deficiency for our menopausal woes, it's crucial to point out that even at lower levels, estradiol still offers significant benefit, and there's no consensus on how much is enough to avoid brain fog. Transdermal estradiol has shown moderate effects in enhancing cognitive function in some, but negative results in others. Researchers attribute this to a phenomenon referred to as the "critical window theory," arguing that estradiol supplementation within five years of menopause may enhance cognition, but after five years it has no, or even negative, effects. This theory parallels others that suggest that hormone replacement in general is relatively safer and more effective when introduced directly after menopause rather than later on.

Eastern medicine holds that we process emotion and memory in the same area of the body. Can you guess where this may be? Expressions like *heartbroken, heart wrenching*, or *heartfelt* may give you a clue. The heart, or "king of all organs" according to Eastern medicine, determines who and what can proceed through the palace gates. Despite having the authority to make such decisions and do as he pleases, an overwhelmed king is incapable of wielding his power. The human heart is strong enough to pump blood throughout the entire body approximately sixty times a minute, but when emotionally challenged, its powerful ability to circulate blood greatly diminishes.

The heart isn't the only source of brain fog in Eastern medicine; other organs also play a distinct role. Chronic indigestion, allergies, common colds, and/or pain are viable causes because they steal energy away from the heart. An overactive immune system will push more energy than needed out to the surface of the body, forming a strong protective shield but a softer core. A heavy meal may require more energy to digest, taking it away from other deserving areas of the body. Brain fog may also come from relentless pain that constantly sends SOS signals to the brain, demanding more and more of your focus and energy.

While brain fog and circulatory problems may occasionally indicate heart or other organ issues, they are primarily a result of energy imbalance rather than physiological illness. If, after following the steps in this chapter, your symptoms don't improve, I recommend that you consult a professional to rule out other possible causes.

Overcoming brain fog is frequently an uphill battle, leaving us with so many possible sources but nowhere to turn. In the midst of despair, we often look for that "special remedy" or "magic pill" and forget that the solution may actually be closer than we think—within our own mind and body. No matter what the source may be, the first step always begins with our intention and focus on healing. The second is creating an optimum environment for our symptoms to improve.

Let's start by introducing some general tips that have been proven to alleviate brain fog symptoms no matter what body type or accompanying issue(s) you may have.

Tip #1: Relax and Breathe!

The first thought that enters the middle-aged mind when forgetting becomes an issue is "I must be getting older/Alzheimer's/dementia." While this may be the case for a small fraction of women, most of the time it's simply due to feeling overstressed and overwhelmed with obligation and responsibility. Try taking three deep breaths before attempting to remember the forgotten task. If you still don't recall it, then try another three. Still no luck? Just forget it and move on, since chances are that if you don't try too hard to retrieve a memory, it will eventually return. Dwelling on our lack of memory actually makes it worse.

Tip #2: Eat Right for Your Type

The human brain requires a steady flow of minerals, vitamins, and other nutrients in order to function properly. Brain fog could be a result of insufficient brain nutrition and nourishment. One common misunderstanding is the idea that eliminating all carbohydrates improves health. Yes, reducing one's intake of simple carbs like snack foods and sugar could enhance health, but the brain cannot function properly without the help of glucose from complex carbs like whole grains, beans, brown rice, and so forth. Even certain complex carbs, however, may not be compatible with your body type. In my book *Your Yin Yang Body Type* I offer a concise list of foods for each type along with the percentage of each food group to ensure that nutritional requirements are met. I recommend consulting this list and adding or eliminating different foods based on the requirements of your type. Also, keep in mind that excessive consumption of sugar and caffeine interferes with memory in the long run by overstimulating the brain at first but eventually resulting in fatigue and loss of memory.

Tip #3: Enhance Your Sleep Quality

Sleep plays a significant role in consolidating and storing memory. It gives us the ability to press "stop" on the recorder of our day-to-day experiences, which could otherwise drive us crazy, like that song you just can't get out of your head. Deep sleep provides us with a fresh canvas upon which daily memories can be painted. With sleep deprivation, no matter how beautiful a picture we create in our mind, on canvas it just looks like a scribble. Are you having difficulty getting to sleep? Try focusing on the feeling and sound of slowly inhaling and exhaling while you lie in bed. Your breath helps not only to relax the body but also to clear your mind of accumulated daily clutter, and focusing on it in a meditative state could actually produce the same brain waves achieved during healthy sleep. So you don't really have to enter a deep sleep per say to feel rested and ready to go the next morning. Please refer to chapter 7 for more information.

Tip #4: Reduce Toxins in Your Home

Brain fog isn't always a result of insomnia or illness. Other not-so-conspicuous factors like household molds, dust, pet dander, cigarette smoke, and household cleaners may play a significant role in memory loss, fatigue, and lack of focus. While eliminating these from your home may not be easy, especially if you live in a moist climate, have several pets, or are a smoker, all hope isn't lost. Try purchasing an air filter, burning incense (or essential oils), cleaning the house regularly, and/or using natural cleaning/hygiene products.

Tip #5: Exercise to Enhance Flow to Your Brain

Cardiovascular exercise is perhaps the most effective way to improve brain circulation. It also increases endorphin levels, which are said to increase memory formation. Try exercising at least four days a week to optimize your circulation and increase memory. If you haven't exercised in a while, then start slowly, without demanding or expecting too much. Increase the intensity of your workout gradually, choosing a pace that doesn't leave you feeling excessively fatigued or sore for more than forty-eight hours afterward. Are you able to sweat when working out? A flood of endorphins is released within the body as soon as we start sweating, enhancing our health while giving us a euphoric feeling.

Tip #6: Stay Hydrated

A study done in 2013 found that dehydration was one of the most commonly reported brain fog triggers.[2] How could a lack of water intake cause brain fog? The simple answer is gravity. Most of what we put into our body eventually sinks down to the bottom, easily leaving the top half neglected. Drinking about half of your body weight in ounces is usually enough to keep saturated from head to toe. Are you still thirsty and dry after drinking plenty of water? Try adding electrolytes like magnesium and potassium to your water for enhanced absorption.

Tip #7: Take Omega-3 and Vitamin B$_{12}$

Omega-3 and/or vitamin B$_{12}$ deficiency may also contribute to brain fog. Many of my patients with brain fog are deficient in these nutrients since they aren't getting enough from their diet. Please refer to the appendix for a list of omega-3-rich foods. Table 12.1 provides the top vitamin B$_{12}$ foods categorized according to their compatibility with each yin yang body type, along with the recommended consumption level—high, moderate, low, or minimal.

- High—At least one serving a day
- Moderate—Up to five servings a week
- Low—At most three to four servings a week
- Minimal—At most one to two servings a week

TABLE 12.1. TOP SIX FOODS RICH IN VITAMIN B$_{12}$

Food Source	Yang Type A Compatibility	Yang Type B Compatibility	Yin Type A Compatibility	Yin Type B Compatibility	Single Serving Size	Percentage of Daily Recommend Value
Clams	High	Moderate	Low	Minimal	3 oz	1401%
Liver	Low	Minimal	Moderate	High	3 oz	1178%
Crab	High	Moderate	Low	Minimal	3 oz	163%
Red meat (beef)	Low	Minimal	High	Moderate	3 oz	85%
Sockeye salmon	Low	Minimal	High	Moderate	3 oz	80%

For a more comprehensive list of vitamin B₁₂-rich foods, try googling "vitamin B₁₂ foods" and compare your results to the list provided in my other book, *Your Yin Yang Body Type,* to determine whether or not they are compatible with your type.

BRAIN FOG AND YIN YANG BODY TYPES

Brain fog is indiscriminate among the four Sasang body types, striking all who fall into its trap. Yet each type is affected in slightly different ways depending on its stronger and weaker organ systems. Sasang medicine focuses primarily on the influence of our mind—or heart, to be more precise—and its effect on our hormone levels, nervous system, blood circulation, and so on. According to this approach, brain fog is often due to an imbalance of our body type's song nature and/or jung emotion (see table 12.2 on the next page). The song nature, remember, is our day-to-day emotional inclination, while the jung emotion manifests when our song nature isn't balanced.

You might ask, "If brain fog is a result of emotion, then why do so many women experience menopause-related brain fog?" The accumulation of stress, a need for change, and amassing responsibilities may contribute. At this point we either make the necessary changes and adjust our lifestyle or continue to struggle relentlessly. When we discover and balance our song nature, the jung emotion doesn't get the chance to take over and wreak havoc. The clearer our path, or myung, is, the easier it is to live life without distraction, distinguishing what is important and putting aside what isn't. Menopause forces us to discover our ultimate purpose in life and to let go of unnecessary habits while holding on to and enhancing its meaning. Lee Je-ma believed that discovering and carrying out our ultimate purpose, or *chon myung,* is the secret to living a healthy, prosperous, clearly focused, and long life.

Brain fog is the result of accumulated and stagnant energy within our body type's stronger (hyperdeveloped) organs, which are in charge of pumping energy throughout the body. As more and more air enters a bicycle tire, it gets harder to pump. The accumulation of air in the tire can be compared to the buildup of energy within our stronger organs as life progresses, making it harder for newer energy to make its way through.

Why do our stronger organs behave this way? Simply because they are tired, fed up with life's ups and downs, and at the breaking point. In Sasang medicine, this is referred to as *pokbal* (emotion explosion), and it can manifest as brain fog, hot flashes, sudden bursts of anger, sorrow, and so on. Emotional explosion is the result of pent-up, unexpressed emotion. Rather than manifest as an emotional outburst, it may simply lead to physical issues as the body loses its ability to cope. If you are having difficulty focusing and remembering, then reflect on your body type's song nature and make balancing it a priority.

TABLE 12.2. SONG AND JUNG EMOTIONS ACCORDING TO BODY TYPE

Body Type	Song Nature (Predominant Emotion)	Jung Emotion	Effect of Emotional Explosion
Yang Type A	Anger	Sorrow	Exhaustion/ collapse
Yang Type B	Sorrow	Anger	Rage
Yin Type A	Joy	Calmness/ comfort	Laziness/ immobility
Yin Type B	Calmness/ comfort	Joy	Detachment

ESSENTIAL OILS FOR BRAIN FOG

From my experience, the most effective way to address brain fog with herbs is to inhale them. No, I don't recommend stuffing herbs up your nose (although this was among the not-so-appealing treatment methods of the past). Instead, I suggest utilizing the power of essential oils. In Eastern medicine, inhaling eucalyptus to resuscitate an unconscious person was a method used for thousands of years. Studies show that smell is one of the most powerful ways to stimulate the brain because the olfactory (sense of smell) nerve communicates directly with the brain, activating the hippocampus and amygdala, which process memory and emotion. Smell has a direct effect on the emotions, often triggering thoughts of the past. In *The Essential Teachings of Sasang Medicine,* Lee

Je-ma explains that our senses are our closest connection to the heavens, and that certain aromas can enhance health through strengthening this relationship.

Essential oils can be inhaled in several different ways. The key is to inhale as much aroma as possible without irritating your skin or nasal passages. A common method is to place a folded piece of tissue inside a surgical mask doused with 1 to 3 drops of essential oil and wear it for at least thirty minutes a day. Dabbing a drop of essential oil directly under the nostrils is another simple way. Caution! Applying essential oil directly on the skin might cause local skin irritation. To avoid this, I'd recommend that you mix 1 drop of essential oil with 1 ounce of water before applying it the first time, or just stick to the prior method.

YANG TYPE A

By the time the Yang Type A is halfway through with a task, she is already getting started on another one. Multitasking is her strength, but it requires that she be centered and rooted—easier said than done. The overwhelmed Yang Type A will still be eager to take on more responsibility but simply forget the task at hand. She may absent-mindedly throw away the bills even after insisting that she'll take care of them. Her desire to take on several tasks at once is usually a means of avoiding feeling angered when others don't complete them—a trait born from her song nature of anger. Harboring such feelings of anger year after year eventually unleashes intense sorrow from the explosion of her jung emotion, which brings about extreme fatigue, regret, and loss of willpower. Prior to menopause, many Yang Type A women choose to conceal their anger, fearing that it may injure them or others. Others may lash out at any given moment despite attempting to hold back.

In Eastern medicine, the kidneys are associated with long-term memory and the heart with short-term memory. Born with weaker kidneys, the Yang Type A's long-term memory is often affected by emotional and/or physical trauma or illness. Short-term memory loss is more obvious and concerning for most people since it is immediately apparent, but long-term memory loss can easily go unnoticed. What exactly does it mean to lose one's long-term memory? For the Yang Type A it is an emphasis on the here and now and a disregard of the past and future. Long-term relationships and future goals don't matter as much anymore, as she focuses on getting everything done *now*.

Solution
Slow down before it's too late!!

- Join a yoga or other meditation-based class to send energy back down to your vulnerable kidneys.
- Curb your anger by letting things slide without getting irritated.
- Take some "me" time out of your busy schedule to relax, breathe, and clear the clutter from your mind.
- Think and plan before you act.
- Give the remedies below a try.

The following remedies help lift the Yang Type A's brain fog.

 ## Bo He
(Common: Peppermint; Latin: *Mentha piperita*)
As mentioned in chapter 6, field mint soothes and cools the overactive stomach energy of the Yang Type A. It also has a calming effect on the mind, alleviating stress and anger and promoting sleep. A study conducted in 2008 showed that the aroma of peppermint, a close cousin of field mint, exhibits memory-enhancing properties.[3] In Sasang medicine this effect is attributed to its strong aroma, capable of powerfully dispersing energy and enhancing the smooth flow of blood. Like its cousin, peppermint is also calming and can be taken as a tea and/or inhaled to soothe stress and anger. The above study also showed that the scent of peppermint enhanced concentration for tasks requiring sustained visual attention.

Common Uses
Peppermint relieves headaches, throat disorders (swollen and sore throat, tonsillitis, swollen glands), stress, anxiety, insomnia, depression, and brain fog.

Sources

High-quality peppermint essential oil can be purchased from the doTERRA or Piping Rock Health Products websites.

Preparation and Dosage

Douse a tissue with 1 to 3 drops of peppermint essential oil, place it inside a surgical mask, secure the mask with the tissue inside over your mouth and nose. Breathe in and out deeply for at least thirty minutes. Repeat several times a day or as desired, replacing the tissue and adding fresh oil once daily. You may also try dabbing a drop of essential oil directly under the nostrils. Be aware that this method may cause local skin irritation.

Herbal Friend: Jing Jie
(Common: Japanese Catnip; Latin: *Schizonepeta tenuifolia*)

Schizonepeta, also known as Japanese catnip, is commonly used in Sasang medicine to address the Yang Type A's common colds, phlegm, and allergies. Like peppermint, it aromatically disperses blockages of energy, blood, and especially phlegm/mucus in the sinuses and chest. Together with peppermint, it clears away cluttered thoughts, enhancing focus and memory. Add 2 drops of Japanese catnip extract to a folded tissue along with 2 drops of peppermint essential oil, place the tissue inside a surgical mask, and wear it for thirty minutes a day. Refer to the above dosage section for further details. I have yet to locate Japanese catnip essential oil but discovered that an extract manufactured by Hawaii Pharm works just fine for this task.

Peggy, the Mile-a-Minute Yang Type A

Peggy took care of everything from washing the dishes, cleaning the house, and laundry to cooking meals and taking care of the kids. Whenever her husband offered to help, she would insistently refuse. As she approached menopause, Peggy started to forget to do the laundry on Sunday or would leave the dishes in the sink for the next day. Yet whenever her husband took over and kids washed their own dishes, her angry song nature would reveal itself, and she would furiously tell them to rinse better. Eventually she started to forget about special events, which made her feel even angrier when she finally remembered. Once, after realizing she had forgotten her anniversary, she wept uncontrollably for hours, crying herself to sleep and triggering the explosion of her body type's sorrowful jung emotion.

YANG TYPE B

The Yang Type B is driven by her song nature of sorrow, which pushes her to the limits of her capability. Always feeling rushed, she wages a war within to accomplish, achieve, and move forward, all for the sake of reducing or avoiding disappointment. More than anything else, the Yang Type B fears staying still, for this is when sorrow can creep its way in and take over. Speeding down the road in her convertible race car, she is oblivious to all that surrounds her: the beautiful lake, fresh air, and foliage. All she can think of is the destination, which always seems to be miles ahead.

Sa mu (public affairs), correlating with her stronger lungs, gives the Yang Type B an emphasis on the big picture. She naturally devotes her energy toward saving the world before saving her own body or family from starvation. Since forgetting to take out the garbage or to prepare lunch for her children is commonplace, it's only when things get really out of hand that others start to take notice. The menopausal Yang Type B may actually forget to go to the bathroom or feed herself until she is extremely exhausted from malnutrition. Lee Je-ma, a Yang Type B, was spoon-fed by his distressed wife as he drowned himself in his work.

Solution
Don't push yourself too hard!

- Focus on the small picture, placing one foot in front of the other rather than leaping forward.
- Curb your sorrow by letting things slide without feeling depressed and neglected.
- Take some "me" time out of your busy schedule to relax, breathe, and clear the clutter from your mind.

- Find satisfaction with smaller tasks and outsource others that cause excessive stress.
- Give the remedy below a try.

The following is a remedy that lifts the Yang Type B's brain fog.

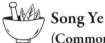 **Song Ye**
(Common: Scots Pine Needles; Latin: *Pinus sylvestris*)

In chapter 10 we discussed how pine nodes are effective in the healing of joint pain, allergies, and colds. Other parts of the pine tree are also beneficial for the Yang Type B, assisting the flow of lung energy throughout the upper body. Here we introduce the cognitive-enhancing properties of pine needles. The Yang Type B's temperament of sadness is often behind cognitive impairment, and since pine is capable of stimulating the flow of lung energy associated with grief, it also enhances her mood. A study in 2015 displayed how Pycnogenol, a trademarked formula that includes a flavonoid found in pine, has significant cognitive-enhancing effects.[4] The strong aroma of pine pierces through the Yang Type B's cluttered mind, stimulating her awareness and her ability to acknowledge her immediate surroundings.

Common Uses
Pine alleviates joint pain (e.g., shoulders, knees), brain fog, allergies, common colds, water retention, and muscle and/or tendon pain.

Sources
Pine essential oil made by NOW Products can be purchased on the Jet and iHerb websites. Rocky Mountain Oils also offers pine essential oil on its website.

Preparation and Dosage
Place a folded piece of tissue with 1 to 3 drops of pine essential oil within a surgical mask. Secure the mask with the tissue inside over your nose and mouth and breathe in and out deeply for at least thirty minutes. Repeat several times a day or as desired, replacing the tissue and adding fresh oil once daily. You may also try dabbing a drop of essential

oil directly under the nostrils. Be aware that this may cause local skin irritation.

Willow, the Brain-Fogged Yang Type B

"Willow! Are you even listening to me?" her friend asked as Willow simply stared into space. Unbeknownst to her friend, Willow's mind wasn't in an empty haze. Instead, she was processing her thoughts as they raced through her mind like musical notes, vibrating through the concert hall of her brain to the sound of a Mozart piano concerto. "Wait . . . what?" Willow replied, as if snapped back into her body by the shock of her friend's voice. These episodes occurred on and off for years, as Willow preoccupied herself with powerful thoughts that danced through her head, abruptly twisting, twirling, rising, and falling, powered by a deep sense of gloom and despair. She'd often write her thoughts down just to get them off her shoulders, occasionally showing her friends, only to receive a blank stare in return. It may have been a math problem that was plaguing her, or an innovative way to produce fuel-efficient car engines. Her friends described her as a dreamer, a mad scientist, a genius, an eccentric, morbid, or just simply bizarre. Despite these insightful moments driven by her song nature of sorrow, Willow just wanted to be more like her friends and able to relax without the constant sound of thoughts angrily buzzing through her mind.

YIN TYPE A

Distraction is born from the yang types' desire to stay active and not being busy enough, but for the yin types it stems from being overwhelmed and a desire to slow down. The Yin Type A's song nature of joy gives her a deep-rooted wish to be free of obligation, rules, and chores. Yet her affinity for dang yo, or group orientation, keeps her from completely disengaging. When she is pushed too far without meeting the needs of her joyous song nature, the Yin Type A chooses comfort over anything else, sacrificing work, relationships, and responsibilities—

a sign of her exploding jung emotion. Brain fog may be a result of her mind going on vacation, leaving memory and focus behind. The menopausal Yin Type A is no stranger to obligation, since by this point she may have reared children, cooked countless meals, washed innumerable loads of laundry, and held down a job.

The Yin Type A's liver bites off more than it can chew, hoarding energy, blood, minerals, fat, emotion, and so forth. With such an absorbent liver, she clings to the past and present, taking in her surroundings and experiences, struggling at times to let them go. Her stress from dealing with traffic, a broken coffee machine at work, or an irate client on the phone simply builds up to the point where there is no room for remaining thoughts. This is where things get funky and the Yin Type A starts to lose her focus and memory.

Solution

Keep your mind active!

- Focus on the big picture and escape getting stuck on the details.
- Avoid letting your desire for relaxation keep you from challenging your body and mind.
- Take aerobic classes, walk the treadmill, or engage in other cardiovascular activities to enhance flow to your brain.
- Switch gears and keep your mind occupied, stimulated, and flowing by doing other things such as crossword puzzles, Sudoku, and/or other brain-stimulating games.
- Give the remedies below a try.

The following remedies help lift the Yin Type A's brain fog.

 ### Xun Yi Cao
(Common: Lavender Oil; Latin: *Lavandula angustifolia*)

In Eastern medicine Xun Yi Cao (meaning "grass with fragrant clothes"), or lavender oil, is known for its strongly aromatic attire. No matter where or when you come in contact with lavender, there's no doubt that it will impress you with its penetrating scent. This highly aromatic property makes lavender an effective herb to address the

Yin Type A's stubborn respiratory issues like chronic allergies and persistent common colds. Eastern medicine associates this with the ability to strengthen the lungs and assist their ability to disperse energy throughout the upper body. Lavender is one of the most well-known and best-researched essential oils, boasting significant effects in general mood enhancement and improving mental health, memory, and cognitive function.[5] Sasang medicine holds that the lungs control the flow of energy to the brain and that stimulation of the Yin Type A's weaker lungs with aromatic substances like lavender can enhance brain activity.

Common Uses
Lavender alleviates brain fog, common colds, allergies, sore throat, skin rashes, rubella, dizziness, and headaches.

Sources
Lavender essential oil made by NOW Products can be purchased in natural food stores and on the Jet and iHerb websites. Piping Rock Health Products and Bulk Apothecary also offer pure lavender oil on their websites.

Preparation and Dosage
Place a folded piece of tissue doused with 1 to 3 drops of lavender essential oil within a surgical mask. Secure the mask with the tissue inside over the nose and mouth and breathe in and out deeply for at least thirty minutes. Repeat this process several times a day or as desired, replacing the tissue and adding fresh oil once daily. You may also try dabbing a drop of essential oil directly under the nostrils. Be aware that this may cause local skin irritation.

Herbal Friend: An Shu
(Common: Eucalyptus Oil; Latin: *Eucalyptus globulus*)

The intense sensation of eucalyptus essential oil bursting through the sinuses after one sniff is enough to convince anyone of its therapeutic effect. In Eastern medicine direct insertion of eucalyptus oil into

the nose via a straw was traditionally used to resuscitate the unconscious. Applied together, lavender and eucalyptus make a strong
yet fragrantly pleasant remedy for brain fog, drowsiness, and general malaise. Place a folded piece of tissue doused with 1 to 3 drops
of lavender essential oil and 1 to 3 drops of eucalyptus essential oil
within a surgical mask. Secure the mask with the tissue inside over
the nose and mouth and breathe in and out deeply for at least thirty
minutes. Refer to the above dosage section for further details.

Angie, the Day-Dreaming Yin Type A

A typical day of Angie's life consisted of rushing her kids out of the
house, gulping down two cups of coffee, hastening off to work, dealing
nonstop with clients, cooking dinner after returning home, and then
. . . It's all a blur from that point onward. Angie used to enjoy family
time, watching movies, and cuddling with her husband, but now it was
hard for her to focus on anything. Her mind would relentlessly wander
off or just draw a complete blank. She started to notice this more
often during the day and found herself overlooking her responsibilities
at work. With her boss's recommendation, Angie decided to take a
short vacation, and strangely enough, after only a day at the beach,
Angie's brain fog abruptly lifted! Yet as soon as she returned to work,
there it was, ready to grab her. Little did Angie know that her jung
emotion—associated with the desire for comfort—was taking over
and that her health was at stake if she didn't soon rediscover her joyous song nature.

YIN TYPE B

The Yin Type B's song nature of comfort is the basis for her every action.
"How comfortable is this chair?" "Is he a warm and cozy guy?" "Does
that restaurant have a relaxing atmosphere?" Such questions constantly
flow through the mind of a Yin Type B, and when life gets chaotic, she
easily zones out, in search of a comfortable place deep within the quiet
corners of her mind. For the unbalanced Yin Type B, comfort can only
be found when she is disengaged, alone, and at home. Without striking

a balance between feeling comfortable at home and in the company of others, her brain fog can easily become an everyday hindrance as her mind retreats further into a fantasy world.

The Yin Type B's stronger kidneys constantly yearn for peace and quiet, but in a busy and often chaotic world, this is hard to achieve. A weaker digestive system adds to the challenge, making it difficult for her to digest not only food but experiences, too. Unlike the Yin Type A, it isn't excessive liver absorption of emotion and food that gets her in trouble but the kidneys' desire to stay away from them and not get involved. Even with half the responsibility of other body types, the Yin Type B may feel as if she has too much on her plate and decide to shut others out and ignore her basic needs. She'll easily forget what to say when standing in front of others or overlook important social commitments.

Solution
Engage before it's too late!!

- Take life at your own pace and avoid getting overwhelmed.
- Challenge yourself to socialize, but don't lose track of comfort.
- Enjoy the comfort you feel while alone, but don't get carried away by it. The more you retreat, the less you will feel inclined to socialize with others.
- Many Yin Type Bs are extremely sensitive and self-critical. Acknowledge, remember, and appreciate your type's needs, even if other types don't agree or share the same values.
- Give the remedies below a try.

The following remedies help lift the Yin Type B's brain fog.

 ## An Xi Xiang
(Common: Benzoin Oil; Latin: *Styrax benzoin*)
As we saw in chapter 6, benzoin is referred to as An Xi Xiang, or "peaceful rest fragrance," and is often used as an oil to uplift the spirit, elevate the mood, and promote emotional harmony. Lee Je-ma credits An Xi Xiang with the ability to clear the body of pathogens and toxins while balancing the heart and mind. Along with other Yin Type B

herbs, this one also supports the digestive system, making it easier for the Yin Type B to digest life's challenges and transform them into a source of strength and well-being. The easily overwhelmed Yin Type B's brain fog is usually a result of indigestion of not just food, but life in general, which can be attributed to her weaker spleen energy.

Common Uses
Benzoin clears the mind, enhances concentration, calms and uplifts emotions, and relieves digestive and respiratory disorders.

Sources
Bulk Apothecary offers benzoin essential oil on its website.

Preparation and Dosage
A few drops of benzoin oil may be dabbed onto a cotton ball and rubbed beneath the nostrils to clear the sinuses or onto the abdomen up to three times a day to promote digestion. You may also try folding a piece of tissue doused with 1 to 3 drops of benzoin oil within a surgical mask. Secure the mask with the tissue inside over the nose and mouth and breathe in and out deeply for at least thirty minutes. Benzoin oil may also be dabbed onto the wrists as a fragrance or burned with a diffuser or oil burner as an aroma.

Caution
Although benzoin is used as an ingredient in medicinal teas, it is usually ingested only under the care of a professional. Most sources warn against ingesting it and recommend it for topical use only. Yet even topically, this potent medicinal has plenty of healing power. The application of essential oils directly onto the skin may produce localized skin sensitivity, such as rashes or redness. Try diluting the first few applications of benzoin with small amounts of water until your skin gets used to it. If your skin is not irritated, then try applying it directly.

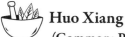 **Huo Xiang**
(Common: Patchouli Oil; Latin: *Pogostemon cablin*)
Also mentioned in chapter 6, patchouli is used as a tea to clear the sinuses, support the digestive system, and balance the flow of energy

throughout the body. Its aromatic fragrance can be inhaled to stimulate the function of the Yin Type B's weaker spleen and pick up her mood, enhance memory, and clear away cluttered thoughts. Yin Type Bs in particular benefit from patchouli because its warm nature strengthens their weaker spleen and helps the stomach break down and assimilate foods.

Common Uses
Patchouli alleviates indigestion, allergies, common colds, congestion, coughing, shortness of breath, lack of appetite, depression, and brain fog.

Sources
Patchouli essential oil made by NOW Products can be purchased on the Jet and iHerb websites. Another quality product is provided by Plantlife.

Preparation and Dosage
A few drops of patchouli oil may be dabbed onto a cotton ball and rubbed underneath the nostrils to clear the sinuses, or onto the abdomen up to three times a day to promote digestion. You may also try folding a piece of tissue doused with 1 to 3 drops of benzoin and 1 to 3 drops of patchouli oil within a surgical mask. Secure the mask with the tissue inside over the nose and mouth and breathe in and out deeply for at least thirty minutes.

Linda, the Pipe-Dreaming Yin Type B

A career as a novelist served Linda well, since she could stir up fictional scenarios within her mind at the drop of a hat. But when it came to publisher deadlines, her productivity would always abruptly diminish. Instead of satisfying such obligations, she'd sit in front of her computer, vacantly staring at the screen for hours until she had no choice but to give up. Sometimes she'd drift off into a place within the depths of her imagination, free from obligation, time constraints, or human interaction. Here she always felt an incredible sense of tranquility, but she felt more at odds with reality and its social responsibilities the more time she spent there. Caught between two worlds, Linda's life was a constant balancing act between satisfying a thirst for retreat and fulfilling the requirements of daily life.

Continuing the Voyage

Useful Resources for
Your Menopausal Journey

Anchored and ballasted with further knowledge about your body type and what to do if your ship sails astray, you're almost ready to navigate through the rest of your journey. But before you set sail again, there are a few pointers I'd like to share.

Even after reading this book, you may have lingering questions about your yin yang body type, which is often revealed only after persistent self-reflection and trial and error. You may also still be wondering how to address a particular menopausal condition. While this book attempts to encompass the basics of Sasang medicine and menopause, it cannot replace the expert advice of a qualified Sasang practitioner. Thus, if you wish further guidance regarding your yin yang body type, you may try one or more of the following options:

- My first book, *Your Yin Yang Body Type*, provides a detailed overview of Sasang medicine, introducing the four body types and compatible foods, herbs, and exercises, along with body-type-specific remedies for ten common ailments, such as headaches, indigestion, stress, and so forth.
- Log on to sasangmedicine.com and visit our discussion forum, which covers various topics from discovering your yin yang body type to addressing specific health concerns. Simply click "Sasang

Discussion Forum" on the main menu to view the discussions. If you have a pressing question that is not already addressed there, you may register to open a new discussion. I review this forum regularly and will post a response to your inquiry.

- Log on to sasangmedicine.com and click on one of the "Contact Us" icons to sign up for a direct consultation with me. This is a convenient way to access guidance in discovering your yin yang body type and to receive one-on-one assistance with a particular health condition.

- While in most cases you can determine your yin yang body type as laid out above, you may also contact my clinic to make an appointment for an accurate assessment of your body type and help with your particular menopausal transition. Along with the methods described in this book, Sasang practitioners also utilize a vast array of clinical diagnostic protocols such as pulse taking, skin-texture analysis, and voice-tone assessment to determine your body type and prescribe appropriate treatment. More information about our clinic can be found on the Harmony Acupuncture and Herbs website. You may contact us:

Harmony Acupuncture and Herbs
21730 Willamette Dr.
West Linn, OR 97068
Tel: (503) 722-5224
website: www.harmonyclinics.com

CURRENT SASANG
AND MENOPAUSE RESEARCH

Despite its firm establishment and popularity in Korea, Sasang medicine is still in its infancy in the West, with a limited amount of material available in English. Information on Sasang medicine that is currently scattered throughout the internet can be located by typing "Sasang medicine," "four constitutional medicine," or "Korean constitutional medicine" in any major search bar. Research in Sasang medicine has recently appeared in English-language journals. The PubMed website, hosted by the National Institutes of Health, provides one of the largest collections of published medical research worldwide, including several Sasang medical studies translated into English. The Sasang medicine website (sasangmedicine.com), updated frequently, is another source of Sasang medical studies published in the English language.

The latest menopause-related research can be easily accessed through websites such as ScienceDaily, endocrineweb, News Medical, and the National Institutes of Health by typing "menopause" in the search bar. The former two websites are a bit less technical, with articles that summarize recent studies, whereas the latter provide research abstracts containing statistical outcomes.

MENOPAUSE SUPPORT SERVICES

There's a plethora of menopause support groups on the web, each having its own focus and underlying theme. At Menopause ChitChat women can reflect and openly share thoughts about their menopausal journey. HealthBoards provides a huge list of menopause-related discussions and insights. Some hospitals within the United Stated provide menopause outreach programs, such as Red Hot Mamas, that inform menopausal women about the latest treatments and provide a place to share their experiences and get feedback. For other support groups near you, try searching for "[your town or city and state] menopause support groups" on the web and see what comes up.

TO YOUR HEALTH!

No matter how thorough I strive to be, there's always more to discuss about Sasang medicine and menopause. Even after publishing this book, I'll probably think of at least a dozen more things that I would wish to include. But rest assured, *Yin Yang Balance for Menopause* contains enough information to help you on your journey. With the knowledge of your body type and how to balance your strengths and weaknesses, you'll make it through unscathed and stronger. I hope, from the bottom of my heart, that *Yin Yang Balance for Menopause* reinforces the wind behind your sails.

Five Nutritional Guidelines for Optimum Menopausal Health

Abundant and often conflicting information on the internet and in books/magazines makes the decision of what and how much to eat during and after menopause a tough call. As we have discussed throughout this book, for the yang types, consuming cool-natured food supports their hypodeveloped liver and kidney energies, and for the yin types, warmer foods nourish the lungs and spleen. I recommend reading the "Eating Right for Your Yin Yang Body Type" chapter of my first book, *Your Yin Yang Body Type,* for more insight into food energy and suggested intake guidelines for hundreds of body-type-specific foods.

Rather than get into too much detail here, I am keeping things simple by presenting five research-supported nutrients that are beneficial for menopausal health. Each section begins with one or more studies supporting the consumption of a particular food/mineral and ends with a table that categorizes it according to its compatibility with each of the four yin yang body types, along with its recommended level of consumption, designated as "high," "moderate," "low," or "minimal." The following list provides a definition for each of these levels. When available, the researched therapeutic single-serving size of each particular food/mineral is included.

- High—Body-type compatible; at least one serving a day
- Moderate—Nutritionally beneficial but not body-type compatible; up to five servings a week
- Low—Little nutritional value and not body-type compatible; at most three to four servings a week
- Minimal—Neither nutritionally beneficial nor body-type compatible; at most one to two servings a week

The suggested intake of each nutrient in this appendix is based primarily on your yin yang body type, rather than on general symptomatic presentation or age-related guidelines. Even though soy is considered to have the highest plant-based estrogen content, for example, it isn't compatible with Yin Type Bs even if they are estrogen deficient. Soy, said to stimulate the kidneys in Sasang medicine, may congest the Yin Type B's hyperdeveloped kidney system, but it is perfect for the hypodeveloped kidneys of the Yang Type A, providing health benefits far beyond those of estrogen. In short, the foods listed in this appendix support the overall health of each yin yang body type, with the added benefit of their menopause-related attributes.

Each food/nutrient is also given a single-serving amount in the far right column of the table. Single-serving amounts typically fluctuate according to the source, sometimes making this a topic of confusion. The amounts listed in the tables below are body-type-specific and based primarily on the Sasang guidelines set forth in this appendix, only occasionally coinciding with other sources.

Although several of the nutrients below are available in supplement form, this information wasn't included for the sake of encouraging readers to incorporate actual food sources into their diet. If you are especially deficient in a particular nutrient, then supplementing with concentrated amounts, under the guidance of a nutritionist, physician, or naturopath, may be necessary.

PHYTOESTROGENS

Estrogen levels within the body decline significantly during menopause no matter which body type you are. This process often takes the body by surprise as it frantically attempts to adjust. To make this transition easier and avoid the potential side effects of synthetic hormone replacement, more and more women are turning to plant-based estrogens. Astonishingly, these estrogens are so similar to human estradiol that the body doesn't know the difference! Phytoestrogens are divided into two major categories; isoflavones and lignans. Soybeans are rich in isoflavones, while flaxseed, whole grains, legumes, fruits, and vegetables are adequate sources of lignans.

An interest in phytoestrogen research in the West followed the discovery that Asian women reported relatively fewer occurrences of hot flashes and osteoporosis than American women. The average Japanese diet consists of 50 to 200 milligrams of phytoestrogens daily, primarily from miso and tofu.[1]

Hot Flashes

Because of its high content, soy is the most researched of all phytoestrogen sources. Studies have demonstrated its effect in reducing hot flashes. One study involving the daily consumption of a phytoestrogen-rich diet (80 grams tofu, 400 milliliters of soy drink, 1 teaspoon of miso, and 2 teaspoons of linseeds daily) boasted a 50 percent reduction of hot flashes. As an added benefit, participants also reported decreased vaginal dryness.[2]

Red clover, also rich in phytoestrogens, has been the subject of several hot flash studies. Researchers were puzzled about why one study performed in 2003 reported a decrease in hot flashes in 75 percent of participants, while another, in 1992, showed no significant effect.[3] I believe this can be explained by differences in population, since these studies were conducted in different countries, and body-type ratios vary according to geographical location. Red clover has a warm to hot nature, compatible only with the yin types.

Disease Prevention

According to a study published in 2002, phytoestrogens may also play a significant role in preventing cardiovascular disease and high cholesterol.[4] A thorough review of over a hundred phytoestrogen studies found substantial evidence of phytoestrogens' ability to prevent osteoporosis if started during or directly after menopause.[5]

Foods Sources of Phytoestrogens

While soy, most compatible with the Yang Type A, has the greatest amount of phytoestrogens, several foods that are associated with other types have significant quantities too. Table A.1 lists foods with the highest amounts of phytoestrogens. (Refer to page 339 for a list of compatibility-level definitions.)

TABLE A.1. FOODS RICH IN PHYTOESTROGENS

Food Source	Yang Type A Compatibility	Yang Type B Compatibility	Yin Type A Compatibility	Yin Type B Compatibility	Single-Serving Size
Soy	High	Moderate	Low	Minimal	1 cup of soymilk; ½ cup of tofu, tempeh, soybeans, or soy meats
Red clover	Minimal	Low	Moderate	High	Not available
Tempeh	Low	Minimal	High	Moderate	½ cup (4 oz)
Flaxseed	Low	Minimal	High	Moderate	2 tbsp. (15 g)
Sesame seeds	Low	Minimal	High	Moderate	⅓ cup (36 g)
Fenugreek	Minimal	Low	Moderate	High	3.5 oz (100 g)
Oats	Low	Minimal	High	Moderate	½ cup (78 g)
Barley	High	Moderate	Low	Minimal	½ cup (92 g)
Lentils	Low	Minimal	High	Moderate	½ cup (96 g)
Alfalfa	Low	Minimal	High	Moderate	1 cup (33 g)
Mung beans	High	Moderate	Low	Minimal	½ cup (52 g)
Apples	Minimal	Low	Moderate	High	1 apple
Carrots	Low	Minimal	High	Moderate	2.8 oz (80 g)
Pomegranates	Minimal	Low	Moderate	High	1 pomegranate
Fennel	Minimal	Low	Moderate	High	½ cup (44 g)
Anise	Minimal	Low	Moderate	High	1 tsp. (2.1 g)
Kudzu	Low	Minimal	High	Moderate	Not available
Mint	High	Moderate	Low	Minimal	2 tsp. (1.5 g)

Be Aware

Although phytoestrogens are relatively safe, especially if you follow the above guidelines, be aware of digestion-related issues, such as constipation, diarrhea, bloating, or flatulence. I recommend reducing your intake or eliminating these foods entirely if acute symptoms occur. Some professionals believe that excess intake of isoflavones may have an inhibitory effect on the thyroid, decrease mineral absorption, reduce the effects of tamoxifen (breast cancer treatment), and/or produce allergic reactions.[6] Consuming each phytoestrogen source according to your yin yang body type significantly reduces potential risks.

BORON

Boron, a precursor for bodily production of estrogen, is also considered an essential nutrient (not produced within the body) for humans, contributing to cell growth and integrity. Boron promotes the reuptake and proper metabolism of calcium, magnesium, and phosphorus within the body, preventing loss through urine. Deficiency of these nutrients is implicated in osteoporosis. Luckily, boron is abundant in a variety of fruits and vegetables, and deficiency is rare. A daily 3-milligram dose of boron has been credited with increasing levels of estrogen in postmenopausal women.[7]

Foods Sources of Boron

The daily recommended intake of boron is only 15 to 20 milligrams, which is easily provided by consuming any of the foods listed in table A.2 (page 343) according to the suggested quantities. A single serving of almonds, for example, contains 2.5 milligrams, while 100 grams of prunes has 25.5 milligrams. (Refer to page 339 for a list of compatibility-level definitions.)

Be Aware

If any of the foods in table A.2 are included in your diet, then additional boron supplementation isn't recommended. Even though dosages of up to 4 grams of boron a day were reported without incident, anything above this amount is considered toxic. For some individuals

0.5 gram/day for fifty days caused minor digestive distress.[8] The chance of indigestion is greatly reduced when consuming boron-rich foods associated with your yin yang body type.

TABLE A.2. FOODS RICH IN BORON

Food Source	Yang Type A Compatibility	Yang Type B Compatibility	Yin Type A Compatibility	Yin Type B Compatibility	Single-Serving Size
Chickpeas	Low	Minimal	High	Moderate	½ cup (82 g)
Almonds	Low	Minimal	High	Moderate	1 oz (¼ cup)
Bananas	High	Moderate	Low	Minimal	1 banana
Walnuts	Low	Minimal	High	Moderate	1 oz (¼ cup)
Avocado	Low	Minimal	High	Moderate	1 avocado
Broccoli	Moderate	High	Minimal	Low	1 cup (91 g)
Prunes	Low	Minimal	High	Moderate	3 pcs (25 g)
Oranges	Generally easy to digest but best for the Yin Type B				1 orange
Red Grapes	High	Moderate	Low	Minimal	1 cup (32 grapes)
Apples	Minimal	Low	Moderate	High	1 apple
Raisins	High	Moderate	Low	Minimal	1.4 oz (40 g)
Pears	Low	Minimal	High	Moderate	1 pear

NATURAL PROGESTERONE

Progesterone is often overshadowed by its sister hormone, estrogen, which decreases more rapidly during and after menopause. Although not as abrupt, progesterone levels also decline significantly throughout this phase. Lower levels of progesterone are directly related to peri- and postmenopausal insomnia, depression, anxiety, weight gain, fatigue, headaches, joint/muscle pain, sensitivity to touch, and/or a lack of interest in sex. In early perimenopause, estrogen levels temporarily spike, leaving progesterone in the dust. This is referred to as "estrogen dominance" and is sometimes characterized by excessive fluid retention, bloating, and moodiness. If you are experiencing any of the symptoms related to estrogen dominance or progesterone deficiency, it may be time to test your hormone levels. If you have exceedingly low levels and experience these symptoms, then a conversation with your physician about natural sources of oral or topical progesterone may be of benefit.

Foods Sources of Progesterone

The foods listed in table A.3 (page 345) encourage the production of progesterone in your body and might help alleviate symptoms of non-acute progesterone deficiency and/or complement the effects of other approaches. (Refer to page 339 for a list of compatibility-level definitions.)

OMEGA-3 FATTY ACIDS

Omega-3 is an essential fatty acid, meaning that it cannot be produced within the body but is necessary for our survival. Fish with high levels of oil have the most omega-3 fatty acids, yet other sources are also available (see table A.4 on page 347). Even though reducing excess dietary fat is a vital part of any weight-loss routine, eliminating all fatty foods can produce adverse effects. Essential fatty acids are responsible for a variety of cell functions, including the regulation of inflammatory response and intercellular communication. Supplementing with omega-3 is one way to ensure that we are consuming enough fatty acids when on a low-fat diet. Omega-3 has also been praised for its ability to reduce inflammation and bone loss after menopause.

The omega-3 discussion wouldn't be complete without the inclusion of its counterpart, omega-6, which is also responsible for regulating inflammation but less related to hot flashes and metabolism. The modern diet tends to go overboard with omega-6, which is present in vegetable oils (e.g., canola, safflower, and corn oils), while skimping on omega-3, primarily obtained from fish oil. Some argue that an imbalance of the omega-6 to omega-3 ratio may be the reason why so many foods we eat today instigate inflammatory responses.[9] Excess omega-6 intake has also been linked to various chronic inflammatory diseases such as arthritis and tumor growth.[10]

TABLE A.3. FOODS RICH IN NATURAL PROGESTERONE

Food Source	Yang Type A Compatibility	Yang Type B Compatibility	Yin Type A Compatibility	Yin Type B Compatibility	Single-Serving Size
Egg yolk[†]	High	Moderate	Low	Minimal	1 egg yolk
Cow milk*	Moderate	High	Minimal	Low	1 cup (4 oz)
Soy milk[†]	High	Moderate	Low	Minimal	1 cup (4 oz)
Chicken[†]	Minimal	Low	Moderate	High	½ chicken breast
Red meat	Low	Minimal	High	Moderate	½ steak; 1 hamburger
Shellfish[‡]	High	Moderate	Low	Minimal	6 mussels; 4 oysters; 8 clams
Turkey[†]	Minimal	Low	Moderate	High	¼ turkey breast
Yams[‡]	Low	Minimal	High	Moderate	1 yam
Walnuts[†]	Low	Minimal	High	Moderate	¼ cup (1 oz)
Potatoes[†]	Low	Minimal	High	Moderate	1 potato
Chickpeas[‡]	Low	Minimal	High	Moderate	½ cup (82 g)
Pumpkin*	Low	Minimal	High	Moderate	½ cup (85 g)
Soy*	High	Moderate	Low	Minimal	1 cup of soymilk; ½ cup of tofu, tempeh, soybeans, or soy meats
Kale*	High	Moderate	Low (raw), High (cooked/steamed)	Minimal (raw), Moderate (cooked/steamed)	1 cup (67 g)

*These foods are rich in magnesium, which helps restore hormonal balance.
[†]These foods are rich in vitamin B$_6$, which encourages the production of progesterone.
[‡]These foods are rich in zinc, required by the body to produce progesterone.

Depression and Hot Flashes

A study in 2011 concluded that supplementing with omega-3 fatty acids is relatively safe and effective in the reduction of depression and hot flashes in postmenopausal women. Participants were given 2 grams of open-label fatty acids daily for eight weeks.[11] Another study including 120 perimenopausal women also showed a significant reduction in hot-flash frequency and intensity after an eight-week trial.[12]

Metabolic Syndrome

A recent study of eighty-seven women age forty-five and older with high blood pressure, high triglycerides, and high insulin resistance examined the health effects of omega-3 supplementation and dieting. Researchers separated participants into two groups: one with dieting alone and one with dieting plus omega-3 supplementation (900 milligrams a day). While both groups showed a significant reduction in body mass and waist circumference after the six-month study, the latter group showed additional reduction in blood pressure, triglycerides, and insulin resistance.[13]

Foods Sources of Omega-3

The foods listed in table A.4 are rich in omega-3 fatty acids. (Refer to page 339 for a list of compatibility-level definitions.)

Be Aware

Omega-3 fatty acids may cause thinning of the blood in some folks, so consult your physician if you are taking anticoagulant drugs. Indigestion and gas are common side effects of omega-3 fatty acids but are usually avoided by sticking to your body-type-specific foods. I'd recommend reducing your intake of omega-3-rich foods if, despite following the guidelines presented in this appendix, you still experience indigestion. If ever you notice indigestion after eating a body-type-compatible food, try retaking the yin yang body type test to confirm your type.

TABLE A.4. FOODS RICH IN OMEGA-3

Food Source	Yang Type A Compatibility	Yang Type B Compatibility	Yin Type A Compatibility	Yin Type B Compatibility	Single-Serving Size
Salmon	Low	Minimal	High	Moderate	2–3 oz
Mackerel	High	Moderate	Low	Minimal	4 oz
Sardines	Low	Minimal	High	Moderate	1 can (3.75 oz)
Trout	Low	Minimal	High	Moderate	3 oz
Tuna	High	Moderate	Low	Minimal	3 oz
Walnuts	Low	Minimal	High	Moderate	¼ cup
Pumpkin seeds	Low	Minimal	High	Moderate	1½ cups
Tofu	High	Moderate	Low (raw), moderate (cooked)	Minimal (raw), moderate (cooked)	½ cup (4 oz)
Flaxseed*	Low	Minimal	High	Moderate	2 tbsp.
Chia seed	Low	Minimal	High	Moderate	2 tbsp.
Hempseed	Minimal	Low	Moderate	High	2 tbsp.
Soybean oil	High	Moderate	Low	Minimal	1 tbsp.

*While fish is the main source of omega-3, flaxseed is the best-known plant source, followed by chia seed and hempseed. Flaxseed oil was shown to lower cholesterol in postmenopausal women in Arjmandi et al., "Whole Flaxseed Consumption."

VITAMIN D3 AND CALCIUM

Vitamin D3 has two major menopause-related functions: calcium absorption and mood enhancement. Actually, without vitamin D3, our bones lack the ability to absorb calcium altogether. The most effective way to enhance vitamin D3 production in the body is to expose it to sunlight. Food offers another source, and there's a lot to choose from (see table A.5 on page 350). Vitamin D3 production from sunlight is also responsible for promoting joy and happiness.

The signs and symptoms of a vitamin D3 deficiency may be vague and difficult to detect. Moderate to severe deficiency often results in

SAD, fatigue, and general body and bone aches. You can determine vitamin D₃ and other vitamin deficiencies by taking a blood test, referred to as 25(OH)D, performed by a professional or by purchasing a kit online and sending a blood sample to the lab.

Keep Magnesium in Mind

With so much emphasis on calcium for bone health, its mineral cousin magnesium rarely gets the attention it deserves. Magnesium plays an essential role by assuring the strength and firmness of bones and converting vitamin D to its active form. Excessive calcium supplementation without adequate magnesium intake can result in deficiency. A 2:1 ration of calcium to magnesium consumption is recommended. Calcium supplements routinely adhere to this ratio, but double-check the label just to be safe. Significant levels of both calcium and magnesium can be found in various types of nuts, seeds, and fish. Try googling "magnesium-rich foods" to find out more.

Osteoporosis

Studies show that, in general, neither calcium nor vitamin D₃ supplementation alone is capable of counteracting the effects of osteoporosis, yet taken together they moderately increase bone mass. The benefits of higher doses may not outweigh the risks, since it was also discovered that calcium supplementation (1,000 milligrams of calcium carbonate per day) contributes to a higher frequency of kidney stone formation.[14] Consuming these nutrients in liquid form, or from the foods listed in tables A.5 and A.6 (pages 350–51), greatly decreases the risk of kidney stones. Yet increased mineral intake should always be accompanied with adequate water consumption (half your body weight in ounces) to ensure ample kidney flow.

Before we shove aside the potential for vitamin D₃ supplementation to increase bone mass, let's consider a situation where it showed significant benefit. Conducted during a typically dark winter at a latitude of 42 degrees, a study providing 249 otherwise healthy menopausal women with a year's supply of vitamin D (500 international units) demonstrated that supplementation alone significantly increased bone mass during late winter—a time when bone-mass loss is common among women living in this area.[15] If you live in an area lacking in sunlight, you may need to increase your intake of vitamin D to prevent bone-mass loss.

Vitamin D and Depression

A study including 448 male and female participants showed that increased intake of vitamin D significantly reduced depression.[16] Participants were given extremely high doses of vitamin D (20,000 to 30,000 international units), very difficult to replicate by simply increasing intake via food. If you are diagnosed with depression and vitamin D deficiency, it might be necessary to supplement with higher amounts under the supervision of a trained professional.

Foods Sources of Vitamin D₃ and Calcium

Are you prone to fatigue, sadness, achiness, immune-related issues (e.g., frequent colds or flu), and/or moodiness during the darker months of the year? Try adding the vitamin D_3 sources listed in table A.5 (page 350) to your diet. The recommended vitamin D_3 daily intake for women ages fifty-one to seventy is 600 international units, and after the age of seventy it increases to 800 international units. Because of their tendency to lose bone mass more quickly, the menopausal yang types need up to 1,200 milligrams a day of calcium compared to only 750 milligrams a day needed by the yin types.

The foods listed in table A.5 are rich in vitamin D_3, and those listed in table A.6 are chock-full of calcium. (Refer to page 339 for a list of compatibility-level definitions.)

TABLE A.5. FOODS RICH IN VITAMIN D$_3$

Food Source	Yang Type A Compatibility	Yang Type B Compatibility	Yin Type A Compatibility	Yin Type B Compatibility	Single-Serving Size	Percentage of Daily Recommend Value
Cod liver oil	High	Moderate	Low	Minimal	1 oz	700%
Herring	Low	Minimal	High	Moderate	1 oz	115%
Whole milk	High	Moderate	Low	Minimal	1 cup	24%
Mushrooms (maitake)	High	Moderate	Low	Minimal	1 cup (diced)	196%
Sockeye salmon	Low	Minimal	High	Moderate	3 oz	111%
Sardines	Low	Minimal	High	Moderate	1 can (3.75 oz)	5%
Halibut	High	Moderate	Low	Minimal	3 oz	233%
Almond milk	Low	Minimal	High	Moderate	100 g	10%

TABLE A.6. FOODS RICH IN CALCIUM

Food Source	Yang Type A Compatibility	Yang Type B Compatibility	Yin Type A Compatibility	Yin Type B Compatibility	Single-Serving Size	Percentage of Daily Recommend Value
Figs	Low	Minimal	High	Moderate	4 figs	8%
Oranges	Generally easy to digest but best for the Yin Type B				1 orange	5%
Almond milk	Low	Minimal	High	Moderate	1 cup	24%
Bok choy	Low	Minimal	High	Moderate	1 cup (diced)	16%
Beans (white)	Low	Minimal	High	Moderate	12 g	5%
Yogurt (Greek)	Generally easy to digest (warmed for yin types and chilled for yang types)				3 oz	25%
Almonds	Low	Minimal	High	Moderate	1 oz (¼ cup)	6%

TABLE A.6. FOODS RICH IN CALCIUM (cont.)

Food Source	Yang Type A Compatibility	Yang Type B Compatibility	Yin Type A Compatibility	Yin Type B Compatibility	Single-Serving Size	Percentage of Daily Recommended Value
Dandelion greens	High	Moderate	Low (raw), high (cooked/ steamed)	Minimal (raw), moderate (cooked/ steamed)	103 mg	10%
Collard greens	High	Moderate	Low (raw), high (cooked/ steamed)	Minimal (raw), moderate (cooked/ steamed)	1 cup	5%
Broccoli	Moderate	High	Minimal	Low	1 cup	4%
Soy milk	High	Moderate	Low	Minimal	1 cup	6%
Kale	High	Moderate	Low (raw), high (cooked/ steamed)	Minimal (raw), moderate (cooked/ steamed)	1 cup (67 g)	10%
Shrimp	High	Moderate	Low	Minimal	4 oz	7%
Cow milk	Moderate	High	Minimal	Low	1 cup (4 oz)	30%
Tofu	High	Moderate	Low (raw), moderate (cooked)	Minimal (raw), moderate (cooked)	½ cup (4 oz)	25%
Adzuki beans	High	Moderate	Low	Minimal	½ cup	13%
Black-eyed peas	Low	Minimal	High	Moderate	½ cup	2%
Sardines	Low	Minimal	High	Moderate	1 can (3.75 oz)	35%

Notes

INTRODUCTION

1. Arrien, *Second Half of Life,* iv.
2. As quoted in King, "Once Upon a Text," 25.
3. Kaufert et al., "Women and Menopause."

2. DISCOVERING YOUR YIN YANG BODY TYPE

1. Koo et al., "Feature Selection."
2. Carré and McCormick, "In Your Face."
3. Passini and Norman, "Universal Conception."
4. Shifren et al. "Sexual Problems."
5. Rosen et al., "Correlates of Sexually Related Personal Distress."

4. FIRE ABOARD: HOT FLASHES

1. Mayo Clinic Staff, "Hot Flashes."
2. Gold et al. "Longitudinal Analysis."
3. Brown et al., "Do Japanese American Women?"
4. Crandall, "Low-Dose Estrogen."
5. Loprinzi et al., "Venlafaxine in Management of Hot Flashes."
6. Ockene et al., "Symptom Experience."
7. Carmody et al., "Mindfulness Training."
8. Huang et al., "Randomized Controlled Pilot Study."
9. Irvin et al., "Effects of Relaxation Response."
10. Fu et al., "Effect of Bamboo Leaves Extract."
11. Choi et al., "Standardized Bamboo Leaf Extract."
12. Osmers et al., "Efficacy and Safety."
13. Jiang et al., "Black Cohosh Improves Objective Sleep."

5. SEALING THE PORTHOLES: OSTEOPOROSIS

1. Norton, "Calcium Supplements."
2. Warensjö et al., "Dietary Calcium Intake."
3. Gambacciani and Vacca, "Postmenopausal Osteoporosis."
4. "Hormone Replacement Therapy (HRT)."
5. Cranney et al., "Meta-Analyses of Therapies."
6. Ibid.
7. Komulainen et al., "HRT and Vit D."
8. "Facts and Statistics."
9. Park, "Eight Health Benefits."
10. Esposito and Kotz, "How Much Time?"
11. "How Do I Get the Vitamin D My Body Needs?"
12. Wolf et al., "Reducing Frailty."
13. Chan et al., "Randomized Prospective Study."
14. Ken Jorgustin, "Top 100 High ORAC Value Antioxidant Foods." Modern Survival Blog, July 18, 2017; updated August 29, 2018.
15. Lim and Kim, "Dried Root of *Rehmannia*."
16. Mei, Mochizuki, and Hasegawa, "Protective Effect of Pycnogenol®."
17. Nakchbandi, "Osteoporosis and Fractures."
18. "Benefits of Cinnamon in Arthritis."
19. Yang, Tie, and Yuyu, "Effects of Tuber Fleeceflower."

6. WOMAN OVERBOARD: THE DEPTHS OF DEPRESSION

1. American Psychiatric Association, *Diagnostic and Statistical Manual,* 356.
2. McCann and Holmes, "Influence of Aerobic Exercise."
3. Lee, "After Menopause."

7. NO WAKE ZONE: IMPROVING YOUR SLEEP

1. American Psychiatric Association, *Diagnostic and Statistical Manual,* 356.
2. Polo-Kantola et al., "When Does Estrogen Replacement Therapy?"
3. Cao et al., "Acupuncture for Treatment of Insomnia."
4. Pegoraro et al., "Gene Expression."
5. Yi et al., "Involvement of Serotonin Receptors."
6. Yeh et al., "Suan Zao Ren Tang as an Original Treatment."
7. Seo et al., "*Zizyphus jujuba.*"

8. MINDING THE WATERLINE: URINARY HEALTH

1. Emmons and Otto, "Acupuncture for Overactive Bladder."
2. Wagman, *The Essential Teachings of Sasang Medicine,* 340.
3. Shin and Huh, "Effect of Intake of Gardenia Fruits."

4. Yang, "New Study."

5. Dhingra et al., "Possible Involvement."

6. Oh and Chung, "Antiestrogenic Activities."

7. Armanini et al., "History of the Endocrine Effects."

8. Ofir et al., "Inhibition of Serotonin."

9. Somjen et al., "Estrogen-Like Activity."

10. Narayanan et al., "Oral Supplementation."

11. Matheson, Mainous, and Carnemolla, "Association between Onion Consumption and Bone Density."

9. UNTANGLING THE FISHING NET: UTERINE FIBROIDS

1. "Uterine Health."

2. Holden-Lund, "Effects of Relaxation."

3. Kondo, Takano, and Hojo, "Suppression of Chemically and Immunologically Induced Hepatic Injuries."

4. Varpe et al., "Evaluation of Anti-Inflammatory Activity."

5. Zhao et al., "Antiatherogenic Effects."

6. Tsuiji et al., "Inhibitory Effect of Curcumin."

7. Bai et al., "Efficacy and Tolerability of a Medicinal Product."

10. SHOULDERING THE ROPES: FROZEN SHOULDER

1. Kuptniratsaikul et al., "Efficacy and Safety of *Curcuma domestica* Extracts."

2. Bourne and Rice-Evans, "Bioavailability of Ferulic Acid."

3. Wang et al., "Effect and Mechanism of Senkyunolide I."; Liu et al., "Phthalide Lactones from *Ligusticum chuanxiong*."

11. ROCKING THE BOAT: LIBIDO

1. National Council on Aging, *Healthy Sexuality*.

2. North American Menopausal Society, "Decreased Desire."

3. Wickman, "Androgen Therapy in Women."

4. Zhang and Yang, "Testosterone Mimetic Properties of Icariin."

12. SAILING THROUGH THE MIST: BRAIN FOG

1. "Six Possible Causes of Brain Fog."

2. Ross et al., "What Is Brain Fog?"

3. Moss et al., "Modulation of Cognitive Performance."

4. Belcaro et al., "The COFU3 Study."

5. Uehleke et al., "Phase II Trial"; Degel and Köster, "Odors"; Jimbo et al., "Effect of Aromatherapy."

APPENDIX: FIVE NUTRITIONAL GUIDELINES
FOR OPTIMUM MENOPAUSAL HEALTH

1. Elkind-Hirsch, "Effect of Dietary Phytoestrogens."
2. Knight, Howes, and Eden, "Effects of Promensil."
3. Jeri and de Romana, "Effects of Isoflavone Phytoestrogens"; Maskarinec, "Effect of Phytoestrogens."
4. De Kleijn et al., "Dietary Intake of Phytoestrogens"; Anthony, Clarkson, and Williams, "Effects of Soy Isoflavones"; Arjmandi et al., "Whole Flaxseed Consumption."
5. North American Menopause Society, "Role of Soy Isoflavones."
6. Taylor, "Best Natural Estrogen Sources."
7. Nielsen et al., "Effect of Dietary Boron."
8. Nielsen, "Boron in Human and Animal Nutrition."
9. Hooper et al., "Risks and Benefits of Omega-3 Fats."
10. Smith, "Nutritionally Essential Fatty Acids."
11. Freeman et al., "Omega-3 Fatty Acids for Major Depressive Disorder."
12. Lucas et al., "Effects of Ethyl-Eicosapentaenoic Acid Omega-3 Fatty Acid Supplementation."
13. Tardivo et al., "Effects of Omega-3 on Metabolic Markers."
14. Jackson et al., "Calcium Plus Vitamin D Supplementation."
15. Dawson-Hughes et al., "Falconer G. Effect."
16. Jorde et al., "Effects of Vitamin D Supplementation."

Bibliography

American Psychiatric Association. *Diagnostic and Statistical Manual of Mental Disorders*. 4th ed. Washington, D.C.: American Psychiatric Association Publishing, 2000.

Anthony, M. S., T. B. Clarkson, and J. K. Williams. "Effects of Soy Isoflavones on Atherosclerosis: Potential Mechanisms." *American Journal of Clinical Nutrition* 68, no. 6 (1998): 1390S–93S.

Arjmandi, Bahram H., Dilshad A. Khan, Shanil Juma, et al. "Whole Flaxseed Consumption Lowers Serum LDL-Cholesterol and Lipoprotein(A) Concentrations in Postmenopausal Women." *Nutrition Research* 18, no. 7 (1998): 1203–14.

Armanini, D., C. Fiore, M. J. Mattarello, J. Bielenberg, and M. Palermo. "History of the Endocrine Effects of Licorice." *Experimental and Clinical Endocrinology and Diabetes* 110, no. 6 (2002): 257–61.

Arrien, Angeles. *The Second Half of Life: Opening the Eight Gates of Wisdom*. Boulder, Colo.: Sounds True Publishing, 2007.

Bai, W., H. H. Henneicke-von Zepelin, S. Wang, et al. "Efficacy and Tolerability of a Medicinal Product Containing an Isopropanolic Black Cohosh Extract in Chinese Women with Menopausal Symptoms: A Randomized, Double Blind, Parallel-Controlled Study versus Tibolone." *Maturitas* 58, no. 1 (2007): 31–41.

Belcaro, G., M. Dugall, E. Ippolito, S. Hu, A. Saggino, and B. Feragalli. "The COFU3 Study: Improvement in Cognitive Function, Attention, Mental Performance with Pycnogenol° in Healthy Subjects (55–70) with High Oxidative Stress." *Journal of Neurosurgical Sciences* 59, no. 4 (Dec. 2015): 437–46.

"Benefits of Cinnamon in Arthritis." The Superfoods (website).

Bommer, S., P. Klein, and A. Suter. "First Time Proof of Sage's Tolerability and

Efficacy in Menopausal Women with Hot Flushes," *Advances in Therapy* 28, no. 6 (June 2011): 490–500.

Bourne, Louise C., and Catherine Rice-Evans. "Bioavailability of Ferulic Acid." *Biochememical and Biophysical Research Communications* 253, no. 2 (1998): 222–27.

Brown, D. E., L. L. Sievert, L. A. Morrison, A. M. Reza, and P. S. Mills. "Do Japanese American Women Really Have Fewer Hot Flashes Than European Americans?: The Hilo Women's Health Study." *Menopause* 16, no. 5 (2009): 870–76.

Carmody, J. F., S. Crawford, E. Salmoirago-Blotcher, K. Leung, L. Churchill, and N. Olendzki. "Mindfulness Training for Coping with Hot Flashes: Results of a Randomized Trial." *Menopause* 18, no. 6 (2011): 611–20.

Cao, H., X. Pan, H. Li, and J. Liu. "Acupuncture for Treatment of Insomnia: A Systematic Review of Randomized Controlled Trials." *Journal of Alternative and Complementary Medicine* 15, no. 11 (2009): 1171–86.

Carré, Justin M., and Cheryl M. McCormick. "In Your Face: Facial Metrics Predict Aggressive Behaviour in the Laboratory and in Varsity and Professional Hockey Players." *Proceedings of the Royal Society B: Biological Sciences* 275, no. 1651 (Nov. 22, 2008): 2651–56.

Chan, K., L. Qin, M. Lau, et al. "A Randomized Prospective Study of the Effects of Tai Chi Chun Exercise on Bone Mineral Density in Postmenopausal Women." *Archives of Physical Medicine and Rehabilitation* 85, no. 5 (2004): 717–22.

Chandra, P., L. L. Wolfenden, T. R. Ziegler, et al. "Treatment of Vitamin D Deficiency with UV Light in Patients with Malabsorption Syndromes: A Case Series." *Photodermatology, Photoimmunology and Photomedicine* 23, no. 5 (2007): 179–85.

Choi, S., M. S. Park, Y. R. Lee, et al. "A Standardized Bamboo Leaf Extract Inhibits Monocyte Adhesion to Endothelial Cells by Modulating Vascular Cell Adhesion Protein-1." *Nutrition Research and Practice* 7, no. 1 (2013): 9–14.

Crandall, C. "Low-Dose Estrogen Therapy for Menopausal Women: A Review of Efficacy and Safety." *Journal of Women's Health* 12, no. 8 (2003): 723–47.

Cranney, A., G. Guyatt, L. Griffith, et al. "Meta-Analyses of Therapies for Postmenopausal Osteoporosis. IX: Summary of Meta-Analyses of Therapies for Postmenopausal Osteoporosis." *Endocrine Reviews* 23, no. 4 (2002): 570–78.

Dawson-Hughes, B., G. E. Dallal, E. A. Krall, S. Harris, and L. J. Sokoll. "Falconer G. Effect of Vitamin D Supplementation on Wintertime and Overall Bone Loss in Healthy Postmenopausal Women." *Annals of Internal Medicine* 115, no. 7 (1991): 505–12.

Degel, J., and E. P. Köster. "Odors: Implicit Memory and Performance Effects." *Chemical Senses* 24, no. 3 (1999): 317–25.

De Kleijn, M., Y. T. van der Schouw, P. Wilson, D. E. Grobbee, and P. Jacques. "Dietary Intake of Phytoestrogens Is Associated with a Favorable Metabolic Cardiovascular Risk Profile in Postmenopausal U.S. Women: The Framingham Study." *Journal of Nutrition* 132, no. 2 (2002): 276–82.

Dhingra, D., P. Joshi, A. Gupta, and R. Chhillar. "Possible Involvement of Monoaminergic Neurotransmission in Antidepressant-Like Activity of *Emblica officinalis* Fruits in Mice." *CNS Neuroscience and Therapeutics* 18, no. 5 (May 2012): 419–25.

Elkind-Hirsch, K. "Effect of Dietary Phytoestrogens on Hot Flushes: Can Soy-Based Proteins Substitute for Traditional Estrogen Replacement Therapy?" *Menopause* 8, no. 3 (May–June 2001): 154–56.

Emmons, S. L., and L. Otto. "Acupuncture for Overactive Bladder: A Randomized Controlled Trial." *Obstetrics and Gynecology* 106, no. 1 (July 2005): 138–43.

Esposito, L., and D. Katz. "How Much Time in the Sun Do You Need for Vitamin D?" U.S. News and World Report (website), July 18, 2019.

"Facts and Statistics." International Osteoporosis Foundation (website). Accessed July 7, 2016.

Freeman, M. P., J. R. Hibbeln, M. Silver, et al. "Omega-3 Fatty Acids for Major Depressive Disorder Associated with the Menopausal Transition: A Preliminary Open Trial." *Menopause* 18, no. 3 (2011): 279–84.

Fu, X., M. Wang, S. Li, and Y. Li. "The Effect of Bamboo Leaves Extract on Hemorheology of Normal Rats" (article in Chinese). *Zhong Yao Cai* 28, no. 2 (Feb. 2005): 130–32.

Gambacciani, M., and F. Vacca. "Postmenopausal Osteoporosis and Hormone Replacement Therapy." *Minerva Medica* 95, no. 6 (Dec. 2004): 507–20.

Ghazanfarpour, M., R. Sadeghi, R. Latifnejad Roudsari, et al. "Effects of Flaxseed and *Hypericum perforatum* on Hot Flash, Vaginal Atrophy and Estrogen-Dependent Cancers in Menopausal Women: A Systematic Review and Meta-Analysis." *Avicenna Journal of Phytomedicine* 6, no. 3 (May–June 2016): 273–83.

Gold, E. B., A. Colvin, N. Avis, et. al. "Longitudinal Analysis of the Association between Vasomotor Symptoms and Race/Ethnicity across the Menopausal Transition: Study of Women's Health across the Nation." *American Journal of Public Health* 96, no. 7 (2006): 1226–35.

Holden-Lund, C. "Effects of Relaxation with Guided Imagery on Surgical Stress and Wound Healing." *Research in Nursing and Health* 11, no. 4 (Aug. 1988): 235–44.

Hooper, L., R. L. Thompson, R. A. Harrison, et al. "Risks and Benefits of Omega-3 Fats for Mortality, Cardiovascular Disease, and Cancer: Systematic Review." *BMJ* 332 (2006): 752–60.

"Hormone Replacement Therapy (HRT)." International Osteoporosis Foundation (website).

"How Do I Get the Vitamin D My Body Needs?" Vitamin D Council (website).

Huang, M. I., Y. Nir, B. Chen, R. Schnyer, and R. Manber. "A Randomized Controlled Pilot Study of Acupuncture for Postmenopausal Hot Flashes: Effect on Nocturnal Hot Flashes and Sleep Quality." *Fertility and Sterility* 86, no. 3 (2006): 700–10.

Hulley, S., D. Grady, T. Bush, et al. "Randomized Trial of Estrogen Plus Progestin for Secondary Prevention of Coronary Heart Disease in Postmenopausal Women." *JAMA* 280, no. 7 (1998): 605–13.

Irvin, J. H., A. D. Domar, C. Clark, P. C. Zuttermeister, and R. Friedman. "The Effects of Relaxation Response Training on Menopausal Symptoms." *Journal of Psychosomatic Obstetrics and Gynecology* 17, no. 4 (Dec. 1996): 202–7.

Jack, Rachael E., O. G. Garrod, and P. G. Schyns. "Dynamic Facial Expressions of Emotion Transmit an Evolving Hierarchy of Signals over Time." *Current Biology* 24, no. 2 (2014): 187–92.

Jackson, Rebecca D., Andrea Z. LaCroix, Margery Gass, et. al. "Calcium Plus Vitamin D Supplementation and the Risk of Fractures." *New England Journal of Medicine* 354 (2006): 669–83.

Jeri, A. R., and C. de Romana. "The Effects of Isoflavone Phytoestrogens in Relieving Hot Flashes in Peruvian Postmenopausal Women." Ninth International Menopausal Society World Congress on Menopause, Yokohama, Japan, 1999.

Jiang, K., Y. Jin, L. Huang, et al. "Black Cohosh Improves Objective Sleep in Postmenopausal Women with Sleep Disturbance." *Climacteric* 18, no. 4 (2015): 559–67.

Jimbo, D., Y. Kimura, M. Taniguchi, M. Inoue, and K. Urakami. "Effect of Aromatherapy on Patients with Alzheimer's Disease." *Psychogeriatrics* 9, no. 4 (2009): 173–79.

Jorde, R., M. Sneve, Y. Figenschau, J. Svartberg, and K. Waterloo. "Effects of Vitamin D Supplementation on Symptoms of Depression in Overweight and Obese Subjects: Randomized Double Blind Trial." *Journal of Internal Medicine* 264, no. 6 (2008): 599–609.

Karlsen, Carol F. *The Devil in the Shape of a Woman: Witchcraft in Colonial New England.* New York: W. W. Norton, 1987.

Kaufert, P., P. P. Boggs, B. Ettinger, N. F. Woods, and W. H. Utian. "Women and Menopause: Beliefs, Attitudes, and Behaviors." *Menopause* 5, no. 4 (Winter 1998): 197–202.

King, Helen. "Once Upon a Text: Hysteria from Hippocrates." In *Hysteria Beyond Freud*, by Sander L. Gilman, Helen King, Roy Porter, G. S. Rousseau, and Elaine Showalter, 25. Berkeley, Calif.: University of California Press, 1993.

Knight, D. C., J. B. Howes, and J. A. Eden. "The Effects of Promensil, an Isoflavone Extract, on Menopausal Symptoms." *Climacteric* 2, no. 2 (1992): 70–84.

Komulainen, M. H., H. Kroger, M. T. Tuppurainen, et al. "HRT and Vit D in Prevention of Non-Vertebral Fractures in Postmenopausal Women: A 5-Year Randomized Trial." *Maturitas* 61, nos. 1–2 (Sep.–Oct. 2008): 85–94.

Kondo, Y., F. Takano, and H. Hojo. "Suppression of Chemically and Immunologically Induced Hepatic Injuries by Gentiopicroside in Mice." *Planta Medica* 60, no. 5. (1994): 414–16.

Koo, I., J. Y. Kim, M. G. Kim, and K. H. Kim. "Feature Selection from a Facial Image for Distinction of Sasang Constitution." *Evidence-Based Complementary and Alternative Medicine* 6, no. 1 (2009): 65–71.

Kuptniratsaikul, V., P. Dajpratham, W. Taechaarpornkul, et al. "Efficacy and Safety of *Curcuma domestica* Extracts Compared with Ibuprofen in Patients with Knee Osteoarthritis: A Multicenter Study." *Clinical Interventions in Aging* 9 (March 2014): 451–58.

Lee, Jane J. "After Menopause, Female Killer Whales Help Pod Survive." National Geographic (website), March 5, 2015.

Lim, D. W., and Y. T. Kim. "Dried Root of *Rehmannia glutinosa* Prevents Bone Loss in Ovariectomized Rats." *Molecules* 18, no. 5 (May 2013): 5804–13.

Liu, L., Z. Q. Ning, S. Shan, et al. "Phthalide Lactones from *Ligusticum chuanxiong* Inhibit Lipopolysaccharide-Induced TNF-Alpha Production and TNF-Alpha-Mediated NF-kappaB Activation." *Planta Medica* 71, no. 9 (Sep. 2005): 808–13.

Loprinzi, C. L., J. W. Kugler, J. A. Sloan, et al. "Venlafaxine in Management of Hot Flashes in Survivors of Breast Cancer: A Randomised Controlled Trial." *Lancet* 356, no. 9247 (2000): 2059–63.

Lucas, M., G. Asselin, C. Mérette, M. J. Poulin, and S. Dodin. "Effects of Ethyl-Eicosapentaenoic Acid Omega-3 Fatty Acid Supplementation on Hot Flashes and Quality of Life among Middle-Aged Women: A Double-Blind, Placebo-Controlled, Randomized Clinical Trial." *Menopause* 16, no. 2 (2009): 357–66.

Maskarinec, Stacey. "The Effect of Phytoestrogens on Hot Flashes." *Nutrition Bytes* 9, no. 2 (2003).

Matheson, E. M., A. G. Mainous, and M. A. Carnemolla. "The Association between Onion Consumption and Bone Density in Perimenopausal and Postmenopausal Non-Hispanic White Women 50 Years and Older." *Menopause* 16, no. 4 (Jul.–Aug. 2009): 756–59.

Mayo Clinic Staff. "Hot Flashes." Mayo Clinic (website). Accessed October 21, 2016.

McCann, I. L., and D. S. Holmes. "Influence of Aerobic Exercise on Depression." *Journal of Personality and Social Psychology* 46, no. 5 (1984): 1142–47.

Mei, L., M. Mochizuki, and N. Hasegawa. "Protective Effect of Pycnogenol® on Ovariectomy-Induced Bone Loss in Rats." *Phytotherapy Research* 26, no. 1 (Jan. 2012): 153–55.

Moss, M., S. Hewitt, L. Moss, and K. Wesnes. "Modulation of Cognitive Performance and Mood by Aromas of Peppermint and Ylang-Ylang." *International Journal of Neuroscience* 118, no. 1 (Jan. 2008): 59–77.

Nakchbandi, I. A. "Osteoporosis and Fractures in Liver Disease: Relevance, Pathogenesis and Therapeutic Implications." *World Journal of Gastroenterology* 20, no. 28 (2014): 9427–38.

Narayanan, A., M. S. Muyyarikkandy, S. Mooyottu, K. Venkitanarayanan, and M. A. R. Amalaradjou. "Oral Supplementation of Trans-Cinnamaldehyde Reduces Uropathogenic *Escherichia coli* Colonization in a Mouse Model." *Letters in Applied Microbiology* 64, no. 3 (Mar. 2017): 192–97.

National Council on Aging. *Healthy Sexuality and Vital Aging: Executive Summary.* Washington, D.C.: The National Council on Aging, 1998.

Nielsen, F. H. "Boron in Human and Animal Nutrition." *Plant and Soil* 193, no. 2 (1997): 199–208.

Nielsen, F. H., C. D. Hunt, L. M. Mullen, and J. R. Hunt. "Effect of Dietary Boron on Mineral, Estrogen, and Testosterone Metabolism in Postmenopausal Women." *FASEB Journal* 1, no. 5 (Nov. 1987): 394–97.

North American Menopause Society. "Decreased Desire." North American Menopause Society (website), 2008.

North American Menopause Society. "The Role of Soy Isoflavones in Menopausal Health: Report of the North American Menopause Society/Wulf H. Utian Translational Science Symposium in Chicago, IL (October 2010)." *Menopause* 18, no. 7 (Jul. 2011): 732–53.

Norton, Amy. "Calcium Supplements Tied to Kidney Stone Risk in Study." HealthDay, October 13, 2015.

Ockene, J. K., D. H. Barad, B. B. Cochrane, et al. "Symptom Experience after Discontinuing Use of Estrogen Plus Progestin." *JAMA* 294, no. 2 (2005): 183–93.

Ofir, R., S. Tamir, S. Khatib, and J. Vaya. "Inhibition of Serotonin Re-Uptake by Licorice Constituents." *Journal of Molecular Neuroscience* 20, no. 2 (2003): 135–40.

Oh, S. M., and K. H. Chung. "Antiestrogenic Activities of *Ginkgo biloba* Extracts." *Journal of Steroid Biochemistry and Molecular Biology* 100, nos. 4–5 (Aug. 2006): 167–76.

Osmers, R., M. Friede, E. Liske, J. Schnitker, J. Freudenstein, and H. H. Henneicke-von Zepelin. "Efficacy and Safety of Isopropanolic Black Cohosh Extract for Climacteric Symptoms." *Obstetrics and Gynecology* 105, no. 5, pt. 1 (May 2005): 1074–83.

Park, H., G. L. Parker, C. H. Boardman, M. M. Morris, and T. J. Smith, "A Pilot Phase II Trial of Magnesium Supplements to Reduce Menopausal Hot Flashes in Breast Cancer Patients," *Support Care in Cancer* 19, no. 6 (June 2011): 859–63.

Park, Rebecca. "Eight Health Benefits of Vitamin D and How to Get More of It." Remedies for Me (website), July 22, 2018.

Passini, F. T., and W. T. Norman. "A Universal Conception of Personality Structure?" *Journal of Personality and Social Psychology* 4, no. 1 (1966): 44–49.

Pegoraro, M., E. Picot, C. N. Hansen, C. P. Kyriacou, E. Rosato, and E. Tauber. "Gene Expression Associated with Early and Late Chronotypes in *Drosophila melanogaster*." *Frontiers in Neurology* 8, no. 6 (May 2015): 100.

Polo-Kantola, P., R. Erkkol, H. Helenius, K. Irjala, and O. Polo. "When Does Estrogen Replacement Therapy Improve Sleep Quality?" *American Journal of Obstetrics and Gynecology* 178, no. 5 (May 1998): 1002–9.

Rosen, R. C., J. L. Shifren, B. U. Monz, D. M. Odom, P. A. Russo, and C. B. Johannes. "Correlates of Sexually Related Personal Distress in Women with Low Sexual Desire." *Journal of Sexual Medicine* 6, no. 6 (2009): 1549–60.

Ross, A. Catharine, Christine L. Taylor, Ann L. Yaktine, and Heather B. Del Valle. *Dietary Reference Intakes for Calcium and Vitamin D.* Washington, D.C.: National Academy Press, 2011.

Ross, A. J., M. S. Medow, P. C. Rowe, and J. M. Stewart. "What Is Brain Fog? An Evaluation of the Symptom in Postural Tachycardia Syndrome." *Clinical Autonomic Research* 23, no. 6 (2013): 305–11.

Seo, E. J., S. Y. Lee, S. S. Kang, and Y. S. Jung. "*Zizyphus jujuba* and Its Active Component Jujuboside B Inhibit Platelet Aggregation." *Phytotherapy Research* 27 (2013): 829–34.

Shifren, J. L., B. U. Monz, P. A. Russo, A. Segreti, and C. B. Johannes. "Sexual Problems and Distress in United States Women: Prevalence and Correlates." *Obstetrics and Gynecology* 112, no. 5 (2008): 970–78.

Shin, J. S., and Y. S. Huh. "Effect of Intake of Gardenia Fruits and Combined Exercise of Middle-Aged Obese Women on Hormones Regulating Energy Metabolism." *Journal of Exercise Nutrition and Biochemistry* 18, no. 1 (Mar. 2014): 41–49.

"Six Possible Causes of Brain Fog." Healthline (website), June 14, 2017.

Smith, William L. "Nutritionally Essential Fatty Acids and Biologically Indispensable Cyclooxygenases." *Trends in Biochemical Sciences* 33, no. 1 (2008): 27–37.

Somjen, D., E. Knoll, J. Vaya, N. Stern, and S. Tamir. "Estrogen-Like Activity of Licorice Root Constituents: Glabridin and Glabrene, in Vascular Tissues In Vitro and In Vivo." *Journal of Steroid Biochemistry and Molecular Biology* 91, no. 3 (2004): 147–55.

Taku, K., M. K. Melby, F. Kronenberg, M. S. Kurzer, and M. Messina. "Extracted or Synthesized Soybean Isoflavones Reduce Menopausal Hot Flash Frequency and Severity: Systematic Review and Meta-Analysis of Randomized Controlled Trials." *Menopause* 19, no. 7 (July 2012): 776–90.

Tardivo, A. P., J. Nahas-Neto, C. L. Orsatti, et al. "Effects of Omega-3 on Metabolic Markers in Postmenopausal Women with Metabolic Syndrome." *Climacteric* 18, no. 2 (April 2015): 290–98.

Taylor, Deila. "The Best Natural Estrogen Sources for Post Menopausal Women." LiveStrong (website), August 14, 2017.

Thurston, R. C., J. A. Blumenthal, M. A. Babyak, and A. Sherwood. "Emotional Antecedents of Hot Flashes during Daily Life." *Psychosomatic Medicine* 67, no. 1 (Jan.–Feb. 2005): 137–46.

Tsuiji, K., T. Takeda, B. Li, et al. "Inhibitory Effect of Curcumin on Uterine Leiomyoma Cell Proliferation." *Gynecological Endocrinology* 27, no. 7 (2011): 512–17.

Uehleke, B., S. Schaper, A. Dienel, S. Schlaefke, and R. Stange. "Phase II Trial on the Effects of Silexan in Patients with Neurasthenia, Post-Traumatic Stress Disorder or Somatization Disorder." *Phytomedicine* 19, nos. 8–9 (2012): 665–71.

"Uterine Health." Office on Women's Health, womenshealth.gov, updated March 16, 2018.

Varpe, S. S., A. R. Juvekar, M. P. Bidikar, and P. R. Juvekar. "Evaluation of Anti-Inflammatory Activity of *Typha angustifolia* Pollen Grains Extracts in Experimental Animals." *Indian Journal of Pharmacology* 44, no. 6 (2012): 788–91.

Wagman, Gary (trans.). *The Essential Teachings of Sasang Medicine: An Annotataed Translation of Lee Je-ma's Dongeui Susei Bowon.* London: Singing Dragon, 2016. [Original *Dongeui Susei Bowon* published 1891.]

Wang, Y. H., S. Liang, D. S. Xu, et al. "Effect and Mechanism of Senkyunolide I as an Anti-Migraine Compound from *Ligusticum chuanxiong.*" *Journal of Pharmacy and Pharmacology* 63, no. 2 (2011): 261–66.

Warensjö, E., L. Byberg, H. Melhus, et al. "Dietary Calcium Intake and Risk of Fracture and Osteoporosis: Prospective Longitudinal Cohort Study." *BMJ* 342 (2011): d1473.

Wickman, Julie. "Androgen Therapy in Women." *US Pharmacist* 39, no. 8 (2014): 42–46.

Wolf, S. L., M. X. Barnhart, N. G. Kutner, et al. "Reducing Frailty and Falls in Older Persons: An Investigation of Tai Chi and Computerized Training." *Journal of the American Geriatrics Society* 44, no. 5 (1996): 489–97.

Wu, W. H., L. Y. Liu, C. J. Chung, H. J. Jou, and T. A. Wang. "Estrogenic Effect of Yam Ingestion in Healthy Postmenopausal Women." *Journal of the American College of Nutrition* 24, no. 4 (Aug 2005): 235–43.

Yang, C. U. I., W. U. Tie, and L. I. U. Yuyu. "The Effects of Tuber Fleeceflower Root on Bone Metabolism in Mice." *Chinese Journal of Osteoporosis* (2004). (Accessed on the CNKI website.)

Yang, Sarah. "New Study Finds Kelp Can Reduce Level of Hormone Related to Breast Cancer Risk." UC Berkeley News (website), February 2, 2005.

Yeh, C. H., C. K. Arnold, Y. H. Chen, and J. N. Lai. "Suan Zao Ren Tang as an Original Treatment for Sleep Difficulty in Climacteric Women: A Prospective Clinical Observation." *Evidence-Based Complementary and Alternative Medicine* (2011): 673813.

Yi, P. L., C. P. Lin, C. H. Tsai, J. G. Lin, and F. C. Chang. "The Involvement of Serotonin Receptors in Suanzaorentang-Induced Sleep Alteration." *Journal of Biomedical Science* 14, no. 6 (Nov. 2007): 829–40.

Zhang, Z. B., and Q. T. Yang. "The Testosterone Mimetic Properties of Icariin." *Asian Journal of Andrology* 8, no 5 (2006): 601–5.

Zhao, J., C. Y. Zhang, D. M. Xu, et al. "The Antiatherogenic Effects of Components Isolated from Pollen Typhae." *Thrombosis Research* 57, no. 6 (1990): 957–66.

Ziaei, Saeideh, Anoshirvan Kazemnejad, and M. Zareai. "The Effect of Vitamin E on Hot Flashes in Menopausal Women." *Gynecologic and Obstetric Investigation* 64, no. 4 (2007): 204–7.

Index

Each of the remedies provided in the preceding chapters may have other properties beyond the condition they are listed under. Be sure to check out the subsection titled "Common Uses" for each herb to find out other hidden benefits. You may also find it helpful to look up each menopause symptom by name and body type in the index. When using this method, make sure to avoid herbs that do not match your body type or situation.

acceptance, 124, 262
acupuncture/acupressure
 for depression, 172–73
 DU2 point, 227
 for frozen shoulder, 279–81
 for hot flashes, 128–30
 HT8 point, 201
 HT9 point, 130
 for insomnia, 200–202
 LI1 point, 280
 LIV2 point, 128–29, 202
 LIV3 point, 261
 LU9 point, 279–80
 PC8 point, 173
 REN6 point, 226–27
 SJ1 point, 281
 ST44 point, 129–30
 UB66 point, 227–28
 for urinary health, 226–28
 for uterine fibroids, 260–61
anger. *See also* emotions
 Bo He (field mint) to alleviate, 177
 Huang Qin (scullcap root) to resolve, 140
 origin of, 30

 stagnation and, 231
 Yang Type A, 26, 56, 79, 155, 175, 204, 262
 Yang Type B, 58, 79
 Zhu Ye (bamboo leaves) to curb, 176
An Shu (eucalyptus oil), 330–31
anterior body. *See also* emotions
 body types table, 87
 chest, 87, 89–91, 95
 chin, 87, 88–89, 95
 lower abdomen, 87, 93–95
 steps for balancing song, 87–88
 upper abdomen, 87, 91–93
antidepressants, 119–20, 194
An Xi Xiang (benzoin oil), 141–42, 186–87, 332–33
apple cider vinegar, 243–44, 289

Bai Zi Ren (arborvitae seed), 215
bladder exercises, 224–25
bladder issues
 Yang Type A, 230–35
 Yang Type B, 236–41
 Yin Type A, 241–48
 Yin Type B, 248–54

body type tests. *See also* yin yang body
  types
  concluding, 72–73
  emotional and physiological traits
    and, 41–42
  final scores, 73
  menopause-specific indicators,
    42–43, 66–72
  outward appearance and, 38–40
  use of techniques, 37
  which yin or yang type test, 38–42, 53
  yin or yang type test, 37–38, 43–53
Bo He (field mint), 177–78, 324–25
boron, 342–44
brain fog
  breathing and, 318
  causes of, 321–22
  contributing factors to, 315
  defined, 315
  diet and, 318
  essential oils for, 322–23
  example of experience of, 314–15
  exercise and, 319
  hydration and, 319–20
  sleep and, 318–19
  vitamin B$_{12}$ and, 320–21
  Western and Eastern perspectives,
    316–17
  Yang Type A and, 323–26
  Yang Type B and, 326–28
  yin and yang for, 318–21
  Yin Type A and, 328–31
  Yin Type B and, 331–34
breathing
  brain fog and, 318
  dan tian, 131
  hot flashes and, 130–31
  insomnia and, 198

calcium, 144, 349
calcium-rich foods, 151–52, 350–51

calmness, 26, 32–33, 163, 175–76, 252
cervical spine, 96–99
chest, 87, 89–91, 95
chin, 87, 88–89, 95
Chuan Xiong (Szechuan lovage root),
  291–92
Cong Bai (green onion), 253–54

dang yo, 81, 82–83, 89, 181, 267, 305, 328
Da Zao (Chinese jujube), 218–19
depression
  activity and, 172
  acupuncture/acupressure and, 172–73
  balancing predominant emotion
    and, 174
  clarification key, 70–71
  diagnosis criteria, 168
  estrogen and, 169–70
  example of experience of, 167
  exercise and, 172
  feelings and, 172
  major depressive disorder and, 168, 169
  menopause and, 167–68
  statement table, 70
  vitamin D and, 349
  Western and Eastern perspectives,
    169–71
  Yang Type A and, 174–78
  Yang Type B and, 178–80
  yin and yang of, 171–73
  Yin Type A and, 180–84
  Yin Type B and, 184–88
Di Gu Pi (lycium bark), 135
dream remembrance, 192–93
Du Huo (pubescent angelica root), 285

emotions. *See also specific emotions*
  balancing to avoid illness, 75–76
  body quadrants and, 86–107
  hormones and, 9
  hot flashes and, 133

in moving energy, 7, 75
organ association, 7–8
predominant, 25, 26, 76–80, 171
Sasang medicine and, 6, 19
song and jung, by body type, 322
yang, balanced and unbalanced, 77
yin, balanced and unbalanced, 78
energy
  bodily, in Eastern medicine, 121
  emotions in moving, 75
  organ, twenty-four-hour cycle, 122
estrogen
  characteristics of, 20
  decrease in, 20
  depression and, 169–70
  excessive levels of, 22
  hot flashes and, 123
  in monthly cycle, 22
  osteoporosis and, 144–45
  replacement, 118–19
exercise
  brain fog and, 319
  depression and, 172
  hot flashes and, 125–26
  insomnia and, 199, 214
  osteoporosis and, 150–51
  uterine fibroids and, 259–60
eyesight, 34

fatigue, sleep and, 192
fibroids. *See* uterine fibroids
food intake, 126–28
foods
  before bed, avoiding, 199
  boron sources, 342, 343
  calcium sources, 151–52, 349,
    350–51
  hot-flash reducing, 131–32
  isoflavone-rich, 152
  omega-3 sources, 346, 347
  phytoestrogen sources, 341

progesterone sources, 344, 345
  vitamin D sources, 149, 349, 350
frozen shoulder
  acupuncture/acupressure and, 279–81
  Chuan Xiong (Szechuan lovage root)
    for, 291–92
  example of experience of, 274–75
  Hei Mei (blackberries) for, 156
  stretching, 278–79
  using shoulder and, 278
  Western and Eastern perspectives,
    275–76
  Yang Type A and, 283–85
  Yang Type B and, 285–88
  yin and yang of, 276–81
  Yin Type A and, 288–90
  Yin Type B and, 290–92

gaeng nyon gi, 2
Gan Cao (licorice root), 250–52
Gou Qi Zi (goji berry), 205–6
grief, 82, 197, 237, 245, 290, 305

Hai Cao (seaweed), 234–35
Hei Mei (blackberries), 156–57, 235
herbal friends, defined, 113
herbs. *See specific Sasang herbal remedies*
He Shou Wu (fleeceflower root), 165–66
hormones, 19–23. *See also specific*
    hormones
hot flashes
  acceptance and, 124
  acupuncture and acupressure and,
    128–30
  body temperature and, 120
  breathing and, 130–31
  causes of, 116–17
  clarification key, 67–68
  differences of experience, 115–16
  Di Gu Pi (lycium bark) to relieve, 135
  emotions and, 133

estrogen and, 123
ethnicity and, 118
exercise and, 125–26
experience of, 116–18
food intake and, 126–28
foods and vitamins for reducing,
    131–32
Huang Qin (skullcap root) for, 140
insomnia and, 191
intensity in evening, 121
Lu Gen (common reed) for, 137–38
Mu Dan Pi (tree peony) for, 302–3
night sweats versus, 117, 120–21
phytoestrogens and, 340
Sheng Ma (black cohosh) for, 139
statement table, 67
stress reduction and, 123–25
treatments that cause, 118
Western and Eastern perspectives,
    118–22
Yang Type A and, 134–36
Yang Type B and, 136–38
yin and yang of, 122–32
Yin Type A and, 138–40
Yin Type B and, 140–42
Zhi Mu (anemarrhena) for, 135–36
Zhi Zi (gardenia) for, 231–32
Zhu Ru (bamboo shavings) to
    relieve, 137
Huang Qin (skullcap root), 140
Huo Xiang (patchouli oil), 187–88,
    333–34

illness, balancing emotions and, 75–76
insomnia
    acupuncture/acupressure and, 200–202
    Bai Zi Ren (arborvitae seed) for, 215
    bed is for sleeping and, 198
    bedtime before 11 p.m. and, 197–98
    Bo He (field mint) for, 324
    breathing and, 198

clarification key, 71–72
coffee and, 199–200
Da Zao (Chinese jujube) for, 218
defined, 190
difficulty getting to sleep and, 195
difficulty staying asleep and, 195–96
Eastern perspectives on, 194–96
example of experience of, 189–90
exercise and, 199
foods and fluids and, 199
Gou Qi Zi (goji berry) for, 205–6
hot flashes and, 191
hugging a pillow and, 200
"just let go" mantra and, 198
Long Yan Rou (longan fruit) for, 183
Lu Gen (common reed) for, 211
Mai Ya (roasted barley) for, 207
mattress and, 202–3
other symptoms and, 191
Qiao Mai (buckwheat) for, 210
room darkness and, 198–99
routine and, 197
Sheng Ma (black cohosh) for, 139–40
statement table, 71
statistics of, 191
stress and, 191
Suan Zao Ren (sour jujube seed) for,
    214–15
Western perspectives on, 193–94
Yang Type A and, 204–8
Yang Type B and, 208–12
yin and yang of, 196–203
Yin Type A and, 212–16
Yin Type B and, 216–20
Zhi Zi (gardenia) for, 231–32
irritability, 22, 116–17, 138, 178, 229, 248
isoflavone-rich foods, 152

Je-ma, Lee, 15, 74, 89, 111–12, 235,
    321, 322–23
Jiang Huang (turmeric), 268–69, 288–89

Jing Jie (Japanese catnip), 325
Jin Yin Hua (Japanese honeysuckle),
    232–33
joy, 26, 31, 33, 91, 161, 180–81
ju chek, 88–89, 95, 106, 267, 307
Ju Hua (chrysanthemum), 242–43
"just let go" mantra, 198

kidneys, 24, 25, 27, 32–33, 39, 75, 81, 82
kindness, 95–96, 102–3, 106
ko cho, 81, 83–86, 185
kyo wu, 81, 83–86, 185
kyung ryun, 89–91, 95, 96–97, 105–6, 108

laziness, 61, 79, 91
levels of interaction
    dang yo, 81, 82–83, 181, 267, 305, 328
    ko cho, 81, 83–86, 185
    kyo wu, 81–82, 83–86, 185
    overview, 80–82
    sa mu, 81, 82–83, 178, 304, 326
    table, 81
libido
    bringing energy down and, 296–97
    clarification key, 68–69
    example of experience of, 293–94
    expectations and, 297
    lack of, factors contributing to, 296
    Mu Dan Pi (tree peony) for issues of,
        302–3
    pain and, 298–99
    Ren Shin (ginseng root) for
        decreased, 312–13
    statement table, 68
    Tu Si Zi (cuscuta) for lack of, 309
    Western and Eastern perspectives,
        294–99
    Wu Jia Pi (devil's club) for deficient,
        305–6
    Yang Type A and, 300–304
    Yang Type B and, 304–7

yin and yang of, 299–300
    Yin Type A and, 307–10
    Yin Type B and, 310–13
    Yin Yang Huo (horny goat weed) for
        decreased, 308–9
liver, 24, 25, 27–28, 31–32, 33, 39, 79–82
Li Zi (chestnuts), 162–63
Long Dan Cao (gentian root), 265
Long Yan Rou (longan fruit), 183–84
lower abdomen, 87, 93–95
Lu Gen (common reed), 137–38, 179, 211
lumbar spine, 101–4
lungs, 24, 25, 28–29, 33–34, 39, 158,
    208, 277

magnesium, 348
Mai Ya (roasted barley), 207
major depressive disorder, 168, 169
mantra for better sleep, 198, 205, 209,
    213, 217
meditation for better sleep, 205, 209, 218
menopause
    body type and, 12–13
    defined, 13–15
    emotions and, 74–108
    misconceptions of, 5–6, 9
    organ systems and, 27–33
    response to, 7
    senses and, 33–35
    significance of, 2–3
Mindfulness-Based Stress Reduction
    (MBSR), 123–24
Mo Yao (myrrh), 264
Mu Dan Pi (tree peony), 302–3
Mu Gau (Chinese quince), 239–40,
    306–7

natural progesterone, 343–44, 345
night sweats, hot flashes versus, 117,
    120–21
nutritional guidelines, 338–51

omega-3 fatty acids, 344–47
organs. *See also specific organs*
  energies of, 122
  temperatures and body fluids and,
    154
organ systems
  body type determination, 23–27
  functions and body types, 24
  menopause and, 27–33
  senses and, 33–34
osteopenia, 146, 162, 246
osteoporosis
  calcium and, 144
  calcium-rich foods and, 151–52
  estrogen and, 144–45
  example of experience of, 143
  exercise and, 150–51
  genetics and, 146
  Gou Qi Zi (goji berry) for, 205–6
  Hei Mei (blackberries) for, 156
  isoflavone-rich foods and, 152
  Li Zi (chestnuts) for, 162–63
  Long Yan Rou (longan fruit) to help
    prevent, 183
  sodium consumption and, 152–53
  Song Zi (pine nuts) for, 162
  vitamin D and, 148–50, 348–49
  Western and Eastern perspectives,
    147
  Yang Type A and, 154–58
  Yang Type B and, 158–60
  Yin Type A, 160–63
  Yin Type B, 163–66
osteoporotic fractures, 146

pair herbs, 113. *See also* herbal friends
phytoestrogens, 339–42
pokbal (emotion explosion), 322
posterior body. *See also* emotions
  cervical spine, 96–99
  lumbar spine, 101–4

overview, 95–96
  sacral spine, 104–7
  thoracic spine, 99–101
progesterone, 20, 21–22, 343–44,
  345
Ptolemy of Alexandria, 2
Pu Gong Ying (dandelion root), 243
Pu Huang (cattail pollen), 267–68

Qiang Huo (notopterygium root),
  284–85
Qiao Mai (buckwheat), 210

Ren Shin (ginseng root), 312–13
research, current, 336–37
Rou Gui (cinnamon), 142, 164–65,
  251–52, 313
Ru Xuang (frankincense), 263

sacrum, 104–7
SAD (seasonal affective disorder),
  148–49, 348
sadness, 7–8, 56, 59, 71, 75, 155, 178,
  180
sa mu, 81, 82–83, 178, 304, 326
Sasang herbal remedies, 112–14. *See
  also specific herbal remedies*
Sasang medicine
  defined, 15–16
  diet in, 153–54
  emotions and, 6, 19
  four levels of interaction, 80–86
  health in, 14
  as herbal approach, 111–14
  key principles in, 27
  premise of, 6–9, 15–16
  sexual health issues in, 295
selective serotonin reuptake inhibitors
  (SSRIs), 169–71, 194
self-confidence and dignity, 282–83
senses, menopause and, 33–35

sex. *See also* libido
  Yang Type A and, 302
  Yang Type B and, 305
  Yin Type A and, 308
  Yin Type B and, 311
Shan Zha (hawthorn fruit), 219–20
Sheng Di Huang (rehmannia), 157, 303
Sheng Ma (black cohosh), 139–40,
  269
Shi Zi (persimmons), 240–41
sleep. *See also* insomnia
  brain fog and, 318–19
  dream remembrance and, 192–93
  fatigue and, 192
  improving, 189–220
  influences on quality, 203–4
  REM, 193
smell, sense of, 33, 34
sodium consumption, 152–53
Song Jie (Masson pine), 159, 286–87
Song Zi (pine nuts), 162, 246
sorrow, 26, 29, 79, 181, 236
spine, 96–106. *See also* posterior body
spleen, 24–25, 27–28, 30, 34, 39, 64,
  81–82, 217
stagnation, 20, 126, 135, 148, 161, 223,
  231, 299
stress, 26, 123–25, 150–51, 189–91,
  195–96
stress incontinence, 222. *See also*
  urinary health
stretching, frozen shoulder, 278–79
Suan Zao Ren (sour jujube seed),
  182–83, 214–15
support services, menopause, 337
su seung hwa gang ("coolness ascending
  and warmth descending"), 7

taste, sense of, 33–34
testosterone, 20
thoracic spine, 99–101

tolerance, 95–96, 105–6
Tu Si Zi (cuscuta), 309–10

upper abdomen, 87, 91–93
urge incontinence, 222. *See also*
  urinary health
urinary health
  acupuncture/acupressure and,
    226–28
  apple cider vinegar for, 243–44
  bladder exercises, 224–25
  coffee intake and, 225–26
  Cong Bai (green onion) for, 253
  example of experience of, 221–22
  Gan Cao (licorice root) for, 250
  Hai Cao (seaweed) for, 234
  Hei Mei (blackberries) for, 235
  Jin Yin Hua (Japanese honeysuckle)
    for, 232–33
  Mu Gau (Chinese quince) for, 239–40
  Pu Gong Ying (dandelion root) for,
    243
  Rou Gui (cinnamon) for, 251–52
  Shi Zi (persimmons) for, 240
  Song Zi (pine nuts) for, 246
  Western and Eastern perspectives,
    222–23
  Yang Type A and, 229–35
  Yang Type B and, 235–-41
  yin and yang of, 223–28
  Yin Type A, 241–48
  Yin Type B, 248–54
  Yin Xing Yi (ginkgo) for, 247
  Yi Zhi Ren (black cardamom seed)
    for, 254
  Yu Gan Zi (gooseberry) for, 237–38
  Zhi Zi (gardenia) for, 231–32
uterine fibroids
  acupuncture/acupressure and,
    260–61
  causes of, 257

Dang Gui/Dong Quai (angelica root) for, 271

example of experience of, 255–56

exercise and, 259–60

guided imagery and, 260

Jiang Huang (turmeric) for, 268

Long Dan Cao (gentian root) for, 265

massage and, 260

Pu Huang (cattail pollen) for, 267–68

Ru Xuang (frankincense) for, 263

Sheng Ma (black cohosh) for, 269

statistics of, 256

symptoms associated with, 256

Western and Eastern perspectives, 258–59

when to see a professional about, 256

Yang Type A and, 262–64

Yang Type B and, 264–66

yin and yang of, 259–61

Yin Type A and, 266–70

Yin Type B and, 270–73

UV light, 149–50

vitamin D, 147, 148–50, 347, 349, 350

walking, 61, 143, 150, 260

weight gain, 22, 30, 31, 40, 56, 119, 160, 170

wi eui, 95–96, 99–100, 108, 174, 252, 282–84, 286

Wu Jia Pi (devil's club), 159–60, 305–6

Xun Yi Cao (lavender oil), 329–30

yang emotions, 76–77

Yang Type A
anger, 26, 56, 79, 155, 175, 204, 262

aversion to calmness, 175–76

bladder issues, 230–35

body feature score chart, 47

brain fog and, 323–26

chest, 87, 89–91

clarification key, 55–56

cold and insecurity, 186

defined, 18

depression and, 174–78

eyesight, 34

female, 48

frozen shoulder and, 283–85

hot flashes and, 120, 134–36

impulsiveness, 155

insomnia and, 204–8

irritability, 175–76

kindness, achieving/receiving, 102–3

kyo wu, 81, 84, 85–86

lack of joy, 181

mantra for better sleep, 205

meditation for better sleep, 205

metabolism, 56

neck pain and/or weakness, 97–98

oppression sensitivity, 174–75

organ systems and, 24, 25

osteoporosis and, 154–58

outward appearance, 39–40

predominant emotion, 26

sadness, 180

sex and, 302

sleep, 55

statements, 54

stomach, 55

teas for, 205

tolerance, 105–6

upper back pain and/or weakness, 100

urinary health and, 229–35

uterine fibroids and, 262–64

Yang Type B
anger, 58, 79

bladder issues, 236–41

body feature score chart, 47

brain fog and, 326–28

chin, 87, 88–89

clarification key, 58–59

cold and insecurity, 186
defined, 18
depression and, 178–80
female, 49
foods, 180
frozen shoulder and, 285–88
hearing, 34
hot flashes and, 136–38
insomnia and, 208–12
irritability, 178
kindness, achieving/receiving, 103
lack of joy, 181
libido and, 304–7
liver and gallbladder, 58–59
lungs, 158, 209
mantra for better sleep, 209
meditation for better sleep, 209
neck pain and/or weakness, 98
organ systems and, 24, 25
osteoporosis and, 158–60
predominant emotion, 26
sadness, 59, 71, 75, 178
sa mu, 81, 82–83
sex and, 305
sorrow, 236
statements, 57
teas for, 209
tolerance, 106
upper back pain and/or weakness, 100
urinary health and, 235–41
uterine fibroids and, 264–66
Yan Hu Suo (corydalis), 272, 292
yin and yang
   of brain fog, 318–21
   of depression, 171–73
   energy balance, 19
   of frozen shoulder, 276–81
   hormones and, 19–21
   of hot flashes, 122–32
   of insomnia, 196–203
   intermingling of, 18
   of libido, 299–300
   natural phenomenon, 17
   of osteoporosis, 148–53
   theory, 17
   traits, 19
   of urinary health, 223–28
   of uterine fibroids, 259–61
yin emotions, 78
Yin Type A
   angry nature imbalance, 79
   bladder issues, 241–48
   body features, 62
   body feature score chart, 50
   brain fog and, 328–31
   clarification key, 61–62
   cold and insecurity, 186
   dang yo, 81, 83
   defined, 18
   depression and, 180–84
   exercise for better sleep, 213
   female, 51
   food sensitivities, 62
   frozen shoulder and, 288–90
   hot flashes and, 138–40
   insomnia and, 212–16
   irritability, 178
   joy temperament, 79, 80, 161, 241, 267
   kindness, achieving/receiving, 103
   lack of joy, 180–81
   laziness, 61
   libido and, 307–10
   mantra for better sleep, 213
   neck pain and/or weakness, 98
   organ systems and, 24, 25
   osteoporosis, 160–63
   outward appearance, 40
   predominant emotion, 26
   sadness, 180
   sense of smell, 33, 34
   sex and, 308
   sorrow, 181

statements, 60
teas for, 214
tolerance, 106
upper abdomen, 87, 91–93
upper back pain and/or weakness, 100
urinary health, 241–48
uterine fibroids and, 266–70
Yin Type B
  anger and sorrow, 79
  bladder issues, 248–54
  body feature score chart, 50
  brain fog and, 331–34
  calmness, 26, 163, 252
  clarification key, 64–65
  cold and insecurity, 185–86
  comfort, 249–50
  defined, 18
  depression and, 184–88
  diet, 64
  female, 52
  frozen shoulder and, 290–92
  health improvement, 164
  hot flashes and, 140–42
  insomnia and, 216–20
  irritability, 178
  kindness, achieving/receiving, 103
  ko cho, 185
  lack of joy, 181
  libido and, 310–13
  lower abdomen, 87, 93–95
  mantra for better sleep, 217
  meditation for better sleep, 218
  neck pain and/or weakness, 98
  need for peace and quiet, 270
  organ systems and, 24, 25
  osteoporosis, 163–66
  predominant emotion, 26
  sense of taste, 33–34
  sex and, 311

statements, 63
teas for, 218
tolerance, 106
upper back pain and/or weakness,
  101
urinary health, 248–54
uterine fibroids and, 270–73
warming abdomen and, 217
Yin Xing Yi (ginkgo), 247–48
yin yang body types. *See also* body type
  tests; *specific body types*
  brain fog and, 321–22, 323–34
  change and, 26
  depression and, 173–88
  hormones and, 23
  hot flashes and, 133–34
  insomnia and, 203–20
  libido and, 300–313
  organ system determination of,
    23–27
  organ systems and, 24
  osteoporosis and, 153–66
  predominant emotions, 26, 171
  Sasang herbal remedies for, 112
  Sasang medicine and, 1, 4, 13
  senses and, 33–34
  urinary health and, 228–54
  uterine fibroids and, 261–73
Yin Yang Huo (horny goat weed),
  308–9
Yi Zhi Ren (black cardamom seed),
  254
Yuan Zhi (snakeroot), 184
Yu Gan Zi (gooseberry), 237–38

Zhi Mu (anemarrhena), 135–36
Zhi Zi (gardenia), 231–32
Zhu Ru (bamboo shavings), 137
Zhu Ye (bamboo leaves), 176–77